Health Informatics

Valerie Powell • Franklin M. Din
Amit Acharya • Miguel Humberto Torres-Urquidy
Editors

Kathryn J. Hannah • Marion J. Ball
Series Editors

Integration of Medical and Dental Care and Patient Data

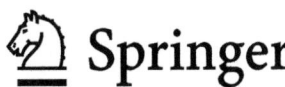

Editors
Valerie Powell, Ph.D., M.S., R.T.(R)
Department of Computer and Information
Systems, Clinical Data Integration Project
Robert Morris University
Moon Township, PA
USA

Amit Acharya, B.D.S., M.S., Ph.D.
Biomedical Informatics
Research Center
Marshfield Clinic Research
Foundation, Marshfield, WI
USA

Franklin M. Din, D.M.D., M.A.
HP Enterprise Services
Global Healthcare, Camp Hill, PA
USA

Miguel Humberto
Torres-Urquidy, D.D.S., M.S., Ph.D.
Department of Biomedical Informatics
University of Pittsburgh, PA
USA

ISBN 978-1-4471-6028-1   ISBN 978-1-4471-2185-5 (eBook)
DOI 10.1007/978-1-4471-2185-5
Springer London Dordrecht Heidelberg New York

British Library Cataloguing in Publication Data
A catalogue record for this book is available from the British Library

© Springer-Verlag London Limited 2012
Softcover reprint of the hardcover 1st edition 2012
Apart from any fair dealing for the purposes of research or private study, or criticism or review, as permitted under the Copyright, Designs and Patents Act 1988, this publication may only be reproduced, stored or transmitted, in any form or by any means, with the prior permission in writing of the publishers, or in the case of reprographic reproduction in accordance with the terms of licences issued by the Copyright Licensing Agency. Enquiries concerning reproduction outside those terms should be sent to the publishers.
The use of registered names, trademarks, etc. in this publication does not imply, even in the absence of a specific statement, that such names are exempt from the relevant laws and regulations and therefore free for general use.
Product liability: The publisher can give no guarantee for information about drug dosage and application thereof contained in this book. In every individual case the respective user must check its accuracy by consulting other pharmaceutical literature.

Printed on acid-free paper

Springer is part of Springer Science+Business Media (www.springer.com)

This volume is dedicated to the patients who, during the time that this book is being published, now require improved integration of healthcare and of patient records to facilitate interdisciplinary communication among their providers in order to assure their well-being and, in some cases, even safeguard their lives. Some of these patients would not now suffer chronic conditions or risks to their lives as severe as they are experiencing if they had had access to an integrated (medical-dental) interdisciplinary healthcare provider workforce earlier in their lives. Two patients who come to mind who needn't have died if they had had access to an integrated care system, are 12-year-old Deamonte Driver who died of a brain abscess in 2007 in Maryland after difficulties locating a dental provider who would accept

Medicaid and then difficulty processing Medicaid eligibility due in part to his family moving residence temporarily to a shelter and also an unnamed Michigan woman who died with severe periodontal disease in 2009, after her state government eliminated adult dental Medicaid benefits while she was recovering from pneumonia and waiting for surgery. May we not lose sight of the "true cost of inaction."

We would also like to dedicate this book to our dear colleague Dr. Heather K. Hill DDS, MS, who passed away earlier this year after a long battle with breast cancer. Dr. Hill was just 37 years old and is survived by her husband and two daughters. She earned a Bachelor of Science in 1996 and a Doctor of Dental Surgery in 2000 from the University of Minnesota and a master's degree in Biomedical Informatics in 2010 from Oregon Health & Sciences University. Dr. Hill's passion for dental informatics was unlimited and she had a great vision for the field. She has left a legacy within the short time that she spent and we are really obliged to her. The field of dental informatics has lost a great leader and a visionary.

Preface

Dentistry Is Medicine – Oral Medicine

Dentistry is medicine–oral medicine. The integration of the discipline of dentistry with the larger community of medicine, in education and in practice, is an imperative. The multi-faceted elements of health care reform, and specifically the mandate to create and implement a comprehensive health information system, has the potential to accomplish the integration that dentistry as been unable, and generally unwilling, to accomplish. The authors of this volume provide important conceptual and logistical foundations for addressing this integration imperative.

Dentistry emerged and developed as an autonomous profession based on the overwhelming prevalence of oral disease, and at a time there were few individuals trained to provide needed treatment. The assumption existed that treating teeth was simply a mechanical endeavor, as no relationship was thought to exist between the health of the teeth and that of the rest of the body. These assumptions must now be challenged. The dental profession has expanded the numbers of dentists, has significantly reduced the prevalence of dental disease, and demonstrated through research that oral health is intimately related to systemic health and well being. The time has come to acknowledge that dentists are physicians of the stomatognathic system, and that their education must be integrated with the education of physicians being trained to care for other functional organ systems; and that oral health care must be included and integrated into the nation's health care delivery system.

Dentistry emerged as a scientific, university-based discipline subsequent to the Carnegie Foundation's report in 1926 edited by William Gies, Dentistry in the United States and Canada. In that report, Gies and his colleagues favored the view that dentistry should become integrated with medicine as a specialty. They argued for an enlarged view of dentistry in which "dental surgeons and dental engineers become oral physicians." The ambivalence of the Gies' committee in believing this was possible is reflected in the statement that "the practice of dentistry should be made an accredited specialty of the practice of conventional medicine, or fully equal to such a specialty in the grade of health service." The Report then concluded that "dentistry cannot now be made a specialty of medicine." This negative assessment of complete integration was probably due to the political culture and climate at the time, no doubt no different than that experienced today. Thus dentistry emerged and developed in the Twentieth Century as an autonomous profession, attempting to be, as the report stated, "fully equal" to a specialty of medicine as a health service.

Dentistry made notable advances in the last century in research and education that resulted in a significant improvement in the oral health of the American people; however, by the last decade of the century it had become increasingly apparent that dentistry could no longer be equal while remaining separate. In 1994, a World Health Organization report Oral Health in for the twenty-first century stated:

The changing disease patterns, the advanced diagnostic and treatment methodologies and the broadening of responsibilities illustrate the need for a new type of oral health professional, someone with special education and skills in the care of the oral and maxillofacial complex. These professionals will have principal responsibility for oral health care, and they may be assisted by specially-trained support personnel. In addition to these generalist oral physicians it is anticipated that the need will remain for specialists.

In early 1995, the Institute of Medicine released the results of its 4 year study of dental education, Dental Education at the Crossroads: Challenges and Change. This landmark study by America's most prestigious science policy body proved to be provocative. While acknowledging the progress dentistry and dental education had made, the report indicated the profession had arrived at a crossroads and transformative changes were required – "the status quo [is], in effect, a path toward stagnation and decline." Significant changes in the environment had and were continuing to occur that made the profession vulnerable. "Dental education and dentistry are made vulnerable by their relative isolation from the broader university, from other health professions, and from the restructuring of health care and financing systems that characterizes most of the health care delivery system." Dentistry had become (and continues to be) isolated organizationally, intellectually, and educationally from medicine, to the detriment of society and the profession.

The recurring theme of the IOM report was one of "closer integration" of dentistry with medicine. The theme was actually emphasized visually in the cover of the report, which was lilac, the academic color of dentistry and forest green, the academic color of medicine. "Dentistry will and should become more closely integrated with medicine and the health care system at all levels: research, education and patient care. The March of science and technology in fields such as molecular biology, immunology, and genetics will, in particular, continue to forge links between medicine and dentistry as will the needs of an aging population with more complex health problems…Government and primary purchasers of health services can be expected to maintain and indeed increase the pressure on health practitioners and institutions to develop more highly integrated and constrained systems of care that stress cost containment, primary versus specialty care, and services provided by teams of professional and other personnel." The profession of dentistry reacted vigorously to the IOM report, generally viewing it negatively and with suspicion. The profession was satisfied with the status quo; dentistry was thriving economically, a perceived prime benchmark of professional success. Organized dentistry rebutted the report with the oft heard expression "dentistry is not medicine." Dental educators, likely influenced by alumni/ae, failed, in general, to respond to the multitude of recommendations of the report, many of which would have resulted in dental education becoming less isolated and more "closely integrated" with medicine.

The environmental issues of the 1990s, affecting health care generally and dentistry specifically, have only resulted in increased pressures for change, both in dental education and dental practice. Arguably, the status quo has been maintained and dentistry is not well-prepared to address the transformations occurring in the nation's health care system. It is possible that the demands for an integrated health information system will prove to be the environmental force that will finally drive the required integration of dentistry with medicine, an integration that has been understood to be an imperative by many since William Gies and his committee advanced the concept in 1926. If so, dentistry will be able to assume its appropriate position as a recognized specialty of medicine, with education and training for the practice of dentistry being alongside individuals studying to participate in other medical specialties; and with dentists finally being understood to be physicians of the stomatognathic system–oral physicians.

Integration of Medical and Dental Care and Patient Data is an important work toward envisioning and realizing the day when dentistry is finally integrated with medicine.

David A. Nash, D.M.D., M.S., Ed.D.
William R. Willard Professor of Dental Education
Professor of Pediatric Dentistry
College of Dentistry
University of Kentucky

Preface

Integrating Medical and Dental Data: More Than a Technical Challenge

This book is about integrating processes and data in medical and dental care. Doing so is a significant challenge in multiple respects: technically, logistically, professionally and culturally. Yet, succeeding at this endeavor is inescapable: As clinicians, we simply owe it to our patients (Baron 2011). We can only improve health if we improve oral and general health at the same time.

The separation of dentistry from medicine is a historical accident. As Dr. Nash explains cogently in his preface, early on "treating teeth was simply a mechanical endeavor, as no relationship was thought to exist between the health of the teeth and that of the rest of the body." Today, we know better. Plenty of studies have shown associations, if not causal relationships, between dental and medical conditions.

Informatics is key to helping healthcare professionals realize the vision articulated in this book. Separating dentistry and medicine has kept things apart that are central to informatics: data, information and processes. Dentists and physicians keep their own records for the same patients, encode patient information using different approaches and rarely communicate about patients. Doing so does not only result in inefficiencies and unnecessary overhead, but also impedes good clinical decision making and patient outcomes. Both may easily understand similar or identical portions of their respective records, such as the medical or medication history. However, clinicians from either field are typically not able to understand information on forms they are not familiar with. For instance, most physicians can not make sense of a tooth chart. Neither can most dentists given a set of medical laboratory tests. So, a crucial question in integrating medicine and dentistry more closely is: How should we communicate?

The answer to this question is primarily a professional and cultural, rather than a technical, one. Exchanging electronic data among dentists and physicians, while not trivial, is a comparatively small problem. To the computer, medical and dental information looks the same – it is just a stream of bits. For clinicians, exchanging information is more complicated. The main challenge is to communicate the information that the other party needs and to ensure that its meaning, as well as its implications, can be understood and acted on. Pediatricians must understand that a diagnosis of early childhood caries requires, among other interventions, nutritional counseling. Dentists, on the other hand, must be familiar with the implications of a range of medical conditions on oral and dental health. Topics of mutual interest and relevance may be most easily understood and considered in dental or medical schools focused on a multidisciplinary, systems approach to patient care. However, such schools are the exception rather than the rule. For the "installed base" of 150,000 dentists and 300,000 physicians other approaches will have to be found.

The best care will be delivered by dentists and physicians together, not separately, as is the case right now. Opportunities to do so abound. Imagine the day when physicians, dentists and other healthcare providers deliver smoking cessation interventions through a seamless and transparent collaboration (McDaniel et al. 2009). Or, when dentists help identify patients with previously undiagnosed, significant medical conditions, such as hypertension, cardiovascular disease, diabetes mellitus, hepatitis and HIV infection (Greenberg et al. 2010). Or, when dentists screen for a whole host of medical conditions using saliva diagnostics (Spielmann and Wong 2011).

Foreshadowing the discussion in this book, we presented a conceptual approach for sharing health information among different clinical disciplines in a paper in 1994 (Schleyer and Eisner 1994). We first considered what information a clinician would need under various circumstances. For instance, in dental emergencies, recently updated medical information relevant to the diagnosis or treatment of the emergency would be useful. Conversely, a recent diagnosis of oral hairy leukoplakia would be of interest to a physician who is working up a patient for a potential infection with HIV. Our concept included the idea of "shareable data" contained in discipline-specific electronic patient records. What data are shared is not static, and depends on the patient, context, goal(s) and which types of clinicians are collaborating on the patient's care. Currently, most clinicians obtain needed information from others through a written or verbal ad hoc consult. This is a cumbersome, error-prone and often slow process. In the electronic world, such information could flow much more easily, efficiently and automatically through the National Health Information Infrastructure or Health Information Exchanges, given appropriate safeguards for security and confidentiality. Standards such as the Continuing Care Record of the American Society of Testing and Materials, adapted to dentistry by the American Dental Association's Standards Committee for Dental Informatics, have begun to address what information should be subject to exchange.

Current settings which implement the exchange of medical and dental information among care providers are few and far between. Three examples are the U.S. Department of Veterans Affairs (VA), HealthPartners in Minnesota and the Marshfield Clinic in Wisconsin, described in this book. The electronic health records of these organizations include both medical and dental data, and provide partially integrated views of these data. Figure 6.3 in Chap. 6 shows a screenshot of Marshfield Clinic's Cattails Dental System that displays information from a patient's medical record in the lower left corner.

The organizations which are working towards realizing the vision articulated in this book are important practical laboratories for what works and what does not. While the VA is limited with regard to its patient population, and HealthPartners and Marshfield serve patients only in specific regions, it would be useful to learn what information clinicians exchange, how they use it, and, most importantly, how doing so influences decision making and patient care outcomes.

As many regional health information networks and health information exchanges have shown, the technical and logistical problems of exchanging health information are solvable. But, how can we help clinicians understand, use and act on received information? Many dental students learn quite a bit about medicine during their studies, but the inverse appears not to be true (Ferullo et al. 2011). We therefore should consider not just how to communicate information, but also how to assist recipients in understanding and using it. Clinical decision support can help by providing additional information and guidance when and where it is needed. However, the majority of research studies in decision support have focused on providing assistance only to individual clinicians. To support closer integration of medical and dental care, this research should be extended to provide collaborative decision support for multiple providers caring for the same patient.

This book is setting out a tall challenge for the health care community. Achieving the vision of integrating medical and dental care requires nothing less than rethinking how we care for our patients as a team of healthcare providers, not as individual practitioners. Can we achieve this vision? Maybe it is good to look at a group that already has done so. In biomedical informatics, physicians, dentists, nurses, pharmacists and members of other disciplines collaborate to advance how we use data and information in healthcare. It is telling that the idea for this book arose from the informatics community – let's hope it can serve as an example for all of healthcare!

Titus K.L. Schleyer, D.M.D., Ph.D.
Associate Professor and Director, Center for Dental Informatics
School of Dental Medicine
University of Pittsburgh

References

Baron RJ. It's time to meaningfully use electronic health records: our patients are demanding it. Ann Intern Med. 2011;154(10):697–8.

Ferullo A, Silk H, Savageau JA. Teaching oral health in U.S. medical schools: results of a national survey. Acad Med. 2011;86:226–30.

Greenberg BL, Glick M, Frantsve-Hawley J, Kantor ML. Dentists' attitudes toward chairside screening for medical conditions. J Am Dent Assoc. 2010;141:52–62.

McDaniel AM, Stratton RM, Britain M. Systems approaches to tobacco dependence treatment. Annu Rev Nurs Res. 2009;27:345–63.

Schleyer T, Eisner J. The computer-based oral health record: an essential tool for cross-provider quality management. J Calif Dent Assoc. 1994;22:57–64.

Spielmann N, Wong DT. Saliva: diagnostics and therapeutic perspectives. Oral Dis. 2011;17:345–54.

Preface

Editors' Preface

This is the story of a simple idea (the mouth is part of the body) and what it means in the context of the complexities in healthcare organization, care delivery, provider education, and care reimbursement, along with recommendations. This volume seeks to optimize the delivery of healthcare by stating why isolated components of healthcare delivery need to work together, by asserting how health information technology (HIT) can help these components collaborate to improve care quality and patient safety, by documenting how existing barriers stand in way of interdisciplinary collaborative practice supported by HIT, and by recommending how to remove such barriers.

Our first reaction could have been, this is too difficult to do. The barriers to bringing dental care and medical care together into a collaborative framework include traditions of practice and education, political considerations, separate insurance or payer structures. The results of this are:

- separate statistical compilations of data for medical and dental conditions and treatment impeding a unified assessment of current conditions,
- separate cultures of practice workflow,
- (in most cases) separated electronic patient records systems for medical and dental practice and often independent goals for software standards (thus also standards that anticipate the potential need to articulate medical and dental patient records),
- negative and unproductive attitudes of some providers in the two domains toward each other,

- health care planning bodies, forums, and commissions that do not include representation from both types of providers,
- laws, regulations, and policies that do not acknowledge a need for collaboration among physicians and dentists in the treatment of a given individual patient within a single time frame,
- separate reimbursement structures, rationales, and plans, and thus also, from a technical standpoint, separate claim streams, impeding development of interdisciplinary state disease registries using performance measures to support care quality improvement and adoption of collaborative care in practices,
- care quality initiatives that, by their various respective structures, are not explicitly tasked with addressing the role of oral health care integrally in patient care, affecting the design and establishment of performance measures for care quality improvement,
- the disquieting perception that, in certain respects, the two domains were drifting further apart in the absence of a common unifying principle for education and cooperation, and,
- ultimately, the circumstance that these conditions are replicated to some extent in societies around the globe, thus affecting the care of patient populations worldwide.

When we thought of the suffering and early mortality faced by large numbers of patients with chronic illnesses and a variety of other conditions, we decided we could not avoid this task. We realized we cannot be afraid to ask questions and identify problems merely because the situation is complex.

All the editors for this volume are health informaticists, meaning that we focus on the application of information technology to health care requirements. We know that in any industry, one must match the program developed, with precision, to the activities in that industry. To develop banking software, we need to understand exactly what kinds of transaction go on in the banking industry that must be represented and processed in the system we envision. If we want to characterize software appropriate for the healthcare industry, we assume we have the skills to formulate an accurate model for that industry. When we examine the healthcare industry, we notice siloization in a number of respects. By siloization, we mean that parts of the practice of healthcare are conducted in isolation from other parts. This isolation of providers from one another carries the attendant risk that the patient may be harmed (or may not receive efficacious care) by dividing up the work into silos, where two care providers **concurrently** address the health needs of a **single individual patient**, without adequate supporting communication to assure that what is done is one "stream" of care activities (administration and prescription of medications, performance of surgeries) will be safe and efficacious while, within the same time frame, care activities proceed in a second "stream." We wonder how healthcare can be optimized under conditions of less-than-adequate articulation of care delivery for a single patient. Therefore we are professionally obligated to call to the attention of the industry we serve, that certain ways of "doing business" stand in the way of getting an optimal result and should be addressed.

Preface   xvii

The most troublesome healthcare siloization for us, although by no means the only siloization present, is that isolating the education of, practices of, and payments to medical and dental providers. To underscore the point that the issues we are addressing are more general than those involved in the separation of medicine and dentistry, we are fortunate to have input from ophthalmology on how eye care imaging could be more effectively used in healthcare.

During this period of time the science and technologies of healthcare are shifting, guided by knowledge of DNA, molecular imaging, and the promise of "personalized healthcare." As we learn what genetics and proteomics can teach us, we become increasingly aware that "pathogen behavior does not consider how human healthcare delivery is structured" and that a team approach is required for optimal care delivery and truly "patient-centered" healthcare.

When we imagined the billions being allocated to health information technology (HIT), we reviewed the maxim of software development, "know what your software is supposed to do before you design and deploy it." We recognized that HIT could not be designed correctly until we had a correct healthcare delivery model. The beginning of the design process is requirements analysis. Establishing software requirements cannot start until a correct model for healthcare delivery is agreed upon, with all significant categories of providers represented at the table. If the current model is faulty, software based on that model is being designed and deployed at great expense and the resulting software, flawed by its omissions, will (in the form of technological inertia) pose a barrier to achieving integrated care in the future. HIT software corrections will subsequently require non-trivial added expenditures to revise not only the software, but also the workflows and organizational structures that match it. Ethically, with regard to the design and specification of healthcare systems, we cannot countenance this and have therefore prepared this volume.

To establish continuity with initiatives which have preceded this book, the first preface by Dr. David A. Nash addresses the need for integration of care, while the second preface, by Dr. Titus K. Schleyer, links this volume with the research and teaching in biomedical and dental informatics which have preceded it.

In order to help assure the appropriate interdisciplinary mix of input, we solicited contributions of varying lengths, knowing that being flexible on length would help attract contributors whose practice demands, administrative roles, and research schedules would otherwise not permit them to participate in this volume.

A brief outline of the coverage of the chapters:

Chapter 1 addresses the rationale for integrating medical and dental care and patient records and presents a timeline to demonstrate the gradually growing awareness of the need for integration.

Chapter 2 focuses on technical and theoretical requirements for establishing the integrated electronic record, including such topics as interoperability, knowledge representation, respective requirements of medical and dental providers, patient identification, and decision support.

Chapter 3 deals with metrics and measurements, including quality measures and the meaningful use concept.

Chapter 4 examines current conditions, covering economic considerations, needs of particular populations, provider viewpoints, biosurveillance, education, and translational research. By looking at how eye care imaging can be more effectively used in health care, this chapter looks beyond the medical-dental relationship toward the more general requirements of care delivery for integration of care and patient records supported by health information technology.

Chapter 5 helps the reader see to what extent integration of medical and dental care and records is or is not "on the radar" in various countries, in order to provide an international perspective. This chapter offers thorough treatment of Mexico and Portugal, with brief coverage of the United Kingdom and Canada.

Chapter 6 portrays a working example of care and data integration in the Marshfield Clinic system across a major part of rural Wisconsin.

Chapter 7 is the conclusion, collecting and highlighting recommendations made in this volume.

The first two appendices present forms and materials from two sources which have explicitly addressed integration of care: the University of Detroit Mercy School of Dentistry (Appendix A) and the Wisconsin Diabetes Mellitus Advisory Group (Appendix B).

In one of the appendices (Appendix C) you will find a cataloging of what we call *contact points* between medical and dental care and research, along with references to relevant clinical literature to each topic. The set of contact points involves a wide range of medical subspecialties as well as great range of specialties in dental care.

Appendix D furnishes a list of online resources with their URLs and the list of abbreviations precedes the prefaces.

Valerie J.H. Powell
Franklin M. Din
Amit Acharya
Miguel Humberto Torres-Urquidy

Acknowledgements

I would like to take this opportunity to express my sincere gratitude to Dr. Titus Schleyer for his continued support, encouragement and guidance through my journey in the field of Dental Informatics. His mentorship and advice has been paramount in aligning my career goals to excel in the field. I would also like to express gratitude to my mentor, Mr. Greg Nycz for his unparalleled support and tremendous encouragement. It is heartwarming to witness and be a key part of the initiatives under his leadership to improve access to high quality health care services for the underserved and to enhance the health of communities in and around the state of Wisconsin. I would also like to thank Dr. Justin Starren for identifying the importance of Dental Informatics to improve oral and systemic health and providing a unique opportunity for me to pursue this field. I would like to thank my colleagues Dr. Joseph Kilsdonk, Dr. Humberto Vidaillet, Dr. Steve Wesbrook, Dr. Murray Brilliant, Dr. Steve Yale, Dr. Fred Eichmiller and Dr. Umberto Tachinardi for their support in various initiatives that are ongoing at Marshfield Clinic to close the chasm between Medicine and Dentistry. I would also like to thank all the authors, experts and reviewers for their significant contributions to this book. I would also want to express my gratitude to my co-editors Dr. Valerie Powell, Dr. Frank Din and Dr. Miguel Humberto Torres-Urquidy for their enthusiasm and perseverance in this undertaking. Finally, I would like to thank the most important person, my wife Rohini who stood by me throughout this endeavor, during which we also became first-time parents to our beautiful daughter, Anoushka. I could not have made it without her unwavering support and encouragement.

Dr. Amit Acharya

I would like to thank the entire staff and fellow students in the Columbia University Bioinformatics Program during my time there. I am the sum total of all their teaching, guidance, leadership, cooperation, competition, and friendship. Each of them is reflected in this volume. I would especially like to thank Dr. Edward (Ted) Shortliffe, the department chair and Dr. John Zimmerman, my advisor. Ted for running a program in which a dreamer can flourish and John for his patience and understanding. I wish to acknowledge the influence of Dr. Robert Ledley, whom I never met. Dr. Ledley was a pioneer in Informatics and proved that a dentist could contribute to the field at the highest level. Lastly I thank my co-author Valerie Powell whose unrelenting belief in the rightness of the cause and forcefulness in advocacy led to numerous advancements, including this book.

Dr. Franklin M. Din

I wish to express my gratitude to my mentors in learning health informatics who helped me grasp the value of integrated health systems, Dr. Charles J. Austin, former president of Texas A&M University in Commerce and author of textbooks on information systems for health services administration, and Dr.med. Wolfgang Giere, retired director of the Medical Informatics Center, Goethe University of Frankfurt am Main and pioneer of European medical informatics, to the many electronic health record professionals in the Veterans Health Administration (VHA) and in WorldVistA who have contributed to my understanding of health information technologies, to my lifelong friend John W. Konnak, MD, who felt that, "if it affects patient care, you have to address it," to my husband, Dr. James C. Powell, who graciously read through manuscripts and provided both corrections and encouragement, to two Registered Dental Hygienists (RDHs) who helped me understand the needs and viewpoints of this important professional group in oral healthcare, Patti DiGangi and Shirley Gutowski, and to our two preface contributors, Dr. David A. Nash, who made real the connection of this project with his "oral physician" concept, and Dr. Titus Schleyer, whose leadership in biomedical and dental informatics and interest in this project have been an encouragement to all of us.

Dr. Valerie J.H. Powell

I wish to express my gratitude to Drs. Lyn Finelli, Anne McIntyre, Elizabeth Neuhaus, and Herman Tolentino from CDC, whose leadership and example furthered my enthusiasm in informatics. I am also grateful to the members of the Public Health Informatics Fellowship Program, always prone to insightful discussions. I am thankful of having as a mentor Dr. Titus Schleyer, at the University of Pittsburgh, a pioneer in the area of Dental Informatics. Additionally, I would like to thank my wife Cristina for her support and suggestions, which definitely improved our manuscripts. Finally, I would like to thank our contributors for their valuable inputs, without which this volume would certainly not have been the same.

Dr. Miguel H. Torres-Urquidy

Contents

1 **Rationale and Need to Articulate Medical and Dental Data**................ 1
Valerie J.H. Powell and Franklin M. Din

2 **HIT Considerations: Informatics and Technology Needs and Considerations** 25
Miguel Humberto Torres-Urquidy, Valerie J.H. Powell,
Franklin M. Din, Mark Diehl, Valerie Bertaud-Gounot, W. Ted Klein,
Sushma Mishra, Shin-Mey Rose Yin Geist, Monica Chaudhari,
and Mureen Allen

3 **Metrics and Measurements** 139
Valerie J.H. Powell, Amit Acharya, Andrea Mahnke,
Franklin M. Din, and Thankam P. Thyvalikakath

4 **Broader Considerations of Medical and Dental Data Integration** 167
Stephen Foreman, Joseph Kilsdonk, Kelly Boggs, Wendy E. Mouradian,
Suzanne Boulter, Paul Casamassimo, Valerie J.H. Powell, Beth Piraino,
Wells Shoemake, Jessica Kovarik, Evan(Jake) Waxman, Biju Cheriyan,
Henry Hood, Allan G. Farman, Matthew Holder,
Miguel Humberto Torres-Urquidy, Muhammad F. Walji, Amit Acharya,
Andrea Mahnke, Po-Huang Chyou, Franklin M. Din, and Steven J. Schrodi

5 **International Perspectives** 299
Miguel Humberto Torres-Urquidy, Jeffrey R. Glaizel, Rodrigo Licéaga-Reyes,
André Ricardo Maia Correia, Filipe Miguel Araújo, Tiago Miguel Marques,
Filipa Almeida Leite, and Angus W.G. Walls

6 **An Integrated Medical-Dental Electronic Health Record Environment: A Marshfield Experience** 331
Amit Acharya, Natalie Yoder, and Greg Nycz

7 **Conclusion and Recommendations** 353
Franklin M. Din and Valerie J.H. Powell

Appendix 363

Index 409

Contributors

Amit Acharya, B.D.S., M.S., Ph.D. Biomedical Informatics Research Center, Marshfield Clinic Research Foundation, Marshfield, WI, USA

Mureen Allen, M.D., M.S., M.A., FACP Medical Informatics Consultant, New Jersey, USA

Filipe Miguel Araújo, D.M.D., M.Sc. Health Sciences Department, Universidade Católica Portuguesa – Campus de Viseu, Porto, Portugal

Valerie Bertaud-Gounot, Ph.D. University Psychiatric Hospital, Rennes, France

Kelly Boggs, M.B.A. Division of Education, Marshfield Clinic, Marshfield, WI, USA

Suzanne Boulter Department of Pediatrics, Dartmouth Medical School, Hanover, NH, USA

Paul Casamassimo, D.D.S., M.S. Division of Pediatric Dentistry, The Ohio State University College of Dentistry, Columbus, OH, USA

Center for Clinical and Translational Research, Nationwide Children's Hospital, Columbus, OH, USA

Monica Chaudhari, M.S., M.M.S./M.B.A. Washington Dental Service, Seattle, WA, USA

Biju Cheriyan, M.B.B.S., D.L.O. Holy Cross Hospital, Kottiyam and Caritas Hospital, Kottiyam, Kerala, India,

Po-Huang Chyou, Ph.D. Biomedical Informatics Research Center, Marshfield Clinic Research Foundation, Marshfield, WI, USA

André Ricardo Maia Correia, D.M.D., Ph.D. Department of the Portuguese Catholic University (DCS-UCP), Dental Medicine, University of Porto (FMDUP), Health Sciences, Porto, Portugal

Mark Diehl, D.D.S. Health Informatics Program, Misericordia University, Dallas, TX, USA

Franklin M. Din, D.M.D., M.A. HP Enterprise Services, Global Healthcare, Camp Hill, PA, USA

Allan G. Farman, B.D.S., Ph.D., M.B.A., D.Sc., Diplomate ABOMR Department of Surgical and Hospital Dentistry, University of Louisville School of Dentistry, Louisville, KY, USA

Stephen Foreman, J.D., Ph.D., M.P.A. Health Economics, Robert Morris University, Pittsburgh, PA, USA

Shin-Mey Rose Yin Geist, D.D.S., M.S. Departments of Biomedical and Diagnostic Sciences and Patient, Management, University of Detroit Mercy School of Dentistry, Detroit, MI, USA

Jeffrey R. Glaizel, D.D.S., RCDS myDDSnetwork, Toronto, ON, Canada

Matthew Holder, M.D., M.B.A. Underwood and Lee Clinic, Louisville, KY, USA

American Academy of Developmental Medicine and Dentistry, Louisville, KY, USA

Henry Hood, D.M.D. Department of Orthodontic, Pediatric and Geriatric Dentistry, University of Louisville School of Dentistry, Louisville, KY, USA

Underwood and Lee Clinic, Louisville, KY, USA

Joseph Kilsdonk, AuD Division of Education, Marshfield Clinic, Marshfield, WI, USA

W. Ted Klein, M.S. Klein Consulting Inc., Ridge, NY, USA

Jessica Kovarik, M.D. School of Medicine, University of Pittsburgh, Pittsburgh, Pennsylvania, USA

Filipa Almeida Leite, M.D. Teotónio Hospital, Viseu, Portugal

Rodrigo Licéaga-Reyes, D.D.S., Ph.D. Department of Oral and Maxillofacial Surgery, Juarez Hospital in Mexico City, Mexico, DF, Mexico

Andrea Mahnke, B.S. Biomedical Informatics Research Center, Marshfield Clinic Research Foundation, Marshfield, WI, USA

Tiago Miguel Marques, D.M.D., M.Sc. Health Sciences Department, Portuguese Catholic University, Porto, Portugal

Sushma Mishra, M.B.A., Ph.D. Computer and Information Systems Department, Robert Morris University, Pittsburgh, PA, USA

Wendy E. Mouradian, M.D., M.S. Department of Pediatric Dentistry, Schools of Dentistry, Medicine and Public Health, University of Washington, Seattle, WA, USA

Greg Nycz, B.S. Family Health Center of Marshfield, Inc, Marshfield, WI, USA

Beth Piraino, M.D. Renal Division, Department of Medicine, University of Pittsburgh Medical School, Pittsburgh, Pennsylvania, USA

Valerie J.H. Powell, Ph.D., M.S., R.T.(R) Department of Computer and Information Systems, Clinical Data Integration Project, Robert Morris University, Moon Township, PA, USA

Steven J. Schrodi, Ph.D. Center for Human Genetics, Marshfield Clinic Research Foundation, Marshfield, WI, USA

Wells Shoemaker, M.D. California Association of Physician Groups, Sacramento, California, USA

Thankam P. Thyvalikakath, B.D.S., M.D.S., M.S., D.M.D. Center for Dental Informatics, School of Dental Medicine, University of Pittsburgh, Pittsburgh, PA, USA

Miguel Humberto Torres-Urquidy, D.D.S., M.S., Ph.D. (candidate) Department of Biomedical Informatics, University of Pittsburgh, Pittsburgh, PA, USA

Muhammad F. Walji, Ph.D. Dental Branch, University of Texas, Houston, Texas, USA

Angus W.G. Walls, B.D.S., Ph.D., FDSRCS School of Dental Sciences, Newcastle University, Newcastle, UK

Evan(Jake) Waxman, M.D., Ph.D. Department of Ophthalmology, University of Pittsburgh, Pittsburgh, PA, USA

Natalie Yoder, B.S. Biomedical Informatics Research Center, Marshfield Clinic Research Foundation, Marshfield, WI, USA

List of Abbreviations

AADE	American Association of Diabetes Educators
AAMC	American Association of Medical Colleges
AAP	American Academy of Pediatricians
ACE	Angiotensin-Converting Enzyme
ACO	Accountable Care Organization
ADA	American Dental Association
ADA	American Diabetes Association
AM	Amalgam
AMA	American Medical Association
ARB	Angiotensin Receptor Blocker
ARRA	American Recovery and Reinvest Act
BDS	Bachelor of Dental Surgery
BioMedGT	Biomedical Grid Terminology
CAD	Coronary Artery Disease
CCD	Continuity of Care Document
CCM	Chronic Care Model
CDA	California Dental Association
CDA	Canadian Dental Association
CDS	Clinical Decision Support
CDT	Current Dental Terminology
CFR	Code of Federal Regulation
CMS	Centers for Medicare and Medicaid Services
COTS	Commercial Off-the-Shelf
CPOE	Computerized physician order entry
CPT	Current Procedural Terminology
CPU	Central Processing Unit
CQM	Clinical Quality Measure
CRF	Chronic renal failure
DDS	Doctor of Dental Surgery
DGES	Dentogingival epithelial surface area
DMD	Doctor of Dental Medicine

DMI	Dental / Medical Integration
DNP	Doctor of Nursing Practice
DO	Doctor of Osteopathy
DoD	Department of Defense
EBICP	Evidence-Based Integrated Care Plan
EDO	Extended Data-Out
EDR	Electronic Dental Record
EHR	Electronic health record
EHT	Electronic health technologies
EMR	Electronic Medical Records
EP	Eligible Professionals
ER/PR	Estrogen Receptor/Progesterone Receptor
ERG	Episode Risk Group
eRx	Electronic prescribing
ESRD	End stage renal disease
FHC	Family Health Center
GMP	General medical practitioners
GH	Group Health Cooperative
HD	Hemodialysis
HF	Heart Failure
HHS	Health and Human Services
HIT	Health Information Technology
HITECH	Health Information Technology for Economic and Clinical Health
HIV	Human Immunodeficiency Virus
HL7	Health Level 7
ICD	International Classification of Diseases
ICD-10	International Classification of Diseases, Tenth revision
ICD-10 CM	International Classification of Diseases, Tenth revision, Clinical modifications
ICD-9	International Classification of Diseases, Ninth revision
ICD-9 CM	International Classification of Diseases, Ninth revision, Clinical modifications
ICU	Intensive Care unit
IDF	International Diabetes Federation
iEHR	integrated Electronic Healthcare Record
IHS	Indian Health Service
IHTSDO	International Health Terminology Standards Development Organization
IOM	Institute of Medicine
IT	Information Technology
LDL	Low Density Lipoprotein
LIS	Laboratory information system
LOINC	Logical Observation Identifiers Names and Codes
LVSD	Left Ventricular Systolic Dysfunction
MCRF	Marshfield Clinic Research Foundation

MD	Medical Doctor
MHD	Medical History for Dentists
MI	Myocardial Infarction
MO	Mesioclussal
MS	Microsoft
MU	Meaningful Use
NCI	National Cancer Institute
NDEP	National Diabetes Education Program
NHIN	National Health Information Network
NIDDK	National Institute of Diabetes and Digestive and Kidney
NIH	National Institute of Health
NQF	National Quality Foundation
OCF	Oral Cancer Foundation
ONC	Office of the National Coordinator
ORN	Osteoradionecrosis
OS	Operating System
OSHRP	Oral and Systemic Health Research Project
PC	Personal Computer
PCMH	Patient centered medical home
PD	Perintoneal Dialysis
PCP	Primary Care Physician
PDSA	Plan-Do-Study-Act
PHC	Personalized Health Care
PHR	Patient / personal health records
POAG	Primary Open Angle Glaucoma
PPO	Preferred Provider Organization
PQRI	Physician Quality Reporting Initiative
RAM	Random Access Memory
ROM	Read Only Memory
SCT	SNOMED CT
SDO	Standards Development Organizations
SGR	Surgeon General's Report
SNODENT	Systematized Nomenclature of Dentistry
SNOMED CT	Systematized Nomenclature of Medicine – Clinical Terms
TFT	Thin film transistor
UI	User Interface
VA	Veterans Affairs
WDS	Washington Dental Service
WDSF	Washington Dental Service Foundation
WHO	World Health Organization

List of Figures

Fig. 1.1	Flow of information in patient care for providers
Fig. 1.2	Open wound size range from 1.24 sq. in. to 3.1 sq. in. adult periodontitis DGES equivalent
Fig. 1.3	Evolving models of support for interdisciplinary communication among medical and dental providers
Fig. 2.1	Signs based on different standards
Fig. 2.2	Presents the sign "Construction ahead" intended to warn drivers that they might encounter an area under construction when driving, used in the UK. Taken out of context, this sign can be jokingly interpreted as the "man with a broken umbrella." In this case, "context" plays a big role in defining meaning, actually changing it completely
Fig. 2.3	Overview of the modeling process
Fig. 2.4	Sequence of models generated to reach a comprehensive representation of healthcare activities
Fig. 2.5	Clinical process or diagnostic-therapeutic cycle appears in the specification
Fig. 2.6	Clinical process as a recursive activity
Fig. 2.7	Model displaying the interactions of the individual with different elements supporting the healthcare delivery process
Fig. 2.8	The Ogden-Richardson's semiotic triangle establishes the different elements that play a role in representing knowledge through concepts
Fig. 2.9	Basic ontology representing clinical information in the form of concepts and their properties as well as the relationships between concepts
Fig. 2.10	Partial view of diseases represented in the ontology of dental emergencies
Fig. 2.11	Partial view of findings represented in the ontology of dental emergencies

Fig. 2.12	Example of disease "Reversible pulpitis" characterized by the relationships in the ontology
Fig. 2.13	Cardiac evaluation and care algorithm for noncardiac surgery based on active clinical conditions, known cardiovascular disease or cardiac risk factors for patients 50 years of age or greater (Fleisher et al. 2007)
Fig. 2.14	Cardiac conditions associated with the highest risk of adverse outcome from endocarditis for which prophylaxis with dental procedures is reasonable (Wilson et al. 2007)
Fig. 2.15	Oncology consult form for cancer patient regarding part or future bisphosphonate therapy
Fig. 2.16	Oral health referral form for cancer patient needing chemotherapy or radiation therapy
Fig. 2.17	GH and WDS approaches to coded patient identifiers
Fig. 2.18	Weak warm body decision flow
Fig. 2.19	PALM IIIc image
Fig. 2.20	PALM Screenshot for booster icon
Fig. 2.21	PALM Screenshot for medical history for dentists application icon
Fig. 2.22	PALM Screenshot for medical history for dentists application
Fig. 2.23	PALM Screenshot for thyroid problem selection
Fig. 2.24	PALM Screenshot for thyroid problem sub-type selection
Fig. 2.25	PALM Screenshot for hyperthyroid general warning
Fig. 2.26	PALM Screenshot for hyperthyroid important warning
Fig. 2.27	PALM Screenshot for prosthetic health valve selection
Fig. 2.28	PALM Screenshot for prosthetic health valve warning
Fig. 2.29	PALM Screenshot for prophylactic antibiotic warning
Fig. 2.30	PALM Screenshot for prophylactic antibiotic dosing for child
Fig. 2.31	PALM Screenshot for prophylactic antibiotic alternative dosing for child
Fig. 2.32	PALM Screenshot for prophylactic antibiotic dosing options selection
Fig. 2.33	PALM Screenshot for high risk patient selection
Fig. 2.34	PALM Screenshot for high risk patient warning
Fig. 3.1	Annual dental visits for children (Pennsylvania)
Fig. 3.2	Assumption that medical health comprises the totality of healthcare
Fig. 3.3	Screenshot of Previser Risk Calculator (PRC) that shows the health history questions PRC asks about to assess patient's risk of periodontal disease.
Fig. 3.4	Screenshot of Previser Risk Calculator (PRC) that shows the disease score ranging from 0 (no disease) to 100 (severe periodontitis) and the risk score ranging from 1 (lowest) to 5 (highest)
Fig. 4.1	Most common chronic US illnesses
Fig. 4.2	Percentage of healthcare spending for individuals with chronic conditions by type of insurance – 2006. Anderson (2010) (Copyright 2010. Robert Wood Johnson Foundation
Fig. 4.3	Per capita healthcare spending and number of chronic conditions – 2006

List of Figures xxxiii

Fig. 4.4	Delivering oral healthcare to a child
Fig. 4.5	Nonproliferative diabetic retinopathy and hypertensive retinopathy
Fig. 4.6	Hypertensive retinopathy
Fig. 4.7	Central retinal vein occlusion
Fig. 4.8	Branch retinal artery occlusion
Fig. 4.9	Branch retinal artery occlusion, fluorescein angiogram
Fig. 4.10	Retinal macroaneurysm
Fig. 4.11	Hypertensive optic neuropathy
Fig. 4.12	Fragile X syndrome
Fig. 4.13	Trisomy 21
Fig. 4.14	Cerebral palsy
Fig. 4.15	Patient with congenital syphilis
Fig. 4.16	GERD-related erosion of enamel and dentinal tissues
Fig. 4.17	Patient on phenytoin
Fig. 4.18	Patient 4 months post-weaning
Fig. 4.19	The adult patient suspected of having Fragile X syndrome
Fig. 4.20	Pectus excavatum
Fig. 4.21	Joint laxity observed in patient with Fragile X syndrome
Fig. 4.22	Four children with autism and one neurotypical child
Fig. 4.23	Patient upon initial examination
Fig. 4.24	Patient after comprehensive treatment
Fig. 4.25	Biosurveillance systems should be cognizant of different kinds of events since this can be linked to issues of public health concern
Fig. 4.26	Biosurveillance system architecture
Fig. 4.27	Information technology – informatics department size at Dental Schools in US
Fig. 4.28	US Dental School IT/informatics department personnel with and without dental informatics (DI) training
Fig. 4.29	Current usage of electronic financial systems and electronic dental records among the responded Dental Schools
Fig. 4.30	Commercial electronic dental records used in the US Dental Schools
Fig. 4.31	Number of years since implementing an EDR at the US Dental Schools
Fig. 4.32	US Dental Schools' plan for applying to medicaid meaningful use incentive program
Fig. 4.33	Communication between EMR and EDR among the responding US Dental Schools
Fig. 4.34	Information categories shared between EDR and EMT in some of the US Dental Schools
Fig. 4.35	Is a polymorphism associated with disease?
Fig. 4.36	The concept of linkage disequilibrium
Fig. 4.37	Technological progress in genomics
Fig. 4.38	Linkage studies vs. association studies to discover disease genes
Fig. 4.39	The synergy between access to care, student competency, and financially sustainable dental education converge around CHC/FQHCs

Fig. 5.1	Breakdown of hospital treatments provided in Mexico by type of institution/source of funding
Fig. 5.2	Breakdown of ambulatory treatments provided in Mexico by type of institution/source of funding
Fig. 5.3	Distribution of governmental medical treatment services by institution
Fig. 5.4	The Mexican Institute of Social Security (Instituto Mexicano del Seguro Social – IMSS) is one of the major health care providers in Mexico
Fig. 5.5	Distribution of dental treatment services by sector
Fig. 5.6	Access to communication technologies in Mexico
Fig. 5.7	Health Information Network in Portugal (RIS)
Fig. 5.8	Newsoft Dente® odontogram (with permission)
Fig. 5.9	Newsoft Dente® periogram (with permission)
Fig. 5.10	Novigest® odontogram (with permission)
Fig. 5.11	Novigest® e-agenda (with permission)
Fig. 6.1	Marshfield Clinic Health Center Complex
Fig. 6.2	Physicians' Dashboard application
Fig. 6.3	Dentists' Dashboard application
Fig. 6.4	Ladysmith Dental Center – Family Health Center of Marshfield, Inc. and Marshfield Clinic's first Dental Center
Fig. 6.5	Unique dental patients at Ladysmith Dental Center after first full year of operation (calendar year 2003)
Fig. 6.6	Dedicated clinical training space at Marshfield Dental Center
Fig. 6.7	Unique dental patients at all of Marshfield Clinic Dental Centers in the 2010 calendar year
Fig. 6.8	Percent of patients in each zip code under 200% poverty who were seen at Ladysmith Dental Center
Fig. 6.9	Key concepts from the discussion panel recorded on flips charts
Fig. 6.10	Overarching themes identified as part of the panel discussion analysis

Chapter 1
Rationale and Need to Articulate Medical and Dental Data

Valerie J.H. Powell and Franklin M. Din

1.1 Separation of the Two Domains and the Need to Re-establish a Holistic View to Healthcare

1.1.1 Separate Healthcare Domains

Since the beginning of modern healthcare, medicine and dentistry have existed as separate healthcare domains. One pathway of care is *oral health care* for the oral cavity and certain associated structures (most notably teeth) – commonly called *dental care* (and less commonly *stomatognathic care*) and is delivered by dental providers (general dentists, periodontists, endodontists, and other specialists with degrees like DDS and DMD). A distinct pathway of *systemic health* care delivers care to the rest of the body – called *medical care* and delivered by medical providers (allopathic physicians, osteopathic physicians, nurse practitioners, etc. with degrees like MD, DO, DN).[1] While this separation appeared to serve well for many years, significant changes in healthcare have occurred and this separation is now obsolete and may be harmful. This artificial division of care into organizational silos ignores the fact that the mouth is part of the body (NIH 2000). Field et al. (2000) characterized

---

[1]There is, of course, a systemic care discipline, otolaryngology (also referred to as ear, nose, and throat or ENT care), which covers much of the same anatomy as is covered by oral health providers, minus the teeth and their supporting structures.

V.J.H. Powell (✉)
Department of Computer and Information Systems, Clinical Data Integration Project,
Robert Morris University, Moon Township, PA, USA
e-mail: powell@rmu.edu

F.M. Din
HP Enterprise Services, Global Healthcare, Camp Hill, PA, USA
e-mail: franklin.din@dbmi.columbia.edu

the phrase "medically necessary dental care" in the following manner with reference to the U.S. Medicare program: "Such a restrictive definition may suggest that periodontal or other tooth-related infections are somehow different from infections elsewhere and imply that the mouth can be isolated from the rest of the body, notions neither scientifically based nor constructive for individual or public health."

The growing understanding of how dental affects medical (systemic) and vice versa suggests that continuation of this separation leads to incomplete, inaccurate, inefficient and inadequate treatment of both medical and dental disease. Dentistry and medicine need to harmonize. To facilitate this change and to assure the highest quality care and safety for patients, this book looks at the issues, the challenges, and recommends specific actions to address specific problems. The essential core improvement to bring medicine and dentistry closer is the integration of medical and dental care and data. Currently many medical records and data exist separate and distinct from dental records and data for the same patient.

This siloization in the U.S. persists despite international recognition of the need for integration of the disciplines. According to the World Health Organization (WHO), "The strategy is that oral disease prevention and the promotion of oral health needs to be integrated with chronic disease prevention and general health promotion as the risks to health are linked." Further, "The objectives of the WHO Global Oral Health Programme, one of the technical programmes within the Department of Chronic Disease and Health Promotion, imply that greater emphasis is put on developing global policies based on common risk factors approaches and which are coordinated more effectively with other programmes in public health. The policy of the WHO Global Oral Health Programme emphasizes that oral health is integral and essential to general health, and that oral health is a determinant factor for quality of life." Also, with regard to health information technology, "The WHO/FDI goals for oral health by the year 2000 urged Member States to establish oral health information systems, and this remains a challenge for most countries of the world. The WHO Oral Health Programme is prepared to assist countries in their efforts to develop oral health information systems which include data additional to epidemiological indicators." (Peterson 2008) According to WHO's "Global goals for oral health 2020," (Hobdell et al. 2003) Goal 2 is "To minimize the impact of oral and craniofacial manifestations of systemic diseases on individuals and society, and to use these manifestations for early diagnosis, prevention and management of systemic diseases," and Objective six states, "To integrate oral health promotion and care with other sectors that influence health, using the common risk factor approach."

The data silos reflect and may actually drive and perpetuate the care silos. Consider a typical work and information flow between a dentist and a physician caring for the same patient who has periodontal disease and diabetes in Fig. 1.1.

The communication between the general dentist, who normally does the initial periodontal screening, and the specialist treating diabetes or stroke is typically indirect, proceeding through the Primary Care Physician (PCP) via the chart, EHR, or relies on the patient's initiative. Any medical specialists (endocrinologists, cardiologists) treating a patient are ordinarily dependent on the patient's primary care physician

Fig. 1.1 Flow of information in patient care for providers

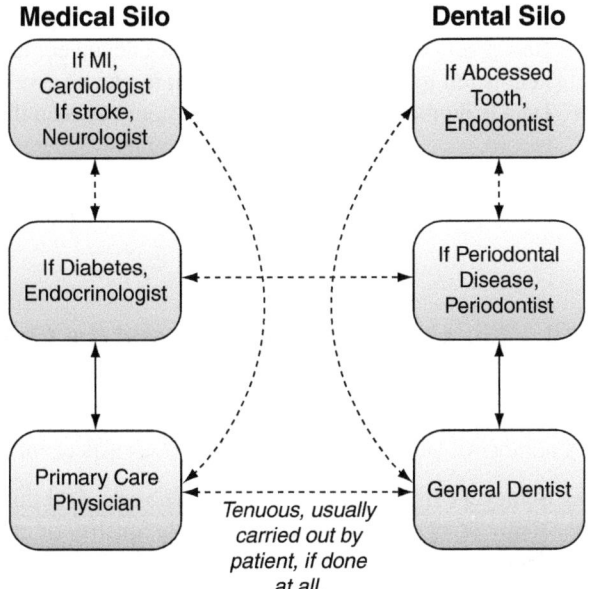

for contact with the providers in the same patient's dental silo. A neurologist treating stroke, for example, who might gain in the processes of diagnosis and treatment from a well-established model of interdisciplinary medical-dental communication, is dependent on the referring PCP for dental information, and that referring PCP might not have a direct channel of communication with the patient's dental provider(s). Fig. 1.1 shows a dotted line (labeled with a question mark) for possible communication between an endocrinologist or diabetologist and periodontist. Unfortunately, they lack a systematic approach to communication with each other. Instead the provider teams (physician and nurse on the medical silo and general dentist and dental hygienist, in the dental silo) must, on their own initiative, obtain the patient's other-silo information. In general this connection must also be regarded as tenuous, as reflected in the dot-dash line. The arrow in the diagram might suggest that the communication is provider-to-provider. In reality, the cross communication is dental provider via patient as active carrier of the message to the medical provider. Unfortunately, providers are ill-prepared to engage at this level of coordination. A well-established model for efficient communication among medical and dental providers who care for the same patient does not ordinarily exist. The exceptions are the University of Detroit Mercy School of Dentistry model (Geist and Geist 2008) and the Wisconsin Diabetes Advisory Group model (WDAG 2011), both with regard to paper charts.

There are many potential intersections in which the medical records can inform the treatment of dental problems and vice versa. Because there is no systematic information exchange at these intersections a number of problems persist that continue to hinder comprehensive patient care.

- Real-time cooperation involving patient care is practically non-existent.
- Best practices guidelines often ignore a dental component to care or that component is left to the whim of the patient to pursue.
- Data is duplicated and often inconsistent between the medical record and dental record.
- The structural barriers to medical – dental communication and care hinder the progress toward complete, patient centered care.

1.2 The Communication Gap and the Collaborative Care Gap (First Two Topics Above)

A number of authors have looked at various aspects of the communication gap:
- Schleyer (Thyvalikakath et al. 2008) observed, "I think the healthcare system has plenty of opportunities to improve the quality of care by simply improving the communication among the people who provide it. However, there are several reasons why this is not happening very much now. Many of them are historical and 'ingrained' in the way each discipline practices, but others are contemporary barriers. … we have to acknowledge that technology is only a piece of the puzzle. It certainly will not be the silver bullet for solving healthcare communication problems. It needs to work hand-in-hand with efforts to (1) augment standards of care to represent the best evidence available; (2) break down professional, systemic, cultural and personal barriers to improved communication; and (3) make the patient the central and focal point of healthcare."
- Dental Education at the Crossroads: Challenges and Change (Field and Jeffcoat 1995), and the Institute of Medicine (IOM) had already recommended closer integration of dentistry with medicine and the health care system as a whole. This IOM report predicted that scientific and technological advances in molecular biology, immunology, and genetics, along with an aging population with more complex health needs, would increasingly link dentistry and medicine, leading to the need for changes in dental education (Sax 2002). From the IOM report: "The report did not call for a single medical/dental profession, but it did conclude that the dental profession will and should become more closely integrated with medicine and the health care system on all levels: education, research and patient care."
- The Midwest Disparities Collaborative in 1998, a diabetes quality improvement initiative using the MacColl Chronic Care Model (CCM), which "aims to create practical, supportive interactions between an informed activated patient and a proactive, prepared clinical team," and rapid Plan-Do-Study-Act (PDSA) cycles from the continuous quality improvement field (Chin et al. 2004). This chronic care initiative included dental care as well as a dilated eye exam, diet intervention, and foot care or foot examination, based on the ADA (American Diabetes

Association) clinical practice recommendations. Chronic care models have been important in integrating dental collaboration in regional and statewide initiatives, of which this is an example. The MacColl CCM was succeeded by the Wagner CCM (Wagner et al. 1996; Wagner 1998; Wagner et al. 2001; Bodenheimer et al. 2002a,b).
- Haughney et al. report on a 3 year study of integration of primary care dental and medical services (Haughney et al. 1998): "This experimental model of health care showed the potential that exists for the coordination and integration of functions between the dental team and the primary care team. Improvement in communication by joint information exchange can be of considerable benefit to patient care. We believe that most of the benefits indicated on this single clinical site could be reproduced in separate locations by the use of integrated record systems and modern methods of information exchange. Integrated primary dental and medical care requires attitudinal change in health care professionals and requires greater emphasis in the education and training of health care professionals in the future."
- Wisconsin Diabetes Advisory Group's (2011) "Wisconsin essential diabetes mellitus care guidelines," describes the Wisconsin Diabetes Prevention and Control Program, and including a chapter on Oral Health and recommendations for interdisciplinary communication (Wisconsin Diabetes Advisory Group 2011). They provide an online interdisciplinary referral form (See Appendix B). The Wisconsin guidelines state: "An oral screening should be performed at diagnosis and at each diabetes-focused visit occurring thereafter. Any positive findings should initiate referral to a dentist or dental specialist to ensure early and prompt diagnosis and treatment. The screening includes an evaluation of the oral cavity for signs of redness, bleeding, halitosis, accumulation of debris around the teeth, gingival recession with exposed root surfaces, separation of teeth, and tooth mobility. People without teeth (edentate) should also receive an evaluation for signs of tissue inflammation or irregularities, white or red lesions, and any change in the fit of their dentures. Physicians, nurses, ancillary healthcare professionals, and caregivers can all perform this evaluation and must reinforce the importance of oral and dental care."
- Aetna's Dental/Medical Integration Program was announced in 2006. According to Dr. Mary Lee Conicella, Aetna Dental's national director of clinical operations "The association between oral health and systemic health is consistently demonstrated in clinical studies, and the findings are positively impacting the treatment and management of patients." Further she said "Specifically, there is a significant body of research that indicates pregnant women and individuals with diabetes or heart disease benefit from early periodontal care. The member outreach program, in conjunction with enhancements to our dental offerings, is designed to motivate these individuals to seek care" (Aetna 2006).
- CIGNA's Oral Health Integration Program^{SM} (OHIP) was announced in 2006. According to CIGNA's announcement (CIGNA 2006), studies "have shown that medical costs for diabetic and cardiovascular patients were significantly lower

when treated for gum disease. Direct and indirect costs for diabetes and heart disease are on the rise." CIGNA announced maternity, diabetes, and cardiovascular oral health programs.
- Dr. George Chiarchiaro, an IHS dentist and project manager for the IHS EDR, said that the new EDR will replace the current one used by IHS and will offer dentists far more options on it than the existing dental record. Dr. Chiarchiaro stated that, "we will interface our new dental record with certain portions of that larger legacy system. One of the interfaces between our new dental software and our existing electronic health record will be to send dental information over to the electronic health record. A physician, or nurse practitioner, pharmacist or physician assistant can open the patient's electronic health record and see what dental procedures have been performed ... they will be able to access that information in the patient's primary health record" (Basu 2006).
- The Scottsdale Project recommended that physicians should screen for periodontal disease; "dentists should work collaboratively with physicians to achieve the best possible patient care outcomes" and identified a need for "a set of guidelines should be developed to define what is important for bidirectional professional communication" (Hein 2007).
- The American Diabetes Association includes "dental referral" and "dental history" in its Standards of Care. (ADA [Diabetes] 2011) Sue Kirkman reported that the two ADAs (American Diabetes Association and American Dental Association) were collaborating on conferences that year (2008) and that "the Professional Practice Committee had just commissioned a technical review of the literature to be jointly written by medical and dental professionals from" both "ADA's" (Kirkman MS, 2008, personal communication; Lamster et al. 2008).
- In 2000, the U.S. Surgeon General released the report "Oral Health in America" to raise awareness of the 'silent epidemic' of dental and oral disease. It concluded that dental caries is the most prevalent infectious disease among American children. While early childhood dental caries emerges within all cultural and economic pediatric populations, oral health disparities are related to socioeconomic status and race/ethnicity, it stated, "As a result of the Surgeon General's report, the American Academy of Pediatrics began a push to examine children's oral health and determine how pediatricians could become involved in addressing the epidemic,' said Huw Thomas, B.D.S., M.S., Ph.D., dean of the School of Dentistry at the University of Alabama at Birmingham." ... In October 2008 the American Academy of Pediatricians (AAP) PEDS 21 Symposium (Pediatrics for the Twenty first Century) focused on oral health and "the Pediatrician's role in Oral Health." From AAP Highlight: More than 40% of children from families at or below the federal poverty line have tooth decay by the time they reach kindergarten. More than 52 million hours of school are lost each year because of dental problems. To combat these and other problems related to dental health, pediatricians are being asked to focus on the oral health of our nation's youth. 'Pediatricians see young infants and children frequently for preventive health

care visits, putting them in an excellent position to identify children at risk for dental health problems, coordinate appropriate care and parent education, and refer affected and high risk children to pediatric dentists,' said Suzanne Boulter MD, pediatrician at Concord Hospital in Concord, NH.

Other authors who deal with the gaps in medical and dental care and data integration as part of a larger understanding include:

- Healthy People 2020 (HHS, Office of Disease Prevention and Health Promotion (Health and Human Services (2010)) includes national objectives in oral health addressing a number of categories for public health improvement, including the need to increase awareness of the importance of oral health to overall health and well-being, to increase acceptance and adoption of effective preventive interventions, and to reduce disparities in access to effective preventive and dental treatment services.
- Oral health in America: a report of the Surgeon General, issued by the Department of Health and Human Services, National Institute of Dental and Craniofacial Research (NIDCR), and National Institutes of Health, in 2000 (NIH 2000).
- In June 2008 the American Association of Medical Colleges published Contemporary Issues in Medicine: Oral Health Education for Medical and Dental Students: Medical School Objectives Project (AAMC 2008).
- In 2009 the International Centre for Oral-Systemic Health was established at the University of Manitoba in Winnipeg.
- In 2010 the U.S. Health Resources and Services Administration (HRSA) announced its new Strategic Plan. For Goal I, on improving access to quality health care and services, Subgoal b called for expanding oral health and behavioral health services and integrating them into primary care settings.

The common theme that binds all these contributions and milestones is the understanding that the patient is negatively affected by the current inability to integrate and harmonize medical and dental care. In many instances, the common needs greatly outweigh the historical separation. For instance, providers in both silos need accurate information on medications prescribed in the other silo (blood thinners, antibiotics, pain medications) and on certain tests ordered in one of the silos. Haughney et al. (1998) reported that "the joint use of patient record systems avoided discrepancies in patient information which would have affected the quality of patient care" and "joint consultations reduced the need for secondary referrals." Geist and Geist (2008) stated, "physicians often do not provide adequate information regarding patients' medical conditions when presented with consultation requests generated by dental students and their instructors about the students' patients."

In the interest of providing a historical view of the initiatives above, the authors have compiled a timeline table, Table 1.1.

This table demonstrates the increasing effort to integrate medical and dental care since Dr. David A. Nash' "Oral Physician" speech in 1994, signifying an increasing awareness of the issue.

Table 1.1 Timeline for integration of medical and dental care and patient data

Year	Milestone(s)
1994	Oral physician speech (Dr. David A. Nash)
1994	*British Dental Journal* reports pilot study
1994	World Health Organization Oral Health Report: *Oral Health for the twenty-first century*
1995	Institute of Medicine Report on Dental Education at the Crossroads
1996	United Kingdom Government White Paper proposes pilot integration schemes
1998	Midwest Disparities Collaborative using Chronic Care Model
1998	*British Dental Journal* reports on 3 year study of integration
2000	Surgeon General Report – Oral Health
2000	*Healthy People 2010* with dental objectives
2003	American Diabetes Association. Clinical practice recommendations
2004	Wisconsin Diabetes Advisory Group, essential diabetes care guidelines
2006	Aetna announces Dental/Medical Integration
2006	CIGNA announces CIGNA Dental Oral Health Integration Programs^{SM} (OHIP) for Maternity, Diabetes, Cardiovascular
2007	New Indian Health Service RPMS Dental System
2007	American Association of Diabetes Educators dental visit measure
2007	Scottsdale Project
2007	World Health Organization global policy for improvement of oral health – World Health Assembly 2007
2008	American Diabetes Association. Standard of Medical Care includes "dental referral"
2008	American Association of Medical Colleges Medical School Objectives Project : Medical and Dental Students Education
2008	American Academy of Pediatricians' statements on oral health for twenty-first century
2008	Health Resources and Services Administration's 7th annual report calls for the "Patient-Centered Medical-Dental Home in Primary Care Training."
2009	International Centre for Oral-Systemic Health was established at the University of Manitoba in Winnipeg, Canada
2010	Healthy People 2020, a set of goals and objectives, was announced by the U.S. Office of Disease Prevention and Health Promotion (ODPHP)
2010	American Academy for Oral-Systemic Health (AAOSH) founded
2010	HRSA Strategic Plan of the Health Resources Services Administration (HRSA) calls for integration of oral health into primary care

1.3 A Broader Look at the Fundamental Healthcare Delivery Model

Some authors have considered these issues and have determined that a broader look at the fundamental healthcare delivery model is in order. The notion of medicine and dentistry as distinct entities must be reconsidered.

Dr. Wendy Mouradian is a leader in the collaborative, interdisciplinary approach to health care, integrating medical and dental care. Dr. Mouradian writes about how she became interested in providing integrated care:

1 Rationale and Need to Articulate Medical and Dental Data

> The biggest influence was when I was the Director of the Interdisciplinary Craniofacial Program at Seattle Children's Hospital where I saw the importance of the dental and oral components of health and the consequences when these were ignored. I also began to appreciate the general medical ignorance of these issues... Then I started to realize that there was an isolation of dentistry in the area of health policy and funding, and as a consequence large gaps in access to dental care. I did a certificate in health care ethics at the UW (University of Washington) and focused on some of these issues in that program. I subsequently went on to work for NIDCR on the Surgeon General's Conference on children and oral health (Mouradian WE, 2008, personal communication).

She indirectly reveals that her interest was preceded by the presence of an interdisciplinary program unit. Not only have interdisciplinary integration and collaborative (medical-dental) care existed prior to the developments of the last 20 years, but there always have been individual providers in both disciplines who have been sensitive to this need for tight collaboration. What has been lacking in health care in the U.S. in general (except in the VA system and in the IHS which have been leaders not only in health information technology, but in integrating care and in implementing preventive and chronic care), is a consistent and generally accepted foundation for communication among these providers for shared patients. In order to establish the proper model for healthcare's future in the U.S., the U.S. requires a model of healthcare that overcomes the "isolation of dentistry in the area of health policy and funding".

Nash (2006), Giddon (2006), Giddon and Assael (2004) have discussed calling dental providers "oral physicians." Giddon points out that "unfortunately, the dental profession, which enjoys what are perceived to be the benefits of independence from medicine, including a higher average salary than physicians – at least when comparing general dentists with primary care physicians in group practice ($174,350 for the general dentist in 2002 and $150,000 for primary care physicians in group practice in 2002) – may not want to incur the bureaucratic disadvantages of managed care and related problems." Nash (2006) cites the oral physician curriculum at the University of Kentucky. Nash writes, "I justified the need for such a transformation based on the significant changes in the environment of dentistry, which I characterized as biological, epidemiological, technological, demographic, professional, and economic." Further Nash states, "changing our name changes nothing of substance," he wants dental education to be reformed and scorns "minor changes" and asserts "separation from medicine may have served the public well in the past. It no longer does."

1.4 Healthcare Education and Preventive Care

In 2008 a report from the U.S. Health Resources and Services Administration (HRSA 2008) called for a "patient-centered medical-dental home," asserting that rapidly "changing dynamics in the U.S. health care environment" were driving "the need for major restructuring of the health care system that highlights disease prevention and comprehensive, coordinated care for chronic diseases." This report urged that "drastic action … be urgently undertaken" to assure an adequate supply of primary care physicians. HRSA's report called for "realignment of our antiquated, inequitable system that pays handsomely for procedures, tests, and specialty services but relatively meager sums for the demanding primary care role of coordinating acute and chronic disease care while delivering preventive care."

HRSA pointed out that in "2004, the American Academy of Pediatrics (AAP), in association with the American Academy of Family Physicians (AAFP), the American College of Physicians (ACP), and the American Osteopathic Association (AOA), defined comprehensive guidelines for the Patient-Centered Medical Home (PCMH) as the central approach to improve health care in the U.S. (Patient Centered Primary Care Collaborative 2007)" Joint Principles of the Patient Centered Medical Home, February 2007 and noted that also in 2004, the American Academy of Pediatric Dentistry (AAPD) formally adopted a policy endorsing the Dental Home (DH) According to HRSA's proposed model, "each patient has a personal physician or dentist who leads a team of clinical care providers and staff who take collective responsibility for delivering comprehensive, coordinated care that addresses all of a patient's health care needs." These statements, as well as the entire HRSA report, make clear that action is needed.

An American Association of Medical Colleges (AAMC) Medical School Objectives Project (MSOP) document states that in a 1995 study, Dental Education at the Crossroads: Challenges and Change, the Institute of Medicine (IOM) (Field and Jeffcoat 1995) had already recommended closer integration of dentistry with medicine and the health care system as a whole: This IOM report predicted that scientific and technological advances in molecular biology, immunology, and genetics, along with an aging population with more complex health needs, would increasingly link dentistry and medicine, leading to the need for changes in dental education. As physicians come to see oral health as a legitimate domain of involvement for their profession, and dentists acquire better understanding of the systemic implications of oral disease, asking the right questions will be as much a matter of perspective as of knowledge and skills. Cultivating such a perspective will require significant change in the curricula of both professions (AAMC 2008), as well as attention to the topics satisfying continuing education requirements for physicians, nurses, dentists, and dental hygienists.

Hein (from Scottsdale Project) states that "in spite of the growing acceptance within the dental community, it cannot be assumed that the medical community is aware of the research to support the effect of periodontal disease on local and systemic inflammation" (Hein et al. 2007).

Thus, in addition to integration of records, there is a need to sensitize the medical community to the dental contribution to systemic health and a converse need to sensitize the dental community to dental contribution to systemic health. The simple recognition of the importance of the other side to overall health is a big step toward acceptance of the integration of medical and dental records.

DePaola and Slavkin (2004) wrote: "In essence, the SGR [Surgeon General's Report, NIH (NIH 2000)] articulated and documented that the mouth is connected to the body, that oral and systemic diseases and disorders can be associated, that oral diseases and disorders can compromise health and well-being over the human lifespan, and that disparities exist in oral health and disease patterns." Among the critical educational needs they cite are: "increase interdisciplinary perspective/practice; and improve our students' ability to relate to and address the overall health of the patient."

An example of a course meeting the AAMC initiatives is "A New Oral Health Elective for Medical Students" (Mouradian et al. 2006). However, according to Rafter et al. (2006), "At a recent conference evaluating dental education (Santa Fe Group) participants determined that an important factor responsible for the difficulties in dental education was the 'silo' approach so commonly found in health education: 'By their reliance on independent curricula, faculty, facilities and research programs, 'silos' contribute to the isolation of health professional training programs.'"

1.5 Progress Toward, Complete Patient-Centered Care – Clinical Considerations

We have painted a relationship between systemic and oral health and disease. Any effort to integrate medicine and dentistry data must reflect the reality of the actual disease. The specifics of some of the more important diseases that impact patients that concern both dentists and physicians are introduced below. For more details on such diseases, please refer to Sects. 2.3, 2.4 and Appendix C.

1.5.1 Diabetes, Cardiovascular Disease and Periodontal Disease

According to Mealey and Rose (2008), "the presence of periodontal diseases can have a significant impact on the metabolic state in diabetes. Diabetic subjects with periodontitis have a sixfold higher risk for worsening of glycemic control over time compared to diabetic subjects without periodontitis. Periodontitis is also associated with an increased risk for diabetic complications. In one study, 82% of diabetic patients with periodontitis experienced one or more major cardiovascular, cerebrovascular or peripheral vascular events during the study period of 1–11 years, compared to only 21% of diabetic subjects without periodontitis."

Professor Edward P. Heinrichs (Periodontics and Preventive Care, School of Dental Medicine, University of Pittsburgh) recently suggested comparing the aggregate "open wound" of periodontitis to an open wound ranging (on the mean) from 1.24 sq. in. to 3.1 sq. in. (the dentogingival epithelial surface area or DGES), according to Hujoel et al. (2001) To visualize the seriousness of periodontitis see Fig. 1.2.

Robert Nelson (NIH/NIDDK) writes, "Recent studies suggest even greater complexity in the relationship between periodontal disease and diabetes. These studies report striking relationships between periodontal disease and the development of the macro- and microvascular complications of diabetes – in particular cardiovascular

Fig. 1.2 Open wound size range from 1.24 sq. in. to 3.1 sq. in. adult periodontitis DGES equivalent

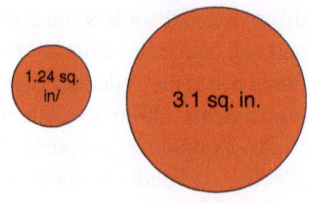

and kidney disease. Whether these relationships are due primarily to the hyperglycemia that typically accompanies periodontal disease or to other mechanisms remains to be determined. Some proposed mechanisms for the link between periodontitis and the complications of diabetes include chronic systemic inflammation associated with increased circulating cytokines and inflammatory mediators, direct infection of the vasculature extending beyond the oral cavity, an autoimmune response to the chronic periodontal infection that leads to endothelial dysfunction, or common susceptibility factors that lead to increased susceptibility to periodontal disease and to vascular diseases simultaneously. Perhaps several or all of these mechanisms are involved" (Nelson 2008).

Ample research literature exists documenting the role of inflammation that are common to periodontal diseases and other systemic diseases (Cochran 2008; Genco 2008; Graves 2008; Ordovas and Shen 2008; Serhan 2008; Van Dyke and Kornman 2008; Wilson 2008).

1.5.2 Prenatal Care, Periodontal Disease and Low Birth Weight

Kushtagi et al. (2008) stated, "the association of low birth weight neonates with high health care costs and high infant mortality has been well established." In a study of 150 women with appropriate variables controlled for, "the presence of periodontal infection was found to be significantly higher in women who delivered low birth weight neonates compared with the control group." Dasanayake et al. (2008) recommend that "because treatment of periodontal disease during pregnancy is both safe and effective, nurses, nurse practitioners, and nurse midwives who care for mothers and infants can play an important role in educating pregnant women about oral health. Because nearly two-thirds of pregnant women do not receive dental care during pregnancy, nursing professionals can counsel pregnant women to seek dental care during pregnancy. If mothers understand that there is a potential link between the bacteria in their mouth, their health, pregnancy outcomes, and the health of their infant, they may be more receptive to and interested in seeking dental care." Michaliwicz et al. (2006) confirm the safety of periodontal care during pregnancy. Vettore et al. (2008) describe "the relationship between periodontitis and preterm low birth weight." McGaw (2002) cautioned that "Prospective studies, and eventually interventional studies, will be necessary before periodontitis can be considered as a causal factor for PLBW."

1.5.3 Post Radiation Osteonecrosis (ORN) and Bisphosphonate Caused Osteonecrosis (ONJ)

Jolly (2004) writes, "Osteoradionecrosis (ORN), also known as postradiation osteonecrosis (PRON), is a serious, debilitating and deforming potential complication of radiation therapy for the treatment of cancer of the head and neck. It has been defined as a necrosis or death of the bone of the mandible or maxilla that may occur following radiation therapy for cancer in the oral and peri-oral region. It is known to occur when bones, in this case the mandible and/or maxilla, are directly in the field of radiation."

According to Ronald P. Strauss (AAMC 2008), "Nothing prepared me for the destruction that I witnessed on Mr. J's jaw caused by osteoradionecrosis. His jaw bone melted away on the X-rays until he had a fractured mandible, all because he had radiation treatment for oral cancer years ago." After detailing Mr. J's condition, Strauss continued, "Even years after the original cancer treatment, [patients] may be at risk for radiation-associated dental caries and osteoradionecrosis. It is critical that the dentist and the oncology team communicate closely about the care of patients who have had head and neck radiation treatment for oral or pharyngeal cancer."

Recently, there have been reports of osteonecrosis of the jaws (ONJ) in cancer patients receiving concomitant anticancer therapy (chemotherapy, steroid therapy, or head and neck radiotherapy) and an intravenous (IV) bisphosphonate (Damato et al. 2004; Child et al. 2011). There are multiple recognized conditions and risk factors associated with the development of osteonecrosis (not limited to the jaws) in cancer patients (Marx 2003; Migliorati 2003; Ruggiero et al. 2004). Potential liability in the cases involving biphosphonate gives another reason why dentists need to be linked into medical information. A dentist may not be the one who prescribes a given biphosphonate but may very well be the first one to observe the complication.

1.5.4 Oral Cancer Screening; Tobacco and Betel Use Screening and Oral Cancer Prevention

Dental providers are now performing oral cancer screenings for cancers of the head, neck, and mouth. According to an online page from the Oral Cancer Foundation (OCF 2009), in addressing dental providers, "For general dental practitioners OCF believes your responsibility is at minimum creating awareness, and being involved in opportunistic discovery of suspect tissue through routine screening of your entire patient population, and referral for second opinion or biopsy when appropriate. For dental specialists such as oral surgeons and periodontists, as well as oral medicine specialists, it is providing second opinions, and when requested or when you believe necessary, performing biopsy of any suspect area."

Macpherson et al. (2003) examined the trade-offs (in the UK) between seeking more routine dental visits to improve oral cancer screening, as a dental check-up would support early detection, and getting general medical practitioners (GMP) to play more of a role in oral cancer screening. Macpherson et al. stated that "a high proportion of GMPs (87%) indicated they routinely made enquiries of their patients in relation to smoking habits" and yet reported only "19% of dental respondents routinely made enquiries into smoking habits, with a further 49% doing so 'occasionally.'" Thus the health professional (dental), perhaps most appropriately in a position to do oral cancer screening, appears not to be as engaged in this aspect of health promotion, even though tobacco use is regarded as a high risk behavior for oral cancer. In Asia, betel quid (BQ) chewing has a role corresponding to that of tobacco chewing in North America. Zhang and Reichart (2007) report that in mainland China, oral "diseases associated with BQ chewing are oral sub mucous fibrosis (OSF), oral leukoplakia (OL) and oral cancer."

1.5.5 Eating Disorders Screening

DeBate and Tedesco (2006) describe how general dentists can play a role in preventing eating disorders: the "dentist, in particular, has a uniquely important and valuable role with respect to assessment of oral and physical manifestations [of anorexia nervosa and bulimia nervosa]. ... Despite this crucial role, few dentists are engaged in eating disorder specific secondary prevention."

1.5.6 Pediatric Care

Dentists can be particularly important to the success of pediatric care. Chu et al. (2007) document referrals by non-dentist providers for oral health care. Mouradian (Mouradian et al. 2003, 2004; Mouradian and Corbin 2003) has been a pioneer and strong advocate for collaborative medical/dental approaches to pediatric oral health care. Mouradian (Mouradian et al. 2004) writes, it "is clear that oral health disparities cannot be addressed without collaborative efforts between dentistry and medicine and other health professions." According to Riter et al. (2008), "Dental disease, the most prevalent chronic disease of childhood, affects children's overall health and ability to succeed. Integrating oral health into routine well-child checkups is an innovative and practical way to prevent dental disease. The Washington Dental Service Foundation (WDSF) is partnering with Group Health Cooperative, a large integrated delivery system, and other providers in Washington State to change the standard of care by incorporating preventive oral health services into primary care for very young children." Other information on interdisciplinary approaches to pediatric dentistry can be found in Mabry et al. (2006) and Douglass et al. (2005).

1.5.7 Oral Hygiene and Respiratory Infections

Yoneyama et al. (1996) point out the role of oral hygiene in reducing respiratory infections in "elderly bed-bound nursing home patients." According to Scannapieco (Scannapieco and Rethman 2003), "recent evidence has suggested a central role for the oral cavity in the process of respiratory infection. Oral periodontopathic bacteria can be aspirated into the lung to cause aspiration pneumonia. The teeth may also serve as a reservoir for respiratory pathogen colonization and subsequent nosocomial pneumonia. Typical respiratory pathogens have been shown to colonize the dental plaque of hospitalized intensive care and nursing home patients. Once established in the mouth, these pathogens may be aspirated into the lung to cause infection. Other epidemiologic studies have noted a relationship between poor oral hygiene or periodontal bone loss and chronic obstructive pulmonary disease. Several mechanisms are proposed to explain the potential role of oral bacteria in the pathogenesis of respiratory infection:

1. Aspiration of oral pathogens (such as Porphyromonas gingivalis, Actinobacillus actinomycetemcomitans, etc.) into the lung to cause infection;
2. Periodontal disease-associated enzymes in saliva may modify mucosal surfaces to promote adhesion and colonization by respiratory pathogens, which are then aspirated into the lung;
3. Periodontal disease-associated enzymes may destroy salivary pellicles on pathogenic bacteria to hinder their clearance from the mucosal surface; and
4. Cytokines originating from periodontal tissues may alter respiratory epithelium to promote infection by respiratory pathogens."

Azarpazhooh and Leake (2006) describe the role of "aspiration pneumonia," leading to more than 15,000 deaths per year in the U.S., with more than 200,000 cases annually, and states that "among ICU patients, those being mechanically ventilated are particularly susceptible to pneumonia."

1.5.8 Kidney Disease and Periodontal Disease

Fischer et al. (2008) describe periodontal disease as a risk factor for kidney disease. Craig (2008) describes how "renal replacement therapy can affect periodontal tissues, including gingival hyperplasia in immune suppressed renal transplantation patients and increased levels of plaque, calculus, and gingival inflammation and possible increased prevalence and severity of destructive periodontal diseases in end stage renal disease (ESRD) patients on dialysis maintenance therapy. Also, the presence of undiagnosed periodontitis may have significant effects on the medical management of the ESRD patient. … periodontitis may be a covert but treatable source of systemic inflammation in the ESRD population." Bayrakter et al. (2007), reported in a study that more plaque and calculus and bleeding on probing were found in the hemodialysis (HD) than in the control group. This evaluation is complex, as HD patients might receive anticoagulation therapy, affecting bleeding, and the altered serum calcium-phosphorus balance possible in ESRD patients. Bayraktar et al. (2007a, 2007b) point out that oral health care for CRF (chronic renal failure) patients should begin "before the beginning or at least within 1 month of their first dialysis treatment," as without oral health maintenance "oral pathologies and infections could jeopardize the opportunity to receive a successful kidney transplant." For more on kidney disease and oral health, see Sect. 4.2.2.

There are many other diseases that affect medical and dental care, like herpetic infections, Vitamin deficiencies. It is not the goal of this section to provide a comprehensive accounting of diseases that affect systemic and oral health. Rather it is meant to clearly convey to the reader that diseases rarely stay limited to oral or systemic domains. As author Powell remarked, "all attempts to keep oral pathogen confined to the mouth have failed miserably."

1.6 Data Inconsistency

The Department of Defense (DoD) leads in medical/dental integration. Part of the reason for their focus is due to the fact the DoD has been aware since 1977 that as many of 10% of dental records of active duty personnel could have discrepancies when compared with their medical records (Lewis et al. 1977). In a group of 100 randomly selected active duty personnel at Walter Reed Medical Center, "eleven discrepancies of major medical significance were found." Discrepancies between medical and dental records is due largely to the reliance on patient reports from treatment in the other discipline, rather than on an integrated electronic record system. Selzer and McDermott (1999) reported that "of patients who completed the same medical history questionnaire twice within a certain time period, 66% had at least 1 significant omission in their history."

According to Lutka and Threadgill (1995), "medical history questionnaires and outpatient medical records of 115 patients were compared. All patients had a medical history of at least 2 years in both records. The dental records were initially reviewed, and patients' responses were compiled; when these were compared with the outpatient medical records, the overall discrepancy rate was greater than 86%. This overwhelming rate of error should make dentists aware that many routinely treated patients have medical conditions that are unknown to providers. Clearly, quality comprehensive care is impossible with inconsistent, perhaps dangerously contradictory records.

Haughney et al. (1998) reported that "the pilot study had revealed, [for 178 joint patients] in a retrospective study, a large number of discrepancies between information contained in the medical records summary and the medical history in dental records." They observed that "the joint use of patient record systems avoided discrepancies in patient information which would have affected the quality of patient care" and "joint consultations reduced the need for secondary referrals." They found that 3 medical records were missing information that was considered important of life threatening and more ominously, 18 dental records were missing similar information. The Table 1.2 below summarizes the discrepancies, based on Haughney et al.

Table 1.2 Medical and dental records discrepancies, based on Haughney et al.

Category	Not on *medical* records	Not on *dental* records	Total
Life threatening	2	4	6
Important	1	14	15
Relevant	20	58	78
Total	23	76	99

1.7 Insurance Claim Silos

The traditional separation and distinction between medical care and dental care is reflected and reinforced in the separate insurance realms (medical vs. dental insurance). This complicates the coordination of care and insurance coverage. This separation is reflected in the sets of codes and terminologies for claims: CPT (for medical care) and CDT (for dental care). A more coordinated approach to insurance should yield significant improvements in patient and public health outcomes like, (a) formally connect the relationship between systemic (medical) and oral (dental) health care streams, (b) reduce disparities of coverage of unserved and underserved populations, (c) better support performance measure assessment and biomedical research. The fact that there are separate insurance frameworks (medical insurance, dental insurance) in health care has important effects.

The situation of having two silos for systemic (medical) and oral (dental) health insurance should be reviewed and analyzed, so that these two silos can be merged into a single health insurance framework, with appropriate attention to (a) the interrelationships between systemic (medical) and oral (dental) health care, including a common terminology to ensure semantic consistency, (b) disparities of coverage, and (c) foundations for performance assessment and biomedical research. There is literature covering oral health disparities in detail (Fisher-Owens et al. 2008; Mouradian et al. 2003, 2004; Mouradian and Corbin 2003; Pyle and Stoller 2003).

The folly of separate insurance coverage is exemplified by Medicare, in which coverage for dental care is completely excluded except for "extractions done in preparation for radiation treatment for neoplastic diseases involving the jaw," and "oral examinations, but not treatment, preceding kidney transplantation or heart valve replacement." (CMS 2005). The protocols surrounding organ transplantation have for years cited the need to remove all active infections, including oral, prior to surgery. However, Medicare has determined that you are allowed to examine but not treat active oral infections in transplant candidates. The Medicare position can be summarized as requiring that inexpensive oral treatment is disallowed prior to a very expensive surgical procedure, which may then be denied on medical grounds in cases where the patient cannot afford dental care. The likelihood of post-surgical complications increases due to the combination of immuno-suppressive drugs and active oral infections. Post surgical complications, especially those that manifest immediate after the surgery are likely to be difficult to resolve, may lead to a reduction in long term prognosis, and is expensive.

While it can be argued that the gaps in dental coverage that exists in Medicare is immaterial to how the rest of the healthcare insurers treat medical and dental coverage, in reality, the size and scope of Medicare and Medicaid means that private insurers must always analyze their plans and coverage in view of Medicare and Medicaid coverage. Medicare and Medicaid serve as the base against which all other coverage is measured. Inclusion of dental care within Medicare is likely to stimulate private insurers, other than Aetna and CIGNA, which have already integrated medical and dental plans, to rethink their policies.

1.8 Evolving from Patient Data Silos to Integrated Technologies

The traditional separation and distinction between medical care and dental care is reflected and reinforced in the separate patient record systems, either sets of (paper) medical charts and (paper) dental charts, or medical (EMR) and dental (EDR) electronic records systems. The models for communication to deliver care are shown in Fig. 1.3.

- Model A, where the patient's recall is a basis for establishing a patient's medical or dental history, uses "SneakerNet," the patient bearing information between the two offices.
- Models B1, B2, B3, and B4 show the use of telephone and fax where employees (clerical or nursing in the medical office; clerical or dental hygiene in the dental office) phone or fax for information and receive a phone call or a fax in return. These models apply where there are only paper systems (B1), where one system uses paper and one is electronic (B2, B3), or where there are two electronic systems and they do not communicate directly with each other (B4).
- Model C is a one-way system designed to assure that the dentist has access to a patient's medical history and medical test results. An implementation of this model is the system used by Healthpartners, Inc., in the Minneapolis, Minnesota, area (Rindal, 2011). Rindal reports that HealthPartners "has medical and dental record systems that serve 25 medical and 15 dental care delivery sites in Minnesota. To support oral healthcare, HealthPartners dental providers can access medical record information (diagnoses, physician office notes, current medications and medical test results). Allowing dental providers access to complete medical information provides the opportunity to improve the quality and safety of dental care for patients with chronic diseases."
- Model D, which was reported in use at one major children's hospital, uses three electronic systems and "pastes" [sic] data from the dental and orthodontic systems into the medical system.
- In integrated Model E1 the medical and dental electronic components are designed to work together, so that dentists have access to a patient's medical history and test results and physicians have access to dental history and test results. With communication flowing in both directions, every provider visit results in vitals being recorded. This model is described in detail in this volume in Chap. 6. Examples of this model are the Marshfield Clinic systems, and the technologies of three U.S. Federally-sponsored healthcare systems, the Indian Health Service (IHS), the U.S. Department of Veterans Affairs (VA), and the U.S. military.

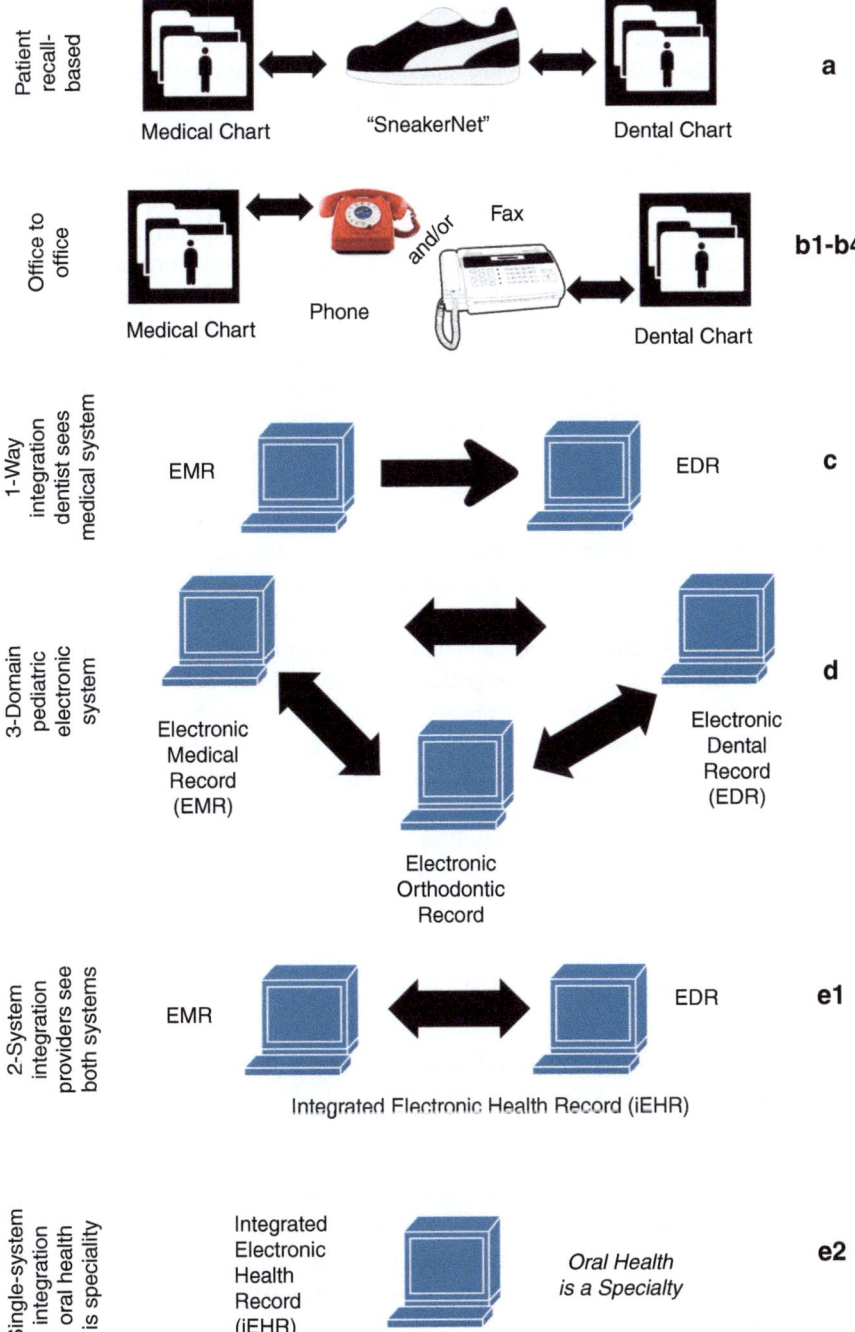

Fig. 1.3 Evolving models of support for interdisciplinary communication among medical and dental providers

- Integrated Model E2 is a single electronic health record system in which Oral Health is simply a specialty. This model implements the "Oral Physician" concept presented initially by Dr. David A. Nash in 1994. A commercial vendor example of this model is offered by Epic. Thomas stated, "While there are special needs for dental, we believe that it is part of a patient's overall health and should be fully integrated with their entire body health record, meaning one medication list, and one source of truth on all diagnoses and treatments. The tools to support the dental specific workflows, such as managing images, documenting easily and quickly on individual teeth notes with shortcuts specific to the most frequent dental terms and flows are the areas that we think can be tailored well, while still on one single encompassing patient record (Thomas T, 2011a, personal communication)." According to Thomas, "in treating a patient record, Epic doesn't segregate dental and medical information in any significant way. While the starting template for documentation for a dentist or oral surgeon will be oriented to teeth, mouth, diagrams, etc. and their answer choices limited to things appropriate for dental, with a click of a button the entire medical record is available. The header shows the patient's allergies, and it's the same list for a dentist, an obstetrician, or an A&E doctor." Thomas continues, "Epic essentially treats dentistry like a specialty. For orthopedics there is a lot of provider-centric content related to bones and joints to speed them along and make documentation easy, in cardiology you have cardiology PACs, images of the heart, documentation specific to stents, and diagnostics for the cath lab. All of these then end up as aspects of a single, comprehensive record. So the patient with a broken ankle, hypertension, and a dental abscess will have in one list the pain meds for the ankle, the hydrochlorothiazide for the heart, and antibiotics for the abscess. The dentist will focus on the images of the patient's mouth, their dental x-rays, and notes from the dental hygienist, but all the rest is still there. The orthopedist will focus on the x-ray of the ankle, however they'll be alerted if they order a pain med that interacts with the patient's heart meds" (Thomas T, 2011b, personal communication).

1.9 Data Standards

The gulf that separates medicine and dentistry is also reflected in the language and codes sets used in each. A few examples:

Current Procedural Terminology (CPT) is the code set used to standardize medical procedure and services, while Current Dental Terminology (CDT) is the code set used to standardize dental procedure and services. There is very little overlap; even the coding format is different. Since the American Medical Association (AMA) controls the CPT and the American Dental Association (ADA) controls the CDT, any attempt at harmonization will require a commitment from the leadership of both Professional Organizations.

Medicine use International Classification of Diseases revision 9 (ICD 9) or 10 to code for medical diagnosis. Dentistry in general does not attempt to standardize dental diagnosis using ICD or any other diagnostic code set.

Systematized Nomenclature of Medicine (SNOMED) is a robust, well known, well-maintained, and comprehensive clinical terminology for Medicine. Its dental counterpart, the Systematized Nomenclature of Dentistry (SNODENT) does not share many of SNOMEDs advantages.

Any attempt at integrating the professional fields will also require an effort to harmonize the language and data structure to match.

1.10 Summary

The link between oral health and systemic health cannot be denied. The separation of dental and medical is no longer defensible or sustainable in modern healthcare. An efficient interdisciplinary communication model is required. However an interdisciplinary agreement on the nature of such communication does not exist. When a periodontist receives a patient referred by a general dentist, it is clear what information should be send to the referring dental provider. In many instances, that same information is not meaningful or useful to a referring primary care physician or endocrinologist providing care for a patient with diabetes. A collaborative medical-dental approach to care would also lead to reciprocal best practice concepts for screening, such as the opportunities for dental providers to screen for eating disorders or oral cancer or for medical providers to screen for oral health as suggested by a number of sources. Providers in both silos sharing care of patients will benefit from accurate information on medications prescribed in the other silo (blood thinners, antibiotics, pain medications) and on tests ordered in one of the silos.

The reader has been introduced to the case for integration as well as some supporting evidence. The following chapters will expand on the ideas presented in this chapter. The core need, the foundation for success, for achieving the integration of the clinical practices is the integration of the records. Dental records must integrate with medical records and medical records must accommodate the needs of dental providers. This extends to all applications, architectures, standards, and advanced functions envisioned in an interoperable healthcare environment.

References

Aetna. Aetna launches program that includes specialized pregnancy dental benefits. Dental Economics; 2006 Nov. 21, 2006 http://www.dentaleconomics.com/display_article/277878/56/none/none/Onlin/Aetna-launches-program-that-includes-specialized-pregnancy-dental-benefit. Accessed 6 Dec 2008.

American Association of Diabetes Educators (AADE) (2007), AADE7 Self Care Behaviors™, at:http://www.diabeteseducator.org/ProfessionalResources/AADE7/. Accessed 10 March 2008.

American Diabetes Association. Standards of medical care in diabetes – 2011. Diabetes Care. 2011;34 Suppl 1:S11–61.

Association of American Medical Colleges (AAMC), Contemporary issues in medicine: oral health education for medical and dental students: medical school objectives project 2008 (AAMC, Washington, DC).

Azarpazhooh A, Leake JL. Systematic review of the association between respiratory diseases and oral health. J Periodontol. 2006;77:1465–82.

Basu S. New IHS dental record will boost patient care through enhanced functions, officials say. U.S. Medicine. July 2006; http://www.usmedicine.com/article.cfm?articleID=1355&issueID=89.

Bayraktar G, Kurtulus I, Duraduryan A, Cintan S, Kazancioglu R, Yildiz A, et al. Dental and periodontal findings in hemodialysis patients. Oral Dis. 2007;13:393–7.

Bayraktar G, Kurtulus I, Duraduryan A, Kazancioglu R, Yildiz A, Bural C, Bozfakioglu S, Besler M, Trablus S, Issever H (2007a) Dental and periodontal findings in hemodialysis patients. Oral Dis 13(4):393–397 doi: 10.1111/j.1601-0825.2006.01297.x.

Bayraktar G, Kurtulus I, Kazancioglu R, Bayrangurler I, Cintan S, Bural C, Bozfakioglu S, Besler M, Trablus S, Issever H, Yildiz A (2007b) Evaluation of periodontal parameters in patients undergoing peritoneal dialysis or hemodialysis. Oral Dis 14(2):185–189 doi: 10.1111/j.1601-0825.2007.01372.x.

Bodenheimer T, Wagner EH, Grumbach K. Improving primary care for patients with chronic illness. JAMA. 2002;288(14):1775–9.

Bodenheimer T, Wagner EH, Grumbach K (2002b). Improving Primary Care for Patients With Chronic Illness, The Chronic Care Model, Part 2 J Amer Med Assoc 288, 15:1909–1914.

Child JA, Davies FE, Wu P, Gregory WM, Bell SE, Szuberti AJ, Navarro-Coy N, Drayson MT, Owen RG, Feyler S, Ashcroft AJ, Ross J, Byrne J, Roddie H, Rudin C, Cook G, Jackson GH, Boyd KD, Morgan GJ. Effect of zoledronic acid (ZOL) versus clodronate (CLO) on skeletal-related events (SRES) in patients (PTS) with multiple myeloma (MM) during intensive (INT), non-intensive (Non-INT), and thalidomide maintenance™ therapies: MRC myeloma IX study results. International myeloma workshop, Paris, 3–6 May 2011. http://www.myeloma-paris2011.com/content/view/15/10/ Accessed 25 Jun 2011.

Chin MH, Cook S, Drum ML, Jin L, Guillen M, Humikowski CA, et al. Improving diabetes care in Midwest Community Health Centers with the health disparities collaborative. Diabetes Care. 2004;27(1):2–8.

Chu M, Sweis LE, Guay AH, Manski RJ. The dental care of U.S. children: access, use and referrals by nondentist providers. J Am Dent Assoc. 2007;138:1324–31.

CIGNA. Oral Health Integration Programs[SM]. 2006. http://www.maricopa.gov/benefits/pdf/2008/CIGNA_Dental/cignadental_oralhealth_ip.pdf. Accessed 25 Jun 2011.

Centers for Medicare and Medicaid Services (CMS). Medicare dental coverage overview. Dec 2005. http://www.cms.hhs.gov/MedicareDentalCoverage/. Accessed 17 June 2011.

Cochran DL. Inflammation and bone loss in periodontal disease. J Periodontol. 2008;79:1569–76.

Craig RG. Interactions between chronic renal disease and periodontal disease. Oral Dis. 2008;14:1–7.

Damato K, Gralow J, Hoff A, Huryn J, Marx R, Ruggiero S, Schudert M, Toth B, Valero, V. Expert Panel* Recommendations for the prevention, diagnosis, and treatment of osteonecrosis of the Jaws. June 2004. http://www.ada.org/prof/resources/topics/topics_osteonecrosis_whitepaper.pdf.

Dasanayake AP, Gennaro S, Henricks-Muñoz KD, Chhun N. Maternal periodontal disease, pregnancy, and neonatal outcomes. Am J Matern Child Nurs. 2008;33:45–9.

DeBate RD, Tedesco LA. Increasing dentists' capacity for secondary prevention of eating disorders: identification of training, network, and professional contingencies. J Dent Educ. 2006;70(10):1066–75.

DePaola DP, Slavkin HC. Reforming dental health professions education: a white paper. J Dent Educ. 2004;68(11):1139–50.

Douglass JM, Douglass AB, Silk HJ. Infant oral health education for pediatric and family practice residents. Pediatr Dent. 2005;27(4):284–91.

Field MJ, Jeffcoat MK. Dental education at the crossroads: a report [Institute of Medicine]. J Am Dent Assoc. 1995;126:191–5.

Field MJ, Lawrence RL, Zwanziger L, editors. Extending medicare coverage for preventive and other services. Committee on Medicare Coverage Extensions, Division of Health Care Services, IOM. Washington, DC: National Academy Press; 2000.

Fisher MA, Taylor GW, Shelton BJ, Jamerson KA, Rahman M, Ojo AO, et al. Periodontal disease and other nontraditional risk factors for CKD. Am J Kidney Dis. 2008;51(1):45–52.

Fisher-Owens SA, Barker JC, Adams S, Chung LH, Gansky SA, Hyde S, et al. Giving policy some teeth: routes to reducing disparities in oral health. Health Aff. 2008;27(2):404–12.

Geist SMRY, Geist JR. Improvement in medical consultation responses with a structured request form. J Dent Educ. 2008;72(5):553–61.

Genco RJ. Clinical innovations in managing inflammation and periodontal diseases: the workshop on inflammation and periodontal diseases. J Periodontol. 2008;79(8s):1609–11.

Giddon DB. Why dentists should be called oral physicians now. J Dent Educ. 2006;70(2):111–3.

Giddon DB, Assael LA. Should dentists become 'oral physicians?' and Yes, dentists should become 'oral physicians'. J Am Dent Assoc. 2004;135:438–49.

Graves D. Cytokines that promote periodontal tissue destruction. J Periodontol. 2008;79:1585–91.

Haughney MGJ, Devennie JC, Macpherson LMD, Mason DK. Integration of primary care dental and medical services: a three year study. Br Dent J. 1998;184(7):343–7.

Health and Human Services, Healthy People 2020 (2010). http://www.healthypeople.gov/2020/default.aspx. Accessed 15 May 2011.

Health Resources and Services Administration. Advisory Committee on training in primary care medicine and dentistry, coming home Rockville, MD: the patient-centered medical-dental home in primary care training. Seventh annual report to the secretary of the U.S. DHHS and to congress, Dec 2008. http://www.hrsa.gov/advisorycommittees/bhpradvisory/actpcmd/Reports/seventhreport.pdf. Accessed 6 May 2010.

Hein C. Lessons learned from Scottsdale, Grand rounds in oral-systemic medicine. 2007. http://www.pennwelldentalgroup.com/display_article/309339/108/none/none/Feat/Lessons-Learned-from-Scottsdale?host=www.thesystemiclink.com. Accessed 15 Jan 2008.

Hein C, Cobb C, Iacopino A. Report of the independent panel of experts of the Scottsdale project, grand rounds supplement; Sep 2007. p. 1–27.

Hobdell M, Petersen PE, Clarkson J, Johnson N. Global goals for oral health 2020. Int Dent J. 2003;53:285–8. http://oralcancerfoundation.org/.

Hujoel PP, White BA, García RI, Listgarten MA. The dentogingival epithelial surface area revisited. J Periodontal Res. 2001;36(1):48–55.

Jolly DE. Osteoradionecrosis, oral health and dental treatment. Dent Assist. 2004;73(2):4–7.

Kushtagi P, Kaur G, Kukkamalla MA, Thomas B. Periodontal infection in women with low birth weight neonates. Int J Gynaecol Obstet. 2008;101:296–8.

Lamster IB, Lalla E, Borgnakke WS, Taylor GW. The relationship between oral health and diabetes mellitus. J Am Dent Assoc. 2008;139 Suppl 5:19S–24.

Lewis DM, Krakow AM, Payne TF. An evaluation of the dental-medical history. Defense Technical Information Center, accession number ADA041260; 1977.

Lutka RW, Threadgill JM. Correlation of dental-record medical histories with outpatient medical records. Gen Dent. 1995;43(4):342–5.

Mabry CC, Mosca NG. Interprofessional educational partnerships in school health for children with special oral health needs. J Dent Educ. 2006;70(8):844–50.

Macpherson LMD, McCann MF, Gibson J, Binnie VI, Stephen KW. The role of primary healthcare professionals in oral cancer prevention and detection. Br Dent J. 2003;195(5):277–81.

Marx RE. Pamidronate (Aredia) and zoledronate (Zometa) induced avascular necrosis of the jaws: a growing epidemic. J Oral Maxillofac Surg. 2003;61:1115–7.

McGaw T. Periodontal disease and preterm delivery of low-birth-weight infants. J Can Dent Assoc. 2002;68(3):165–9.

Mealey BL, Rose LF. Diabetes mellitus and inflammatory periodontal diseases. Curr Opin Endocrinol Diabetes Obes. 2008;15:135–41.

Michalowicz BS, Hodges JS, DiAngelis AJ, Lupo VR, Novak MJ, Ferguson JE, et al. Treatment of periodontal disease and the risk of preterm birth. N Engl J Med. 2006;335(18):1885–94.

Migliorati CA. Bisphosphonates and oral cavity avascular bone necrosis. J Clin Oncol. 2003;21:4253–4.

Mouradian WE, Corbin SB. Addressing health disparities through dental-medical collaboration, part II: cross-cutting themes in the care of special populations. J Dent Educ. 2003;67(12):1320–6.

Mouradian WE, Berg JH, Somerman MJ. Addressing health disparities through dental-medical collaboration, part I: the role of cultural competency in health disparities: training primary care medical practitioners in children's oral health. J Dent Educ. 2003;67(8):860–8.

Mouradian WE, Huebner C, DePaola D. Addressing health disparities through dental medical collaboration, part III: leadership for the public good. J Dent Educ. 2004;68(5):505–12.

Mouradian WE, Reeves A, Kim Sara, Lewis C, Keerbs A, Slayton RL, et al. A new oral health elective for medical students at the University of Washington. Teach Learn Med. 2006;18(4):336–42.

Nash D. Why dentists should become oral physicians: a response to Dr. Donald Giddon's Why dentists should be called oral physicians now. J Dent Educ. 2006;70(6):607–9.

Nelson RG. Periodontal disease and diabetes. Oral Dis. 2008;14:204–5.

NIH. Oral health in America: a report of the Surgeon general. Rockville: U.S. Department of Health and Human Services, National Institute of Dental and Craniofacial Research, National Institutes of Health; 2000.

Oral Cancer Foundation (2009). http://oralcancerfoundation.org/dental/role_of_dentists.htm.

Ordovas JM, Shen J. Gene–environment interactions and susceptibility to metabolic syndrome and other chronic diseases. J Periodontol. 2008;79:1508–13.

Patient Centered Primary Care Collaborative (2007), Joint Principles of the Patient Centered Medical Home, February 2007. http://www.pcpcc.net/content/joint-principles-patient-centered-medical-home. Accessed 15 May 2011.

Peterson PE. World Health Organization global policy for improvement of oral health – World Health Assembly 2007. Int Dent J. 2008;58:115–21.

Pyle MA, Stoller EP. Oral health disparities among the elderly: interdisciplinary challenges for the future. J Dent Educ. 2003;67(12):1327–36.

Rafter ME, Pesun IJ, Herren M, Linfante JC, Mina M, Wu CD, et al. A preliminary survey of interprofessional education. J Dent Educ. 2006;70(4):417–27.

Riter D, Maier R, Grossman DC. Delivering preventive oral health services in pediatric primary care: a case study. Health Aff (Millwood). 2008;27(6):1728–32.

Ruggiero SL, Mehrotra B, Rosenberg TJ, Engroff SL. Osteonecrosis of the jaws associated with the use of bisphosphonates: a review of 63 cases. J Oral Maxillofac Surg. 2004;62:527–34.

Sax HC, editor. Medical professionalism in the new millennium: a physician charter, 2002. Ann Intern Med. 2002;136(3):243–6.

Scannapieco FA, Rethman PR. The relationship between periodontal diseases and respiratory diseases. Dent Today. 2003;22(8):79–83.

Selzer MH, McDermott JH. Inaccuracies in patient medical histories. Compr Ther. 1999;25(5):258–64.

Serhan CN. Controlling the resolution of acute inflammation: a new genus of dual anti-inflammatory and proresolving mediators. J Periodontol. 2008;79:1520–6.

Thyvalikakath TP, Monaco V, Thambuganipalle HB, Schleyer T. A usability evaluation of four commercial dental computer-based patient record systems. J Am Dent Assoc. 2008;139(12):1632–42.

Van Dyke TE. Inflammation and periodontal diseases: a reappraisal. J Periodontol. 2008;79:1501–2.

Van Dyke TE, Kornman KS. Inflammation and factors that may regulate inflammatory response. J Periodontol. 2008;79:1503–7.

Vettore MV, Leal Md, Leão AT, da Silva M, Lamarca GA, Sheiham A. The relationship between periodontitis and preterm low birthweight. J Dent Res. 2008;87(1):73–8.

Wagner EH. Chronic disease management: what will it take to improve care for chronic illness? Eff Clin Pract. 1998;1:2–4.

Wagner EH, Austin BT, Von Korff M. Organizing care for patients with chronic illness. Milbank Q. 1996;74(4):511–44.

Wagner EH, Austin BT, Davis C, Hindmarsh M, Schaefer J, Bonomi A. Improving chronic illness care: translating evidence into action. Health Aff. 2001;20(6):64–78.

Wilson AG. Epigenetic regulation of gene expression in the inflammatory response and relevance to common diseases. J Periodontol. 2008;79(8):1514–9.

Wisconsin Diabetes Advisory Group. Wisconsin essential diabetes mellitus care guidelines. Madison: Wisconsin Diabetes Prevention and Control Program; 2011.

Yoneyama T, Hashimoto K, Fukuda H, Ishida M, Arai H, Sekizawa K, et al. Oral hygiene reduces respiratory infections in elderly bed-bound nursing home patients. Arch Gerontol Geriatr. 1996;22(1):11–9.

Zhang X, Reichart PA. A review of betel quid chewing, oral cancer and precancer in mainland China. Oral Oncol. 2007;43(5):424–30.

Chapter 2
HIT Considerations: Informatics and Technology Needs and Considerations

Miguel Humberto Torres-Urquidy, Valerie J.H. Powell,
Franklin M. Din, Mark Diehl, Valerie Bertaud-Gounot, W. Ted Klein,
Sushma Mishra, Shin-Mey Rose Yin Geist, Monica Chaudhari,
and Mureen Allen

2.1 Achieving Interoperability of Medical and Dental Records

In this chapter, we explore and consider many of the technical, data and knowledge issues that impact electronic health records. These issues include healthcare standards and semantic interoperability, security of applications and data, privacy of information, the ability to identify uniquely a participant across all healthcare

---

M.H. Torres-Urquidy (✉)
Department of Biomedical Informatics, University of Pittsburgh, Pittsburgh, PA, USA
e-mail: mit7@pitt.edu

V.J.H. Powell
Department of Computer and Information Systems, Clinical Data Integration Project,
Robert Morris University, Moon Township, PA, USA

F.M. Din
HP Enterprise Services, Global Healthcare, Camp Hill, PA, USA

M. Diehl
Healthcare Informatics Program, Misericordia University, Dallas, TX, USA

V. Bertaud-Gounot
University Psychiatric Hospital, Rennes, France

W.T. Klein
Klein Consulting Inc., Ridge, NY, USA

S. Mishra
Computer and Information Systems Department, Robert Morris University, Pittsburgh, PA, USA

S.-M.R.Y. Geist
Departments of Biomedical and Diagnostic Sciences and Patient, Management,
University of Detroit Mercy School of Dentistry, Detroit, MI, USA

M. Chaudhari
Washington Dental Service, Seattle, WA, USA

M. Allen
Medical Informatics Consultant, New Jersey, USA

domains, usability and context based information retrieval, and clinical decision support. These generally applicable informatics issues are then examined with a specific focus on the overall goal of integrating medical and dental health information. Thus, we also examine standards specific to dentistry, the data needs of dentists, and clinical dental decision support efforts.

All the benefits of electronic health records depend on the ability of disparate systems to exchange data without loss of meaning, called *semantic interoperability*. With the variety of systems in use, *loss of meaning* can only be prevented by the use of and adherence to standards. These standards deal with communication, data, imaging, the information model and other properties of the healthcare record system. In this section, we provide a primer on the standards involved in achieving a comprehensive healthcare record that is usable across medical and dental domains.

2.1.1 The Role of Standards in Records Integration

Miguel Humberto Torres-Urquidy and Valerie J. Harvey Powell

The development, use and maintenance of standards will definitely play a role in the integration of medical and dental data. In this section, we will briefly review what standards are, as well as their strengths and weaknesses.

Standards are agreements between two or more parties to follow a given set of rules or principles given certain situations. The agreement allows the user of standards to know, in advance, what will occur when interacting with other parties that follow the same standard. More specifically, for healthcare, data standards are defined (Jernigan et al. 2010) as the "…uniform use of common terms and common methods for sharing data…" Again, from this definition, we can derive that agreement or shared understanding is fundamental for making standards useful.

We experience the use of standards every day. Driving on a particular side of the road, initiating a conversation with a greeting or using currency to pay for a service are examples of situations in which a large number of people have agreed to use and follow the same set rules and/or procedures. Using standards bring benefits to those who decide to abide by them. For instance, having the appropriate regional currency allows a person to travel to different parts of the region and conduct transactions efficiently. On the other hand, the use of standards has its costs, related to either development or maintenance. In the case of the early days of currency, in Mesopotamia (Powell 1996), currency could be seen as the representation of grains and the currency value was linked not only to the grains themselves but also to the ability to protect the grains or whether that protection was available. Thus, developing this standard had additional costs than just the simple agreement between trade parties. In modern days, the development, use and maintenance of standards have costs that are not only financial but also cultural, technical and/or political.

It is also important to discuss the objective of standards. Different healthcare data standards have been developed to suit different needs. Traditionally, standards have been divided into those tailored to represent knowledge or "content standards" and those that facilitate data communication or "interchange standards" (Hammond and Cimino 2006). The philosophies behind the development of these two types of standards are different and their applications vary. For instance, an example of content standards is the International Classification of Diseases (ICD). This classification or "system" lets clinicians in different environments to know the diagnosis of the same patient. ICD was originally created to keep track of the reasons for mortality (Jernigan et al. 2010). The use of the standard evolved and the ICD is now used around the world to record not only mortality causes, but also diagnosis used in clinical operations, including documenting patient information and billing. Usually, these standards are referred to as nomenclatures, terminologies or vocabularies. The difference between these names depends usually on the content and objective for which each standard was developed. For instance, the nomenclature (Hammond and Cimino 2006) is defined as "system of terms that is elaborated according to pre-established naming rules" while a terminology is a "set of terms representing the system of concepts of a particular subject field." Other naming conventions include classification systems, dictionaries, thesauruses and ontologies. These systems have the goal to represent knowledge in a structured way.

A different type of standard is used for the exchange of clinical information. Primary examples are the standards produced by the Health Level 7 group (http://www.hl7.org/). This group developed the HL7 Messaging Standard, which enables member organizations to utilize one format to send and receive communications between information systems.

Standards specifying appropriate storage structures for the data will also be important for the area of medical and dental data integration. An example of this type of standard is the ANSI/ADA Specification No. 1000 – Standard Clinical Data Architecture for the Structure and Content of an Electronic Health Record (American Dental Association 2003), which was developed by the American National Standards Institute and the American Dental Association. The ADA continuously produces documents such as specifications and reports that support dental care. These activities are conducted by the Standards Committee in Dental Informatics. Like the ADA, there are several organizations participating in the development of standards.

Fortunately there several standards that are currently in use by both physicians and dentists, and a primary example is DICOM (Digital Imaging and Communications in Medicine) developed by the American College of Radiology and the National Electronic Manufacturers Association (Howerton and Mora 2008) which is used for the electronic exchange of image based information. It will be up to those interested in integrating medical and dental data to identify the appropriate choice of standard depending on the type of information that needs to be transmitted.

2.1.1.1 Challenges

Despite the advances in the development of standards, there are still challenges that need to be addressed when incorporating them. These can result in "unforeseen" issues that may prevent the proper use and transmission of data. For instance, when implementing standards it is necessary to consider issues such as the cultural background, context, costs and other factors that can play a role in their success.

Fig. 2.1 Signs based on different standards

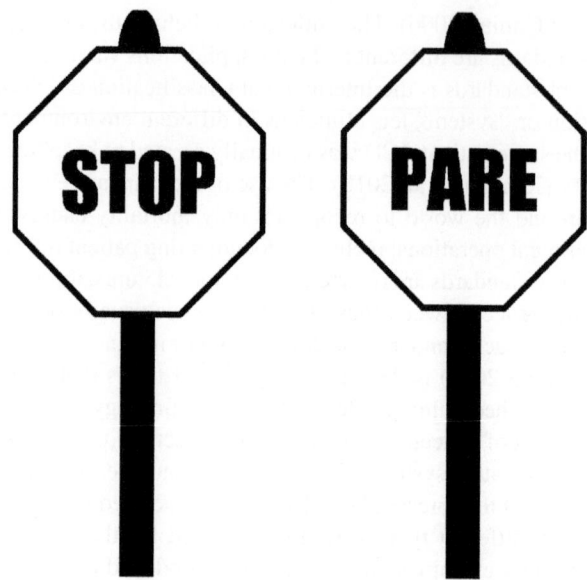

Figure 2.1 presents two signs, made to serve the same goal but based on different standards. Each sign is intended to ask drivers to "STOP." Although both are in the same language (Spanish), different interpretations can lead to problems for a driver who is unfamiliar with the alternative sign. The signs in Spanish read "Alto" and "Pare." Both signs seek to convey the same message to their reader which is "to decrease their speed until the vehicle is no longer moving."

Yet, different countries have different conventions for which sign is commonly used. In most cases, most drivers will understand what they are supposed to do even if they are visitors from a country that uses a different convention. However, in some instances, a driver unfamiliar with one of the words may not know how to interpret the sign, which could cause an accident. In this particular case, the word "Alto" in Spanish also has the meaning of the adjective "tall," adding to the possibility of confusion. Thus, in this case the cultural background plays a role in the interpretation of the standard.

Figure 2.2 presents the sign "Construction ahead" intended to warn drivers that they might encounter an area under construction when driving, used in the UK. Taken out of context, this sign can be jokingly interpreted as the "man with a broken umbrella." In this case, "context" plays a big role in defining meaning, actually changing it completely.

Another challenge with standards is the context in which they are used. We will illustrate this issue by referring to a road sign used in the United Kingdom, and depicted in Fig. 2.7. The sign is used to alert drivers of construction ahead. However, the road sign is also known as "The man with a broken umbrella." If a driver sees the sign, he knows that soon he will encounter a construction area. However, if the same driver is in a party and one jokingly refers to the street sign, the driver understands that the sign's meaning is different.

The former and later examples – the stop sign and the road sign – showcase that, even though was an agreement was made to implement a standard, its interpretation still varies with the context or cultural background. Fortunately, there are solutions to address different interpretation. However, they are costly. In the case of the stop

Fig. 2.2 Presents the sign "Construction ahead" intended to warn drivers that they might encounter an area under construction when driving, used in the UK. Taken out of context, this sign can be jokingly interpreted as the "man with a broken umbrella." In this case, "context" plays a big role in defining meaning, actually changing it completely

sign, the country or regional area could change all their signs for new and unambiguous ones. Afterwards, policy makers would have to retrain the population of the country or regional area to recognize the new sign. The implementation of this solution hinges on the resources the country or regional area has to be able to make this change. Another approach would be to educate all the visiting drivers on what the stop signs mean. In the case of "The man with a broken umbrella," authorities could forbid people misusing the meaning of the sign. Naturally, the problem with this solution is its legitimacy and likelihood of enforcing the rule. Another issue with the sign example is that the signs themselves need to be maintained and someone needs to keep track of the location, use, and the structural condition of the sign.

It is also important to control "expectations" for those implementing standards. Given the issues above, it is possible that two systems that are standard compliant do not communicate. This can lead to misunderstandings and the eventual failure to adopt a particular standard. Yet the challenge here is not the standard itself, but the failure to adopt the appropriate procedures, policies and cultural changes that are necessary to establish communication.

Despite of all these issues, it is highly beneficial to adopt standards and accompanying technologies since the benefits usually surpass the initial costs of adoption. In other parts of this book, we review specific aspects of integrating medical and dental data as well as the particular use of standards that lend themselves naturally to accomplish this integration.

2.1.2 Rationale for Data Standards and Coded Terminologies for Dentistry

Franklin M. Din

The need for Electronic Medical Records (EMR) has been established and social and political forces are coalescing behind the effort. However, the actual implementation lags far behind. It is less the lack of effort and more a lack of understanding of what constitutes an EMR that causes this lag. Many people think an EMR is as simple as taking all the information in a paper record and putting it into a computer: Hard disk replaces paper, keyboard replaces pen, and glowing pixels replace ink. Those that are in the field of Informatics understand that an EMR is a whole new paradigm and thus methods, assumptions, and techniques that apply to paper records may no longer apply. Further, the advantages of digital information are now exposed to the field of medicine. The leveraging of these advantages is evident in many aspect of general life, like national access to the money in your bank account. Similar leaps of functionality are now possible in medicine. However, to get to this new era in health, a fully integrated (works with all data elements within a single application) and interoperable (works with all data elements across all different applications) EMR is required. One of the keys to achieving a fully realized EMR is the related trio of concepts data standardization, controlled vocabularies and clinical terminologies. This paper addresses the issue of data standardization, controlled vocabularies and terminologies as they relate to the Electronic Dental Record (EDR).

2.1.2.1 Purpose

Once all the information in this paper is absorbed, it is hoped that the reader will understand:

- The importance of data standardization, controlled vocabularies and clinical terminologies to integration interoperability of dental and medical data.
- The improvements to clinical care that result from proper use of the three elements (data standardization, controlled vocabularies and clinical terminologies).
- The need to integrate fully terminologies into decision support, allergy and drug contraindication alerts and knowledge discovery processes.
- The need for Commercial Off–the–Shelf (COTS) software developers to plan for the use of such data elements, even if they are not used at the current time.
- The need for dental opinion leaders to promote continually these three elements.

2.1.2.2 Understanding the Need

Data Standardization

An examination of any paper dental record will demonstrate the need for data standards. Let us start with a hypothetical treatment on a patient:
  Upper right first molar received an MO Amalgam restoration.
  This entry could easily be recorded as:

- #3 MO Amalgam
- #3 MO AM
- #3 MO Silver

- #3 MO Amalgam
- 3 MO Tytin®

Any dentist reading any one of these entries knows that they all essentially mean the same thing. To a computer that is limited to text (string) evaluation each one is different. In the case of number 1–3, a computer see 'AM' as different from 'Amalgam' or 'Silver'. The three strings (sequence of alphanumeric characters) are different in each. The computer has no knowledge that they are synonyms. In the case of number 4, there is a space between the '#' character and the '3' character. Again, different strings mean they are different. In the case of number 5, the '#' sign is missing and instead of an indication that this is a generic amalgam, a brand name for the amalgam is used. Again, the computer only knows that the string in number 5 is different from the strings in numbers 1–4. Add misspellings and unusual abbreviations, like 'amalg', and the problem multiplies.

So in order to make the computer understand that any one of the five entries means the same thing (i.e., the same concept) a program would have to have that knowledge built in. A program can have a subroutine that essentially points to a list somewhere in which all five are equated to a common string. Something like:

- #3 MO Amalgam = #3 MO AM
- #3 MO AM = #3 MO AM
- #3 MO Silver = #3 MO AM
- #3 MO Amalgam = #3 MO AM
- 3 MO Tytin® = #3 MO AM

If the dentist enters a '#3 MO Amalgam', the computer substitutes and saves '#3 MO AM'. Thus, we have now standardized the data. The five variations are all equated to one standard string. This list of equivalent strings provides a way for the computer to deal with synonymy.

But what happens if the dentist switches to Brand X amalgam and starts to save his treatment record as '3 MO Brand X'. This new entry matches nothing in the left hand column of the list of synonyms, so again the computer sees a wholly different concept. We have just broken our carefully constructed table of synonyms.

One solution would be to add '#3 MO Brand X' to the list (add "#3 MO Brand X = #3 MO AM"). While this strategy works, every time a new brand is used, another mapping must be generated. This strategy is high maintenance, time consuming, and inefficient. A better way is needed to address this.

Controlled Vocabularies

Is there any real reason that a dental record needs to accommodate all the variations of the treatment, 'upper right first molar with an MO Amalgam restoration'? If a dentist understands that all the possible descriptions, numbers 1–5 above, are equivalent, why do we need to accommodate all? Reducing the number of variations would have real benefits for the EDR and the clinician. It reduces the number of entries that need to be mapped to a common term, and it reduces operator sensory overload and confusion.

You can easily make an argument that number 1–3 are so commonly used that any record keeping system must allow the use of any one. But the use case for number 4 and 5 are less straightforward. The question becomes, in order to keep the number of synonyms to a minimum, what synonym can we eliminate from the list without causing undue problem for clinicians? Clearly number 4 ('#3 MO Amalgam') can be eliminated. We are just reducing the amount of typing necessary to record the treatment.

Number 5 poses a more difficult issue. A case could be made that the brand name is important since different manufacturers have different compositions and knowledge of the composition could be valuable. So there is some value to keeping this entry as is. Since we are now seeking to reduce the number of variations we allow, the question becomes, "Is there any way to keep this information in a way consistent with eliminating the number of choices to choose from?" Yes, if we allow for the use of Brand name as a modifier to one of the three variations that we have already agreed to keep. So now '3 MO Tytin®' becomes '#3 MO AM' with a modifier of "Brand name=Tytin®". By adding a field to modify the term, we have eliminated the problem of including all brand name variants and we have maintained the essential information of '#3 MO AM', which is always important without losing the extra information 'Tytin®'.

We now have a rationale for reducing the number of ways to name the concept of an 'upper right first molar with an MO Amalgam restoration'. By relegating Brand Names to a modifier of the main data element, we are exercising control over the way in which a dentist can complete this data element. We have reduced the number of ways in which this treatment is described from 5 to 3. The dentist is allowed to use 1–3 and the computer saves a single choice.

Our vocabulary is now controlled.

Clinical Terminologies

We have now set up our EDR so that the dentist who wants to record a treatment of 'upper right first molar with an MO Amalgam restoration' has one of three choices to describe the treatment and the computer only saves one description. So all 'upper right first molar with an MO Amalgam restoration' are saved in the computer as '#3 MO AM'. Aren't we done yet?

It is true that within the confines of a single application, we have all we need. Data is standardized and vocabulary is controlled. In this state, the applications are integrated but still do not meet the needs of interoperability.

If we wish to send the information of 'upper right first molar with an MO Amalgam restoration' to another dentist, we cannot be sure that he can read and use the information that we sent. His EDR may not have standardized on the '#3 MO AM'. His software company may have settled on '#3 MO Silver' as the concept. If we send '#3 MO AM', his software must try to interpret this string against his list of synonyms. If '#3 MO AM' is not in the synonyms list, we have failed to share information.

So the controlled vocabulary is still insufficient for true integration and interoperability. One controlled vocabulary is as valid as another is and the harmonization between controlled vocabularies is not standardized. Further, the controlled vocabulary does not provide any information regarding how one concept relates to another. For instance, both caries and periodontal abscess are bacterial diseases, but nowhere in a controlled vocabulary is this information captured. Thus, it is not possible to perform logical analysis of dental terms using only a controlled vocabulary. Using the caries and periodontal abscess example, it is not possible for a computer to include both conditions is a frequency distribution of oral bacterial diseases.

To resolve this issue, we need to progress toward a reference terminology in which:

- *Specificity*: A single concept is established as the base against which all similar terms are equated. One concept with multiple synonymous terms.
- *Relatedness*: Each concept has an explicit relationship to other concepts. Generally the main relationship that give the reference terminology its structure is the "is a" relationship (commonly expressed as type – subtype or parent – child).

These are produced by Standards Development Organizations (SDO), like the International Health Terminology Standards Development Organization (IHTSDO) which produces SNOMED CT and National Cancer Institute (NCI) which produces BiomedGT. These SDOs, within their own well-defined domain of knowledge, construct a data set that can act as a universal representation of medical concepts. To make these concepts useable in any application, they all assign an alphanumeric code to each concept. These codes are the same anywhere in the world. So if '#3 MO AM' is coded '123', then any application throughout the world that understands this code system, will correctly identify '123' as '#3 MO AM'.

The use of coding all concepts has added advantages in that an abstract alphanumeric, '123' is easier to process than a string in which a variant in the string may or may not change the meaning of the concept.

We now have all the elements necessary to make EDRs with interoperability.

We Have Terminologies in Dentistry. Look at CDT. Aren't They Good Enough or Do We Need More?

By now, we hope that you have concluded that a coded terminology is necessary for the future of interoperable electronic records. So this leads to the next issue. What do we really need for an EDR?

Up to this point, we have used the example of '#3 MO AM' because the concept is easy for any Dentist to understand. Further, any dentist also knows that we already have a way to code this concept. Current Dental Terminology (CDT) allows us to code '#3 MO AM' as a combination of the tooth number (which by definition is a terminology) '#3' and the concept of 'MO AM' which is captured in the CDT code of 'D2150'. But that is all we can do with this terminology. The code of '#3' and 'D2150' provides no information about the diagnosis that led to the treatment,

Table 2.1 Dental examination coding

Coded terminology	Coding for "dental exam"
SNOMED CT	34043003 – dental consultation and report (synonym of dental examination)
SNODENT	No coding for a dental examination
LOINC	34045-5 – ORAL EVALUATION EXAM
CDT	D0150 – comprehensive oral evaluation – new or established patient

Table 2.2 Medical history of liver disease

Coded terminology	Coding for "medical history of liver disease"
SNOMED CT	392521001 – history of
	235856003 – liver disease
SNODENT	G-0001 – History of (present illness)
	No code for "Liver Disease"
LOINC	11348-0 – HISTORY OF PAST ILLNESS
	No code for specific illness
CDT	No code for medical history

nothing about the signs and symptoms, nothing about co-morbidities, nothing about the patient's medical status, etc. In any dental record, we would like to capture all clinically relevant information and tooth number and CDT code do not do that. At best, tooth numbering and CDT is incomplete.

The first thing that needs to be decided is what kind of information do we need to capture in a complete dental record? In other words, what is minimal level of information that must be captured in a dental record that allows another dentist to form a complete clinical picture just by reading the record? Secondly, can this minimal information be captured in some coded terminology in order to meet the needs of an EDR?

To answer these questions, let us examine a generic dental visit. The dentist conducts an examination, reviews the medical history, makes a diagnosis, treats the problem and evaluates the treatment for a prognosis. The dentist may also order a prescription and perhaps a lab test. Let us code this generic visit using some existing terminologies that are relevant to dentistry.

Examples of coding for the initial "dental examination" are (Table 2.1):

A patient history is a requirement of a good medical/dental record. Examples of coding a "medical history of liver disease" are (Table 2.2):

Once the examination has taken place, the signs and symptoms along with any descriptive qualifiers are noted. Things like "severe throbbing pain in the lower left jaw." Such statements can be parsed into the individual important components like "severe," "throb", "lower left," "jaw." Each of these can be coded (Table 2.3):

A diagnosis of "caries" for the problem can be coded as (Table 2.4):

A decision is made to perform some procedure to correct the disease or abnormality. As noted in the introduction, treatments can be coded. For "#19 MO amalgam," the coding would be (Table 2.5):

Table 2.3 Coding a patient's complaints

Coded terminology	Coding for "severe throbbing pain in the lower left jaw"
SNOMED CT	29695002 – throbbing pain
	76948002 – severe pain
	255480002 – left lower quadrant
	91609006 – bone structure of mandible
SNODENT	T-11180 – lower jaw bone
	G-A101 – left
	G-A003 – severe
	F-51060 – pain in oral cavity
	No code for "throb"
LOINC	No code for clinical findings
CDT	No code for clinical findings

Table 2.4 Coding for caries

Coded terminology	Coding for "caries"
SNOMED CT	80353004 – simple dental caries
SNODENT	D5-10111 – simple dental caries
LOINC	No code for clinical findings
CDT	No code for clinical findings

Table 2.5 Coding for an MO amalgam

Coded terminology	Coding for "#19 MO amalgam"
SNOMED CT	31196005 – amalgam restoration, two surfaces, permanent
	245658003 – mesial-occlusal
	8962500 – mandibular left first molar tooth
SNODENT	T-54390 – mandibular left first molar tooth
	T-54014 – mesial surface of tooth
	T-54011 – occlusal surface of tooth
	No coding for "amalgam restoration"
LOINC	No code for clinical findings
CDT	D2150 – amalgam – two surfaces, primary or permanent
	No code for tooth #19
	No code for tooth surfaces

Once treatment is performed, there is some evaluation of the "prognosis" of the treatment. The coding would be (Table 2.6):

A drug may be prescribed, like Amoxicillin, 500 mg tablets. And the coding examples are (Table 2.7):

Lab tests can be ordered. For example, a dentist contemplating an extraction may wish to order a PT, PTT or INR for a patient with Liver disease who may have a clotting problem (Table 2.8).

So, if we include the patient personal demographic information as well as the items above, medical history, signs and symptoms, diagnosis, treatment, labs, medications, and prognosis, we have all the needed information to understand the fullness of the office visit.

Table 2.6 Coding for a prognosis

Coded terminology	Coding for "good prognosis"
SNOMED CT	170968001 – prognosis good
SNODENT	No code for prognosis
LOINC	32966-4 – DENTAL PROGNOSIS for a procedure
CDT	No code for prognosis

Table 2.7 Coding for a prescription

Coded terminology	Coding for "amoxicillin, 500 mg tablets"
SNOMED CT	374646004 – amoxicillin 500 mg tablet
SNODENT	No code for drugs
LOINC	25274-2 – AMOXICILLIN 18616-3 – strength
CDT	No code for drugs
Drug codes (Rxnorm, NDC, etc.)	All will code for a drug

Table 2.8 Coding for bleeding control

Coded terminology	Coding for "PT and PTT lab tests"
SNOMED CT	396451008 – PT assay 42525009 – PTT assay
SNODENT	No code for lab tests
LOINC	34529-8 – PT and APTT PANEL
CDT	No code for lab tests

Table 2.9 Extensiveness of code

History and clinical exam	SNOMED CT, SNODENT, LOINC
Diagnosis	SNOMED CT, SNODENT, LOINC
Procedure and treatment	SNOMED CT, CDT, ICD-9
Prognosis	SNOMED CT, LOONC
Medication	SNOMED CT, RxNorm
Labs	SNOMED CT, LOINC

Now the second half of the issue, can these data be coded? Short answer yes, every data element can be coded as evidenced in the examples above. The following table is not definitive but is used merely to demonstrate that there is at least one Terminology to cover an aspect of clinical information (Table 2.9).

The names in the right hand column are names of different terminologies. They are useful for coding a complete dental record. The fact that one or all of these are unknown to you is immaterial to this discussion. The important observation and conclusion from viewing this table is that there is a way to code every pertinent piece of clinical data.

2.1.2.3 Okay, so terminologies and data standards are integral to a complete EDR. Assume that you have a complete EDR with all critical data elements properly coded via one or more Terminology. What is the benefit besides the ability to share the record with another dentist?

Let us start by assuming that a dentist has used a fully realized EDR with coded data elements everywhere for a year. What kinds of benefits accrue to this practitioner?

The best way to analyze this is to compare the fully coded EDR against a standard dental management application in which only CDT codes are maintained. The dentist can generate a lot of knowledge from the EDR data that is nearly impossible to generate from a dental management application. Examples are:

- We wish to analyze root canal treatment utilization. If we are using management software alone, we can do a count of the number of root canal treatments that were performed, the percentage of root canal treatment versus all other procedures, etc. However, there is no way determine how many root canal treatments were the result of periapical abscess versus fractured tooth pulp exposure. With the complete coded EDR, such an evaluation is very straightforward.
- Is there a link between periodontal disease and heart disease? If there is a correlation, what type of periodontal disease at what severity is correlated with what type of heart disease? This analysis is nearly impossible with management software but straightforward with a full EDR. Just query the records in which the code(s) for heart disease and the code(s) for periodontal disease appear for the same patient.
- How about proactive decisions? Suppose the patient has a complex medical history and is taking multiple medications. You have determined that multiple extractions are indicated. What precautions should the dentist take before the extraction, what alterations need to be made to the medication schedule (e.g. stop Coumadin treatment 3 days prior to extraction), and is there a change in prognosis? Decision support that evaluates all these factors automatically would be a great patient safety check. Coded data makes decision support modules possible.

2.1.2.4 The Terminologies Used in the Examples and in the Chart Are a Mixture of Medical, Pharmaceutical and Dental Terminologies. How Do We Determine Which One We Should Use?

A quick look at the table and examples would suggest that dentistry adopt SNOMED CT and forget all the others. SNOMED CT can code most of dentistry. It is not a complete ontology (a structuring of knowledge about things according to their essential qualities) that can fully describe all of medicine and dentistry. Other, more focused terminologies, like LOINC for lab tests, are more comprehensive within a specific domain than SNOMED CT. Thus one of the factors to consider is, "can we sacrifice details for simplicity without losing clinical information?" The true answer to this question requires a careful and detailed analysis of the data requirements for the individual clinical specialty. In our case, the domain is dentistry. This type of analysis is difficult, time consuming, and ultimately may not answer the question.

Since we recognize the every terminology has strength and weakness, a better approach is to use whatever is best for a specific purpose. So using LOINC over SNOMED CT is best for coding of laboratory tests. RxNorm is a better choice over SNOMED CT for drug information. SNOMED CT is the choice for coding of clinical findings. For coding of dental procedures, CDT is the logical choice. This strategy provides the most comprehensive way to code dental information.

2.1.2.5 Outside of CDT and Possibly ICD-9, There Are No EDRs That Incorporate These Terminologies. This Is a Lot of Work to Do. It Is Not Going to Happen in the Near Future

This is precisely the point and the purpose of this position paper. This big effort will take time. However, an old Chinese proverb states, "A journey of a 1,000 miles begins with a single step."

Everything that preceded this section should have convinced you that clinical terminologies are useful and more importantly inevitable. So EDRs, whether custom designed or COTS products, must begin to account for these terminologies in their product. This means that all future software must be designed to accept the coded entries even if the software is not yet prepared to use the coded data elements. In simple terms, the software must account for a clinician selecting a clinical condition and the associated code for that selection. And there must be fields within the database to store this data. The functionality to use this data can be added later. The important thing is to start collecting the coded data as soon as possible.

The actual terminologies to be used are a matter for debate. This author prefers SNOMED CT as the choice for coding of clinical findings, diagnosis, and problem lists. CDT and ICD-9 works well for filing of claims for reimbursement for procedures. LOINC has limited usefulness since dentists rarely order labs tests.

2.1.2.6 Do We Really Need to Share Dental Information with Our Healthcare Brethren?

Dentistry is not separate and distinct from the rest of healthcare. We need to be able to share information with medicine, pharmacy, etc. for patient safety, and treatment efficiencies. There is no reason for patients to have a medical history for a physician and one for a dentist, etc. This occurs because the two professions do not share patient information. In a world with a truly interoperable EDR, pertinent parts of a patient's EMR can be shared with his EDR. For instance, both a dentist and a physician need to know if a patient has liver disease. Having each capture and record, such information is redundant and prone to errors.

Dentists often write prescriptions for their patients. Consider the advantages of electronic prescription order vs. our current paper prescription. As above, there is a time savings and the redundancy of entering demographics and medical history is avoided. The pharmacy can also run the prescription against a knowledgebase of drug-drug interactions prior to dispensing the drug, thus preempting potential harm to the patient.

2.1.2.7 Summary

The full scope of data standards, controlled vocabularies and coded terminologies are beyond this paper. Instead, the hope is that everyone involved with EDRs now understands the importance of this component and that all stakeholders focus their attention to this critical issue. Developers and commercial software vendors must plan to incorporate these data elements in their applications. Purchasers of EDRs must insist that the applications they buy incorporate these elements. And the Dental Informatics community must remain in the lead on these issues.

The Dental Informatics community has special responsibilities. We need to take the lead in spreading the word. This involves meeting with software developers and insisting that our information needs are met. We must act as the opinion leaders and press the agenda in all public forums related to EDRs. We must work within the terminology community to insure that our data needs are an integral part of any decisions by the SDOs. We must ensure that dental organizations, like the American Dental Association (ADA), understand that EDRs are integral to their clinical, research, public health and administrative initiatives. Further, we should provide other dental organizations advice and counsel, as we accept theirs, to insure that we act as partners in our public and professional efforts.

2.1.2.8 Final Thoughts

A case can be made for dentistry to sit out the early efforts in electronic records implementation. Let others make the costly mistakes and once they get things working, then we will join the process. The problem with this "wait and see" approach is that they will make decisions that serve their purposes without regard to the needs of dentistry. These decisions may be detrimental to dentistry. Then we will be in the unenviable position of trying to change the direction of all the others, who are much further advanced, who have undertaken the difficult process of setting and agreeing on standards, and who have committed significant financial expenditures, in order to accommodate our needs or we try to shoehorn a bad solution. A better approach is to engage now, when the difficult issues are being resolved so that our needs are included in any final decision. Better to shape the future than be dictated by the past.

2.1.3 American National Standards for Health Data Integration: Content Development

Mark Diehl

At the 1996 annual meeting of the American Dental Association a resolution was adopted by the House of Delegates stating a vision where a continuum of patient health data, unencumbered by boundaries dictated by profession, specialty or discipline improves the quality of health outcomes, patient safety and economy of care delivery.[1] With this resolution, the American Dental Association became the first and remains the only major health care professional organization to endorse whole-patient integration of patient health data. The Association considers the electronic health record to be a complete collection of patient data, a compilation of an individual's lifetime health conditions and health care from conception through postmortem. This body of patient data is in automated form (i.e. electronic form) rather than an automated conversion of conventional physical paper documents.

The American Dental Association's Standards Committee on Dental Informatics (SCDI) subsequently created a number of standards that implement the House of Delegates 1996 Resolution. Specification 1039 presents a conceptual data model for clinical care. Specification 1000 presents a logical data model for health care data. Both are American National Standards approved by the American National Standards Institute (ANSI) and both address whole-patient data and cross the professional and specialty boundaries traditionally separating medicine, dentistry, and other health care professions. When taken together, along with the companion implementation guide, these standards provide a blueprint for the construction of databases containing whole-patient health data and provide the foundation for semantic interoperability in the exchange of health information. Both the Specification 1039 and 1000 apply to the data tier of health information systems, providing the conceptual and logical data structures for making[2] the patient's health data persistent.

The Specifications 1000, 1039, and related publications are based on current state and federal medico-legal requirements for health records, application of information theory, and the data requirements to support clinical processes and care outcomes. These standards are the only American National Standards that focus on the patient or health care recipient rather than on the management of health records, data exchange or the encounter or business aspects of care delivery.

At the heart of these standards are models that conform to standard information modeling best practices.[3] These standards include a progression of standard information models from a clinical conceptual process model and a clinical conceptual data model to a clinical logical data model. The data entities and attributes presented

---

[1] The American Dental Association House of Delegates Resolution 92H-1996 states this vision of "seamless accessibility of health information throughout all aspects of health care, independent of profession, discipline or specialty, or care delivery environment."

[2] Storing data in the long term.

[3] ASTM 2145–07 Standard Practice for Information Modeling. Available from www.ASTM.org.

Fig. 2.3 Overview of the modeling process

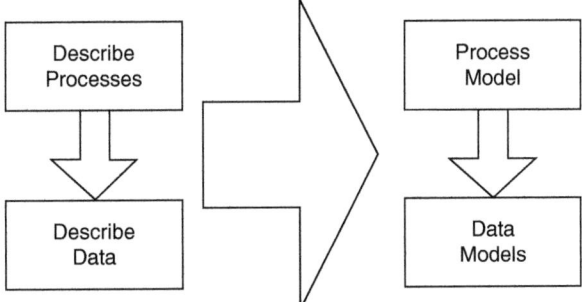

in these standards are those needed to operationalize the processes identified in the process model. Because these data models are derived from a comprehensive, whole-patient clinical process model, the data likewise applies uniformly across professional and specialty boundaries.

Information modeling is an appropriate technique to develop a comprehensive understanding of healthcare processes and the data supporting these processes. The American Society for Testing and Materials (ASTM) standard E2145 for information modeling best practices defines a model as a representation in any form of real or envisioned things or events. Models provide a means to understand structures, processes and concepts where size and complexity renders human perception or comprehension difficult or impossible. Models are valuable tools to explain, analyze or predict processes and structures which currently exist, have existed in the past or may exist in the future. The size, scope, and complexity of the health care delivery environment, along with the complexity of health knowledge and health care processes, makes information models an ideal vehicle to assist human understanding.

2.1.3.1 Modeling Process

As noted in ASTM E2145, information models progress from a description of processes through increasingly detailed descriptions of the data needed to enable these processes. As illustrated below (Fig. 2.3), the data description depends upon a description of the processes that use these data, and the models provide a means to efficiently and effectively describe both processes and data.

This approach predates information system and information theory, going back to the fundamental teachings of the architect Louis Sullivan, "form ever follows function."[4] The *process model* describes the processes and provides the starting point for a conceptual data model. The *conceptual data model* then identifies the

---

[4]Louis H. Sullivan regarded excessively decorative elements as superfluous. Likewise in information modeling, excessive detail and ornamentation contribute little to understanding; rather these serve to complicate design, inhibit comprehension and ultimately defeat the purposes of information modeling. See http://www.famousquotesandauthors.com/authors/louis_h_sullivan_quotes.html and http://en.wikipedia.org/wiki/Louis_Sullivan.

Fig. 2.4 Sequence of models generated to reach a comprehensive representation of healthcare activities

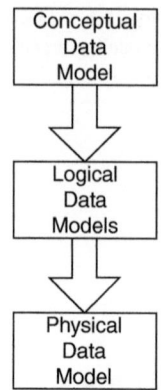

fundamental data items and relationships used by the processes. The conceptual data model is the origin of one or more *logical data models* that expand upon and detail the conceptual data. The logical data models then become the origin of the *physical data model* – a description of the structure of persistent data to be deployed on a specific technology (Fig. 2.4).

This progression of models ensures that the data structure implemented in the system accurately and effectively meets the needs of the processes it supports.

The original Specification 1000 standard was adopted in 2001 and contained descriptions of the process and data models. The Specification 1039 standard expanded upon this description and formalized the process model and derivation of the clinical conceptual data model. Both Specifications employ a structured description using the ANSI standard IDEF notation, IDEF0 for process modeling and IDEF1X for information modeling.[5] The IDEF notation has been successfully used in healthcare activity and data modeling the public and private sector organizations for well over a decade.[6,7]

2.1.3.2 ANSI/ADA Specification 1039[8]

The Specification 1039 establishes a shared understanding of the structure and content of data needed to support healthcare processes. It is the foundation for a variety

---

[5]IDEF methodology described by the National Institute of Standards and Technology, Federal Information Processing Standards Publications 183 Integrated Definition for Function Modeling (IDEF0) and 184 Integrated Definition for Information Modeling (IDEF1X), 23 December 1993. IDEF0 aims at capturing "decisions," "actions" and "activities" and IDEF1X has the goal of modeling data for using it as a resource. These use graphical representations as part of the modeling process.

[6]Bourke, M.K. Strategy and Architecture of Health care Information Systems. New York: Springer. 1994.

[7]United States Department of Defense, Military Health System (MHS) IDEF Process and Data Models used in the MHS Functional Area Model – Activity (FAM-A), and MHS Functional Area Model – Data (FAM-D), various dates.

[8]Available from the American Dental Association, Department of Standards Administration, 211 E. Chicago Ave., Chicago, IL 60611.

Table 2.10 The diagnostic therapeutic cycle

Human decision process	Equivalent healthcare decision process
Observation	Data acquisition
Reasoning	Diagnosis
Planning	Treatment plan
Action	Treatment

of more detailed data representations of clinical information. Specification 1039 also determines the structure and content of clinical data presented in the various types of electronic health and patient records. The Specification document provides descriptions and graphic depictions of those activities and data structures specific to clinical healthcare and population health services. It presents a view of the mainstream of individual and population health and care delivery processes found in the United States, drawing generalities from the activities shared among practitioners and providers. Non-clinical processes and data structures (e.g. administrative, financial, supply chain, etc.) are addressed if they directly relate to personal and population health, and directly support healthcare delivery processes. Important to the reader is that this Specification does not address or establish standards for clinical care. It does not establish standards for the quality, efficacy or effectiveness of clinical practice, the conduct of clinical research, or informatics standards for manufacturing processes in the healthcare supporting industries.

In order to best support healthcare delivery, independent of technology, healthcare profession or specialty, or care delivery environment, the Specification of the clinical conceptual data model applies the "form follows function" approach. This approach first analyzes the fundamental activities shared throughout the delivery of healthcare services.

This analysis creates a *clinical conceptual process model* as a high level structured analysis of the activities shared by care providers in the delivery of health care services. The component detail of the process model is such that it is possible to identify the principal types of data needed to support these activities, but it is only specified until activities of health care providers diverge. The model does not reach the depth of detail where the differences in clinical and business practices require differences in the description of activities and supporting data content and structure. The conceptual process model therefore establishes a clinical foundation for the conceptual data model that directly ties the data structure to clinical process.

All healthcare providers share a common, rational process in performing clinical services, the Diagnostic-Therapeutic Cycle.[9] This process is identical to that employed in other human decision processes, consisting of observation, reasoning and action, as illustrated in the table below (Table 2.10):

---

[9]This Diagnostic-Therapeutic Cycle is variously known by a variety of terms and is widely cited in the medicine texts used in first-year professional education; this is also noted in Van Bemmel, J., and M.A. Musen (Eds.). Handbook of Medical Informatics. 1st edition. Springer. 1997.

In IDEF0 notation, the Clinical Process or Diagnostic-Therapeutic Cycle appears in the Specification as (Fig. 2.5)[10]:

This diagram reflects the four fundamental processes performed in clinical care, and in many other service roles like automotive repair. The first process is to gather information about the case at hand. Component tasks may include performing a physical or clinical examination, use of imaging and physiologic instrumentation, performing histopathology and clinical chemistry studies, etc. Collectively, these produce a body of information that the doctor uses to determine one or more diagnoses and etiologies, as performed in the diagnosis, or data analysis process. One of the possible outcomes of the diagnostic process is the need for additional data, such as a radiographic referral. A differential diagnosis (e.g. Multiple myeloma 0.85, MGUS 0.11, plasmacytoma 0.04) may be the result of the diagnosis process, though commonly providers work from only a single diagnosis. A treatment plan process establishes the intervention plan to address the diagnosis. In complex cases, especially involving coordinated care among multiple professions and specialties, this plan may be constructed in multiple steps, may be revised as needed and may indicate the need for acquisition of additional diagnostic data or performing a subsequent diagnosis step. In the treatment process those interventions identified in the treatment plan are performed. An important note is that outcome assessment is a subsequent performance of this process, where the assessed outcome is the product of the diagnostic process and may indicate the need for subsequent care.

IDEF0 identifies the individual activities and illustrates the relationships among these without showing the sequence in which these are performed. For the clinical process, this is important since the progression of these activities is rarely a single waterfall path, but rather a cascade with branches to previous activities as shown below (Fig. 2.6):

The extensive recursion illustrated above reflects clinical events where a provider may need to return to a previous activity to develop additional data, for example, where during diagnosis the need for data from additional clinical tests becomes evident. This clinical process is continuously repeated over periodically until the course of care is completed.

The arrows in the IDEF diagram are called ICOMs, standing for *Inputs*, *Controls*, *Outputs* and *Mechanisms*. *Controls* are those things that are employed to regulate or constrain the activity. *Inputs* are consumed or changed by the activity and *Outputs* are things created, modified or produced by the activity. Data or information under this notation is always an output or a control – it can never be an input since it the original data or information is never altered or destroyed. The ICOMs, especially the outputs and controls define categories of data to be represented in the conceptual data model. These also approximate the major subject areas in the logical data model derived from the conceptual data model.

---

[10]IDEF0 Diagram from page 30 of the ANSI/ADA Specification 1039.

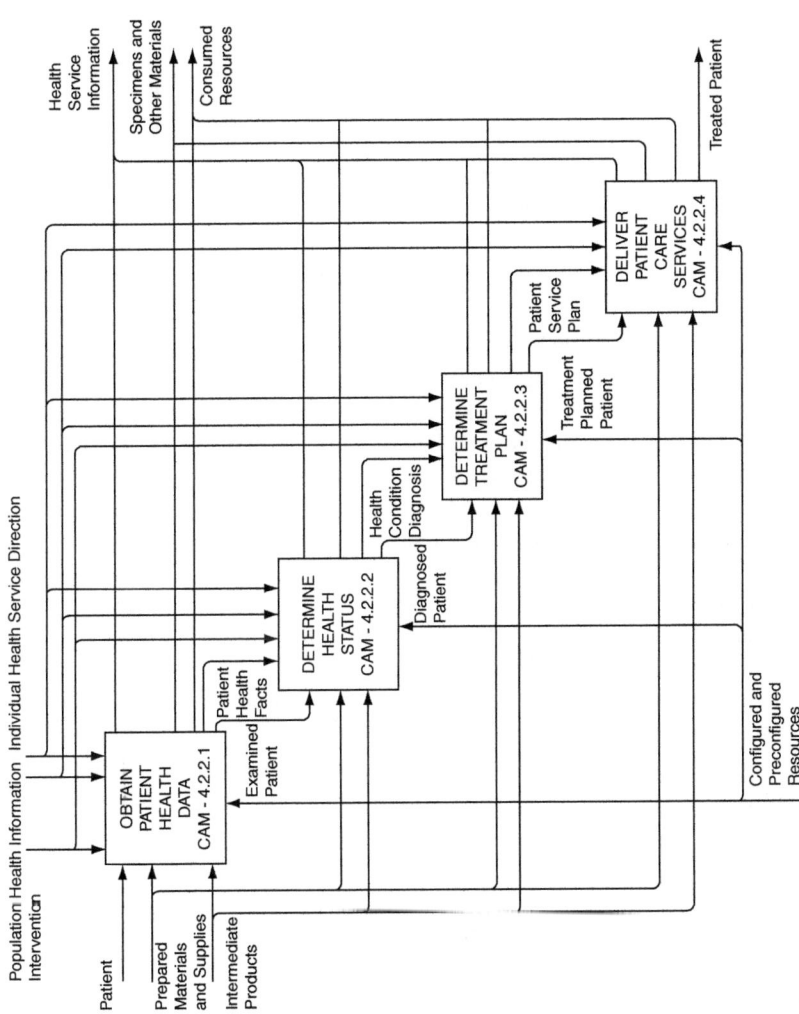

Fig. 2.5 Clinical process or diagnostic-therapeutic cycle appears in the specification

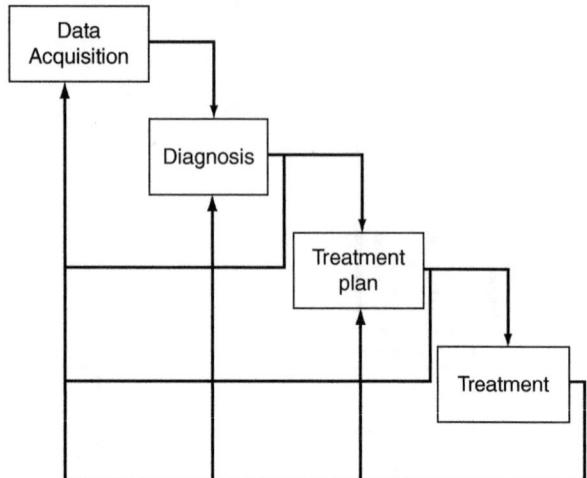

Fig. 2.6 Clinical process as a recursive activity

As shown in the diagram below, the Specification 1039 conceptual data model is centered on the individual, a single person or other living thing (Fig. 2.7).[11]

In this model (Fig. 2.12), every individual has one or more health conditions, defined as their state of health and well being. As noted in the process model diagram shown above, an output of the Obtain Patient Health Data activity is Health Service Information including the body of Health Facts. The data model diagram shows the connection between the Individual and one or more Health Facts generated by that activity. The care provider operates on the assembled body of facts to determine a diagnosis and etiology, and the patient and care provider determine the course of care as a Treatment Plan. This plan may be linked to a desired or intended Health Condition as an expected outcome.

In both the process model and the data model, neither the activities nor data are siloed or compartmentalized by profession or specialty. This conceptual data model serves as the starting point for a clinical logical data model, in the Specification 1000, and becomes one span of the bridge linking the clinical database to the clinical processes it supports.

2.1.3.3 ANSI/ADA Specification 1000

The ANSI/ADA Specification 1000 was approved as an American National Standard by ANSI on February 2, 2001. This standard was initiated in response to the American Dental Association House of Delegates Resolution 92H-1996 previously cited. The origin of this work was the Computer-based Oral Health Record concept model in the mid-1990s. The standard was the culmination of a work effort that created a

---

[11]Other conceptual models are centered on the provider, the procedure or the encounter.

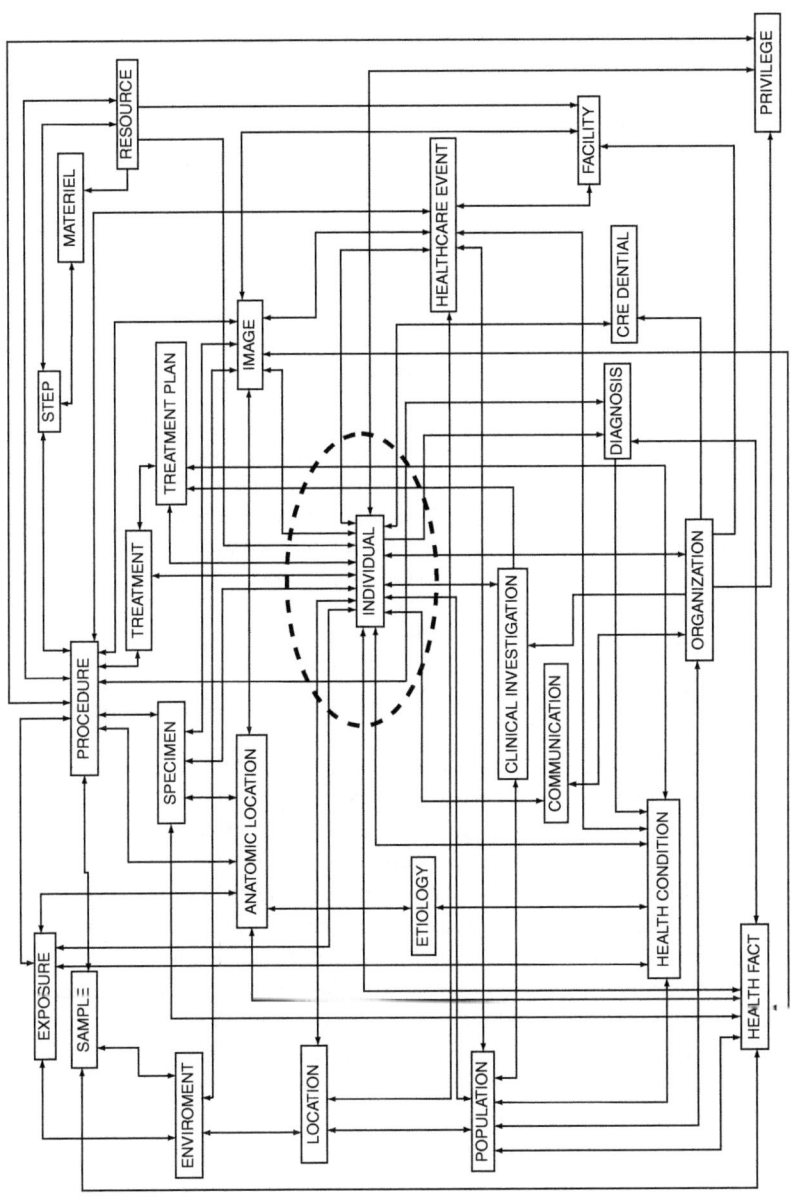

Fig. 2.7 Model displaying the interactions of the individual with different elements supporting the healthcare delivery process

standard health care logical data model based on the COHR Concept Model, and conducted protracted public review of its component subject areas from 1997 through 2000. Revision and updating of the standard and its logical data model began review for consensus in 2008 and was approved by ANSI on February 22, 2010.

The Specification 1000v2 logical data model was developed by expanding upon the Specification 1039 conceptual data model. The numerous 'many-to-many' relationships were broken, additional entities created, and attributes added to the entities to provide detail. Several new subject areas were added to reflect expanding interest in the application of the logical model to health care practice, management and regulation. The Specification logical data model now contains 32 subject areas as identified below:

Individual	Organization healthcare materiel item
Individual characteristics	Provider healthcare materiel
Population	Patient health facts
Population characteristics	Patient specimen
Organization	Patient object
Location	Population health facts
Location associations	Patient health condition diagnosis
Location characteristics	Population health condition diagnosis
Communication	Patient treatment plan
Healthcare event	Treatment plan expected outcome
Health services provider	Population outcome reference
Provider credentials and privileges	Patient health service
Healthcare services	Clinical investigation
Health services objects	Clinical investigation design
Healthcare materiel	Codes and nomenclature
Healthcare materiel item	Reference tables

The concept of 'individual' is used rather than separate entities for patient or care recipient, provider, other interested party, etc. These component roles are type coded in other subject areas and are consistent with the entity-role designation in other standards such as the Health Level Seven Reference Information Model. The term Individual also allows for application to non-human recipients of health services, as in veterinary medicine. Where other industry standard and common data models in medicine and health care are usually from the context of the heath care encounter, the healthcare procedure, or its reimbursement, the context of the Specification 1000 logical data model is the individual and their condition of health and well being. The Individual subject area is, therefore, the key and essential focal point of the Specification. This subject area establishes a standard data structure for the identification of all participants in the health care process.

2.1.3.4 Subject Area Descriptions

The Individual subject area provides a standard structure for the human name that is independent of cultural, geographic tradition, or language constraints. The same data structure is applicable to represent names in the individual's own preferred form. Thus, a person's native Spanish or Asian name structure and content can be represented with the same data structure as readily as with a Western name structure.

Recognizing there is no uniformity internationally regarding the application of a national patient identifier, the Specification allows for a system-assigned identifier or a national identifier is applicable. Any number of alternate patient identifiers, such as motor vehicle operator number or another government-assigned identification number, can be represented. This data structure, where the individual's identification, name, associated detail and characteristics, and health data are in separate entities, readily enables deidentification of health care data for purposes, such as research, implementing data privacy and confidentiality provisions.

The Individual Characteristics subject area presents a structure to record the essential characteristics of an individual as used in patient registration, demographic and epidemiology applications. An Individual may have one or more characteristics represented through a subtyping into eight separate entities by Race, Ethnicity, Language, Religion, Sex Characteristic, Taxonomy, Living Arrangement and Physical Characteristic. Sex Characteristic is preferred over terms such as Administrative Sex, to allow multiple characteristics to be presented (e.g. anatomic sex, sex preference etc.) The Taxonomy enables consistent classification of non-human living things.

The Living Arrangement and Physical Characteristic are new entities added in this revision. The Living Arrangement contains data, such as noting whether an individual lives alone, that may be of importance when planning a course of care. The Physical Characteristic is a collective entity used to contain any number of data items, such as hair color, body mass index etc., that are not generally considered a health fact.

The Population Characteristics subject area has much the same data structure as the Individual Characteristics, allowing for comparison of an individual with one or more populations in which that individual is a member. This relationship provides a data structure that also enables a key and essential element of evidence-based practice where expected outcome is predicted by experience in the appropriate population.

The Organization subject area establishes a standard data structure for the identification of organizations, the relationships among these organizations, and the relationships between the organizations and individuals participating in the health care process. The Location subject area provides a data structure that identifies, names and positions a specific location (geographic, not anatomic) as well as linking that location to individual and organizational occupants.

The Communication subject area creates a standard data structure for communications among individuals and organizations involved in the health care process. This data structure and its reference values are consistent with the Health Level Seven 2.X standards. The Health Care Event subject area reflects that the traditional view of the health care encounter or episode is being challenged by increasing emphasis care delivered outside of the health care facility and the impact of telemedicine and information technology. This subject area reflects that all such health care events share a common set of characteristics, being the junction of all participants of health care services at a point in time, unconstrained by physical co-location.

The Health Services Provider subject area identifies providers, classifies these as either individual providers (doctor, nurse etc.) or an organizational provider (hospital, clinic, private practice etc.), and associates the provider with locations and one or more professional specialties performed at a location.

The Provider Credentials and Privileges subject area establishes a standard data structure to identify and characterize the level of a healthcare professional's expertise obtained through formal training along with any other credentials obtained by that individual. This subject area contains data items used to assign credentials and privileges for both accreditation and certification. It also identifies and characterizes those services and procedures that a healthcare provider is authorized by an organization or other individual to deliver or perform and contains data that characterize a provider such as used in enrollment and credentialing transactions.

The Health Services Objects subject area contains object data, such as video images, of healthcare services and their components such as procedures and steps. These objects may be associated with individuals or organizations, such as a procedure associated with a particular hospital or practitioner. This subject area also provides a data structure to enable a detailed audio/video training module, such as for administration of an anesthetic block or performing a specific incision biopsy.

The Health Care Materiel subject area establishes a standard data structure for those materiel items used in healthcare processes, where the Healthcare Materiel Item subject area links that data with a specific procedure for an individual. The Organization Healthcare Materiel Item subject area contains data structures required to track materiel items within an organization, such as in keeping an inventory of healthcare materiel at clinical locations, routing these items to the point of delivery of care services, and the subsequent recovery and disposition of those items. The Provider Healthcare Materiel subject area contains data structures to enable documentation of a provider's selection of specific materiel items to perform a procedure, reflecting the professional desires of that provider.

Another essential concept in this Specification is the representation of clinical knowledge about the case at hand. The Patient Health Facts subject area creates a structure for patient information that identifies and describes an individual's health facts at a date and time. The term fact as a collective term containing all relevant information items is preferred over separate terms such as finding, observation, symptom, etc., that are subtypes of the parent Fact entity.

The Patient Specimen subject area provides the data structure to document surrogates for that patient, such as excreta, secreta, blood and blood components, tissue, and tissue fluids that have been collected from an individual. The Patient Object subject area presents a data structure to link an image or other representation of an individual's physical structure or process, and handled as a large data stream with associated processes needed to reconstruct the object.

The Population Health Facts subject area presents a structure that organizes and structures population health information as the basis for comparison to an individual's health facts.

The Patient Health Condition Diagnosis subject area establishes a standard data structure for the determination of an individual's health conditions supporting the diagnostic processes performed by a care provider.

The Population Health Condition Diagnosis subject area provides a data structures serving as an evidence-basis or reference for the diagnostic processes used by a care provider to determine an individual's health condition.

The Patient Treatment Plan subject area presents data structures required to support the planning of health care services, presentation to the care recipient, and informed consent by the care recipient. The Treatment Plan Expected Outcome subject area enables the documentation of the desired or expected outcome on which the treatment plan is based. The Population Outcome Reference subject area presents a data structure reference to support the evidence-based logical processes. For example, this could be used to determine the probability of achieving an outcome for an individual, if this is known for the population of which that individual is a member and which presents those same health facts and diagnoses.

The Clinical Investigation subject area provides a data structure supporting clinical investigations in health care research, identifying the participants in a clinical investigation (e.g. investigators, organization, etc.), the type of study population (e.g. control population), and specifies the hypothesis. This can also link the investigation to another study. The Clinical Investigation Design subject area contains data that identifies and details the study methodology or protocol along with specific materiel to be used. This subject area also identifies the subjects participating in the investigation and associates those individuals with the study population.

The Codes, Nomenclature and Reference Tables subject areas are essential to provide reference data for the implementing subject areas, such as individual and population characteristics, clinical components and the supporting services. The Codes and Nomenclature subject area provides a standard data structure to identify, characterize and track over time those reference codes and nomenclature used in the health care process, present these independent of language, and relate codes both within a code system and to codes in other code systems.

2.1.3.5 Conclusion

Implementation of this Specification is addressed in the ANSI/ADA Specification 1027 Implementation Guide. This document shows how to forward engineer the logical data model, optimize the physical data model and create a functioning database that is Specification 1000 compliant. The importance of compliance lies in the benefits of seamless, Standards-compliant data. Such data provides the semantic interoperability that along with the syntactic interoperability of standards such as promoted by Health Level Seven enables individuals to share thought. Without this semantic interoperability, a concept may not be totally understood when conveyed from one person to another, even though the physical communication may have succeeded.

2.1.4 Knowledge Representation and Ontologies

Miguel Humberto Torres-Urquidy and Valerie Bertaud-Gounot

2.1.4.1 Introduction

Intelligent beings are required to construct mental models about their reality since most things that exist are external to them. For instance, a clinician first needs to construct a mental model of the patient's problem before deciding on a particular diagnosis or treatment. This requires clinicians to gather data and make sense of it in a structured way. Depending on the complexity of the task, clinicians use different "tools" to generate this structure. If the problem at hand is relatively simple, they may just ask questions to a patient and store the answers in memory or in a blank sheet of paper. However, as problems become more sophisticated, humans have invented tools to manage this complexity and increase their capability not only to store but also to make sense of large amounts of information. In the past century, the use of computers introduced the concept of electronic databases, and as our understanding on how to use these tools increased we discovered how important it is to structure correctly data and information. Part of this discovery process lead to the adoption of several major approaches to capture meaningfully information. In this section, we will review ontologies as one of several approaches used to structure information. We will provide some definitions, historical background and examples of ontologies that provide a good understanding on how this type of knowledge representation can pave the way for supporting medical and dental data integration.

2.1.4.2 Historical Precedents

Throughout history, there many authors have explored the concept of knowledge representation. Representation of knowledge was one of the preoccupations during the early development of science. Greek philosophers dealt with the concept of being and the representation of knowledge and set precedents for those who would study the topic later on. Aristotle's Metaphysics described how a set of 'Categories' could classify most known entities at the time. In addition, he also pointed out that these categories were not 'composite', that is, "they need to be composed in order to make statements about the nature that can yield affirmation." (Sandholm 2005) Although these categories are debatable, they set the foundation from what is known commonly used as idea of "Concepts" to represent information.

Concepts or ideas are representations of certain thing or element. But what defines a concept? Recently (Campbell et al. 1998), provided a good description of the Ogden-Richardson semiotic triangle (Ogden and Richards 1930). This triangle (Fig. 2.8) provides a framework for characterizing meaning by establishing the relationships between thought, symbols and reality (thus defining a concept).

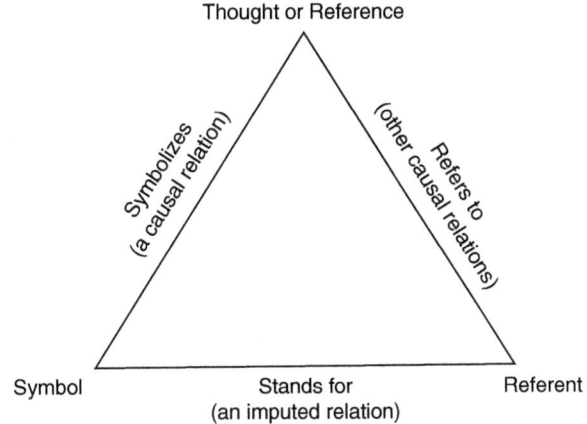

Fig. 2.8 The Ogden-Richardson's semiotic triangle establishes the different elements that play a role in representing knowledge through concepts

As described by Campbell et al., the semiotic triangle identifies the relationships between words, thoughts and things. The triangle explicitly states the relationships where a word (symbol) corresponds to a thought. The word can trigger a thought which is related to an object and vice versa. With this simple diagram, we can determine how information is generally processed by humans and likely by other "smart" entities such as computers. Thus, this triangle can be seen as the base for modern knowledge representation systems, especially those based in the use of concepts. As we will see next, modern Ontologies and Information Models draw extensively on this approach to handle knowledge representation.

2.1.4.3 Ontology

Ontology can be simply defined as a "formal conceptualization of a domain" (Gruber 1993). In simpler terms, we could define an ontology as a group of ideas or concepts that are organized in a meaningful way or structure that can later can be reused to explain or "reason" about a particular subject.

2.1.4.4 Definitions

More formally, the term "ontology" originates from the Greek root "ontos" (being) and "logos" (word) referring "to the subject of existence", i.e. "the study of being as such" (Gasevic et al. 2006). Guarino (1998) defines an ontology as "a particular system of categories accounting for a certain vision of the world." They are also defined as "categories of things that exist or may exist in some domain" (Gasevic et al. 2006). Gruber states that an ontology is "an explicit specification of a conceptualization" (Gruber 1993). Briefly, ontology conceptualizes or defines concepts that represent the whole or a part of reality. Ontologies use concepts in different ways. On occasion, concepts represent not things, but relationships between things.

Using this approach, ontologies manage to capture the meaning of reality in a manageable way. By manageable we refer to the ability to create, maintain and use the knowledge stored in the ontology.

Currently, there are different views and even controversy on how ontologies should be categorized. In this section, we will have more of an applied perspective since the integration of dental and medical data will most likely require utilization of functioning applications that will enable making sense of information in different domains. For a comprehensive review of the different views on ontological work, including the philosophical aspects of knowledge representation, we recommend the reader to review the work of Smith (1998) and others (Staad et al. 2009).

The functional view of ontologies divides them into two major types: (1) content-oriented ontologies, which are likely dealing with a particular area of knowledge and (2) functional ontologies, which traditionally are linked to a particular application and/or are intended to assist solving a particular problem.

2.1.4.5 Components and Structure

Another objective of an ontology is to capture not only the concepts that represent entities in the real world, but also the properties of those concepts. A third goal of an ontology is to represent the relationships between concepts. These relationships can also be concepts. Establishing these relationships alone does not necessarily enable information systems to understand the meaning behind those concepts (this would be a semantic network). To increase their sophistication, advanced implementations of ontologies utilize formal processes or logic to maintain the relationships between concepts valid and tractable. There are different approaches to do this and a popular method is the use of the Web Ontology Language "OWL" in combination with "Description Logics," which we will describe next.

2.1.4.6 Web Ontology Language (OWL) and Description Logics (DL)

OWL is a processing language intended to provide a framework in the form of eXtended Markup Language (XML) statements. With these statements, it is possible to specify the entities that form the ontology and what the boundaries for each entity are. A way to understand how OWL helps constructing and maintaining an ontology is by using the example of a picture puzzle. When beginning to solve a puzzle usually we do not know *where* pieces are supposed to fit. Yet we know *how* pieces are supposed to fit thanks to their shape. As we progress putting the pieces together, a picture starts to emerge and it becomes easier to add more pieces. OWL serves as the standard that defines the shape of the pieces allowing us to integrate concepts into the ontology, and at the same time, making them remain consistent with one another. In other words, OWL assists us in maintaining knowledge integrity. OWL is intended to be machine-readable.

Ontologies are primarily composed by concepts (Fig. 2.9).

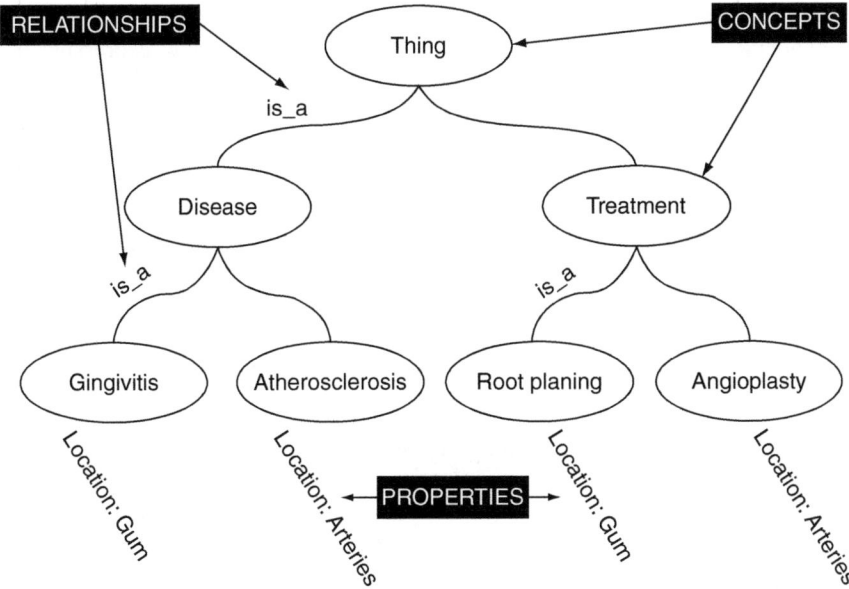

Fig. 2.9 Basic ontology representing clinical information in the form of concepts and their properties as well as the relationships between concepts

Technically, OWL is not used alone but in a combination of group of stacked technologies (World Wide Web Consortium W3C 2011). XML gives the language in which an ontology can be expressed. XML Schema lists a set of constraints in the type of documents and data types that can be expressed. The Resource Description Framework (RDF) gives an emphasis in semantics since it makes available a model for objects and relations. Finally, the RDF Schema allows for specifying the properties and classes.

OWL is known to be available in three "flavors." These flavors permit different levels of expressiveness. OWL *Lite* allows for primarily creating a classification and maintaining simple constraints. For example, this version of OWL is good at rapidly migrating an established thesauri or classification into a formal ontology. OWL *DL* (Description Logics) allows for representing knowledge with "maximum expressiveness while retaining computational completeness (all conclusions are guaranteed to be computable) and decidability (all computations will finish in finite time)" (World Wide Web Consortium 2011). We will talk more about Description Logics in the next section. OWL *Full* allows for "maximum expressiveness" yet without computational guarantees. Software is unlikely to support the features of this version of OWL.

2.1.4.7 Description Logics (DLs)

Description Logics (DLs) can be defined as "… formalisms for representing knowledge (Baader et al. 2004)." The purpose of these is to allow the construction of "intelligent applications" that are capable of uncovering the "implicit consequences of explicitly represented knowledge." In other words, they allow expressing the rules by which concepts will relate/operate with each other. Description Logics build from earlier developed systems for representing knowledge and reasoning such as logic-based formalisms and non-logic-based representations. Logically based representations are powerful and good for handling general-purpose tasks. These systems rely on the use of a variant of first-order predicate calculus. The non-logic representations use ad hoc data structures such as semantic networks and frames. Modern ontologies rely heavily on the use of DLs. Our challenge is to make proper use of this tool to capture the clinical reality.

2.1.4.8 Ontologies in Practice

Ontologies are used for different purposes. Again, the intention of this section is to provide a practical view of ontologies. Next, we are going to provide functional examples, first from the medical perspective, and then examples from the dental domain. In the biomedical domain, ontologies are currently used for supporting research and clinical care. Others (Rubin et al. 2008) provide examples relevant to biomedicine. Here, we mention those that are relevant for integration of medical and dental data:

- *Searching for diverse data*: biomedical literature is complex and filled with intricate descriptions of synonyms, acronyms and abbreviations which make the retrieval of information difficult. Ontologies can serve as smart mechanisms to unify content. The classical example is the Gene Ontology GO which provides a method to identify uniquely functions, processes and products related to gene activity making retrieval of information more coherent.
- *Exchanging data*: transferring information between healthcare entities or systems will be paramount as multidisciplinary teams seek to care for common patients. In biomedicine, an example of the use of ontologies for exchanging data is the handling of Microarray data. Microarrays primarily identify the expression levels of biomarkers for subsequent linkage with clinical conditions. This information is obtained using different platforms which can be represented using the Microarray Gene Expression Data (MGED) Ontology. The MGED Ontology provides a common set of concepts for describing the experimental design enabling the exchange of data.
- *Integrating data*: the modern healthcare environment is increasingly requiring the utilization of data across specialties, providers and geographic domains. A natural choice for supporting this integration is the use of ontologies given their ability to "translate" information with similar meanings but expressed in different contexts. An example is the ontology developed by the Advancing Clinico-Genomic Trials (ACGT) on Cancer project (Smith 2008) to integrate clinical and genetic data from different cancer studies conducted in several research centers. In this project, ACGT Master Ontology was created for "integration for the domains of clinical studies, genomic research and clinical cancer management and care" (Smith 2008).

2.1.4.9 Ontologies in Dentistry

The adoption of ontologies in dentistry is gaining traction primarily among dental researchers. There are several examples of ontologies developed with a specific goal in mind. These include addressing Sjögren syndrome (Long and Goldberg 2006) or for studying Saliva (Ai et al. 2010). These two are good examples on how medical and dental data necessarily need to be integrated in order to support a comprehensive view when providing care and conducting research. In the case of Sjögren syndrome (Long and Goldberg 2006), this is an autoimmune disease that is known for destroying the ability to produce saliva and tears. Yet, the impact of this disease can be systemic, affecting other organs including kidneys and lungs. Thus, it is important to be able to retain information about the whole patient. The other example is the Saliva Ontology (Ai et al. 2010) which aims to support research activities including the development of saliva tests that monitor systemic health and specifically identify diseases. Thus, it is important to support a comprehensive view of the patient's health.

In the case of clinical dental practice, there are several terminologies that are broadly adopted (Leake 2002). The Current Dental Terminology (American Dental Association 1991), International Classification of Diseases-Dental Application (World Health Organization 1994) and the Uniform System of Codes and List of Services (Canadian Dental Association 2001) are used on daily basis. Yet work needs to be done in order to increase utilize their content for integration. A preliminary example is the ontology developed (Torres-Urquidy and Schleyer 2009), to incorporate not only canonical but also an empirical representations of dental knowledge. Their ontology is therefore more likely to bridge the gap between theoretical/textbook concepts and the practical notions used routinely for patient care. Another example of the use of ontologies in dentistry is the case of the Swedish Oral Medicine Web (SOMWeb) system (Falkman et al. 2008) which is intended to support a Community of Practice aimed to improve the communication between experts. In the later case, with the use of technology developments driven by ontological principles, the authors were able to provide better support for the activities and increase the adoption of evidence-based care.

Next, we are going to explore the process for building a Knowledge Base (an ontology) in dentistry. First, we are going to introduce some general procedural concepts, next we are going to review how some of these methods were used (Bertaud-Gounot et al. 2010) to develop an Ontology for Dental Emergencies.

2.1.4.10 Building a Knowledge Base

When building a knowledge base, it is important to understand the processes that help us formalize knowledge. Analysis at several levels (van der Lei and Musen 1991) was introduced:

- "Knowledge level analysis of an application task specifies the behaviors that are required to solve a problem in the world."
- Symbol level analysis "specifies the computational mechanisms needed to model the requisite behaviors."

Subsequently, six steps in the acquisition of expert knowledge (Musen 1988) were proposed when building an intelligent system:

- *Identification*, where the primary themes of the system are characterized;
- *Conceptualization*, in which the identification of ideas occurs. This includes concepts and their relationships. Newell (1982) identified this as the "knowledge-level analysis";
- *Formalization*, which identifies mechanisms for implementing an expert system and transfer the conceptualized knowledge into the rules and parameters of the eventual system;
- *Implementation*, in which the knowledge base is used by a system informs or provide new knowledge in the form of advice;
- *Testing*, in which the system advice is validated by a domain expert and also the knowledge engineer;
- *Revision* of the system, since it is possible that the system does not "behave" as expected due to incorrect representation or modeling of the "facts" and concepts.

However, there is an important consideration that we should face before constructing a new knowledge base, and that is the "Knowledge Acquisition Bottleneck" (Musen 1988). He points out why building knowledge bases or "encoding expert knowledge" is difficult. Several reasons have been discussed including: (1) the inability of experts to communicate and/or (2) "introspect" which create "barriers" for translating and transferring experts' abilities and mental processes to a knowledge base. Thus, during the development process, it is important to remain attentive at issues arising from not establishing the proper communication with subject matter experts.

2.1.4.11 Building the Ontology

There are several approaches for building an ontology. While obtaining knowledge from a subject matter expert can follow the approach presented in the previous section, building an ontology can also be done by using the example of the picture puzzle that we presented before. When first including the content (concepts) that are going to be part of the future ontology we can see these concepts as pieces of a puzzle. In some instances, you may have all the pieces available before starting the assembly of the puzzle, while in others you may only have parts of the puzzle. In this case, the creators of an ontology may know specifically all the information that should be contained in the ontology (for instance, a pre-existing terminology); while in others, the incorporation of new concepts occurs as new information is discovered (this case would apply to the Gene Ontology). As we start assembling the puzzle, some pieces are relatively easy to place given their characteristics. For instance, in a picture puzzle of a map, the position of a piece that contains information on a particular street intersection is almost self-explanatory, while the adjacent pieces should be more or less easy to discern whether they fit or not. On the other hand, if we have a puzzle piece that those not have clearly distinctive features such as part of water or of a park, it will be difficult to identify its final position at the beginning. It will take the arrangement of several pieces before we can be more or less certain of where the piece should go. Similarly, when constructing an ontology and incorporating concepts and relationships between concepts, some concepts will have a clear starting position, others will need repositioning and their relationships reassessed as we incorporate more concepts. With the use of elements such as OWL and Description Logics, information systems help us in identifying the good fit of concepts, making sure that the overall structure of the ontology is consistent with reality. Going back to the puzzle example, OWL and DL serve to set the boundaries and shapes of puzzle pieces, thus making sure that we do not place a rounded piece in a squared segment.

Formally, ontologies can be constructed using a top-down or bottom-up approaches, each with its own advantages and limitations. The top-down approach starts by identifying a predetermined hierarchy. This is useful when the content is already well identified and the structures that are necessary to represent the relationships are well understood. The limitation of this approach is that the incorporation of new or extraneous information may be very difficult since it may require restructuring the whole content.

The bottom-up approach starts by incorporating concepts individually without having predefined structures, the relationships appearing as new concepts are added. This approach provides for more flexibility. Yet, not having a predefined structure can cause the incorporation of new concepts in areas of the knowledge structure, in a way which would not necessarily represent reality appropriately. Having little structure would also make discovering such inconsistencies more difficult.

When constructing the ontology, it is also important to define a preliminary structure that will support the integration of concepts. This definition process is accomplished by using predefined ontologies developed by scientists and philosophers who have worked on identifying what categorizations are applicable to specific types of knowledge. These ontologies are called "top level." Examples of top level ontologies include the Basic Formal Ontology (BFO) (Grenon et al. 2004) and the Descriptive Ontology for Linguistic and Cognitive Engineering (DOLCE) (Gangemi et al. 2002). These provide classifications for concepts according to their inner characteristics. For instance, BFO defines two major categories of concepts: "Continuant" and "Occurrent." A very simple definition for a "Continuant" concept is an entity which exists independent of time. This can be a "heart valve" or a "broken tooth." The alternative would be an "Occurrent" in which concepts refer to entities that only exist with the progression of time, for instance, "pulmonary insufficiency" or "restoring oral function." The top level ontology provides insights into how things should be represented. In addition, the use of top-level ontologies allow for unification between disparate ontologies. When seeking to integrate knowledge from medical and dental databases it should be easier to make the inferences between both databases if the information in both databases use structures that follow ontological principles and both use the same top level ontology.

Note: It is important to clarify that it is possible to use a top level ontology for defining the structure of your "new" ontology and still use a bottom-up approach for constructing the ontology. The key here is that the approach refers to the way in which concepts are incorporated into the structure of the ontology and not necessarily to the structure itself.

The construction of the ontology usually follows the sequence:

- *Defining* the goal of the ontology;
- *Deciding* whether to use a top ontology;
- *Incorporating* concepts into the predefined structure and repeating this process until you are satisfied given the primary goal;
- *Evaluating* whether the ontology is consistent and satisfies the notion of knowledge representation required for the goal.

The construction process itself is usually done by using ontology editors such as Protégé (Noy et al. 2010) or OBO-Edit (Wächter and Schroeder 2010). These editors take care of incorporating the elements described before such as the use OWL-DL. In addition, they provide graphical representations of the ontologies being created. Another feature of these editors is the ability to check for consistency and coherence. As ontologies evolve, the addition of a new concept may make sense when looking at the neighboring concepts and "local" relationships, yet it may incongruent with reality or the tendencies previously set for the rest of the ontology. Finally, these editors also provide additional functionality such as the creation of forms or the ability to export the ontologies into the Web (Noy et al. 2010).

2.1.4.12 Example: An Ontology for Dental Emergencies

Dr. Bertaud-Gounot and colleagues (Bertaud-Gounot et al. 2010) developed an ontology using data collected from the literature and validated with the help of subject matter experts. Their goal was to create an ontology that captures information about dental emergencies. For their process, they obtained articles and extracted concepts that would then be approved by the experts so they would be included in the ontology.

2.1.4.13 Process

The investigators obtained articles from Medline and the Medical and Surgical Encyclopedia (http://www.emconsulte.com/produits/-traites/od1#). Their search included the following keywords: dental emergencies, mouth disease, periodontal disease, pulpitis, and tooth disease. The investigators created summaries from the articles and identified concepts that are relevant for emergency dental care. Once the concepts were identified, they were validated by the clinicians. The investigators used Protégé (Stanford University, CA) as editor and integrated content in an iterative multistep process. In addition, they utilized the Pellet reasoner to check for consistency each time a new concept was aggregated (Fig. 2.10).

Fig. 2.10 Partial view of diseases represented in the ontology of dental emergencies

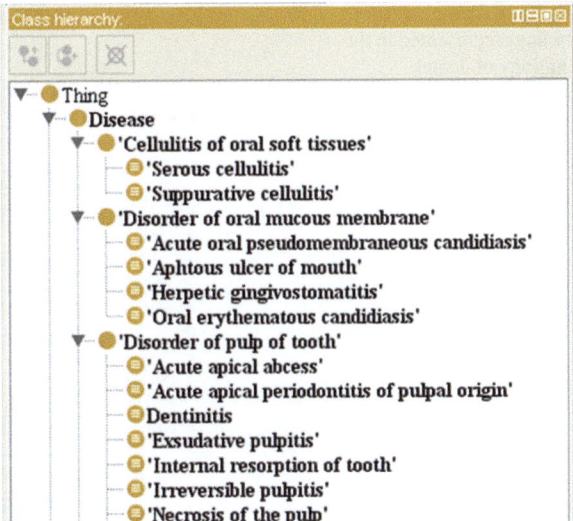

2.1.4.14 Content

The ontology has 202 concepts divided by 28 capturing diseases (Fig. 2.10) and 174 representing findings (Fig. 2.11). The ontology also has 377 restrictions (relations). These relations were established between the diseases and their respective clinical findings (Fig. 2.12).

2.1.4.15 Evaluation

The investigators evaluated the ontology by comparing the concepts and integration of content versus the occurrence of diagnoses found in regular clinical practice. Out of 32 cases, the clinicians' view fully differed from the ontology's in only one case. In addition, the investigators found that the clinicians had partially similar view in 11 cases and identical view in 20 cases of how the information was represented in the clinic and in the ontology.

2.1.4.16 Future of Ontologies in Medical/Dental Care

The need for better representation of patient data is likely to increase since we are now rapidly adopting information technology in all levels of healthcare. This will require making sense of large and disparate volumes of information. Thus, healthcare will have to embrace the adoption of technologies that seamlessly support data integration. Therefore, knowledge representation, and especially ontologies, will likely play a role in supporting this integration.

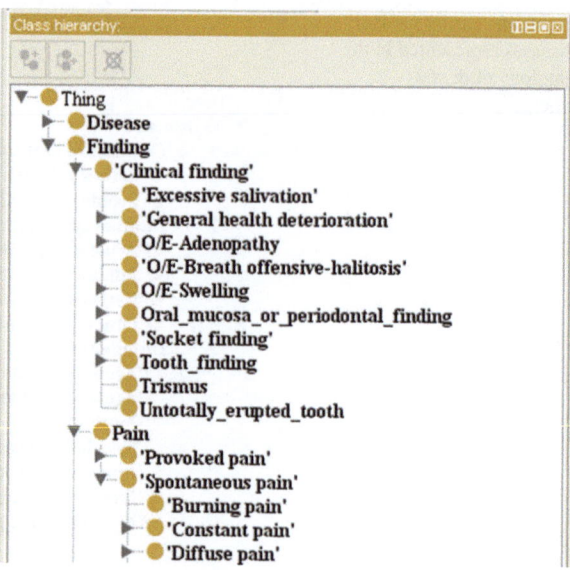

Fig. 2.11 Partial view of findings represented in the ontology of dental emergencies

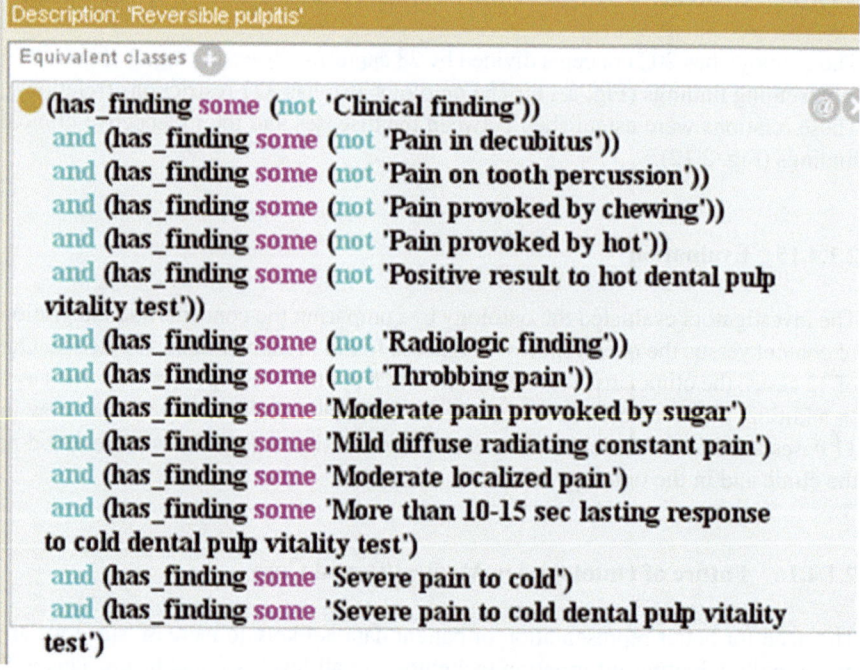

Fig. 2.12 Example of disease "Reversible pulpitis" characterized by the relationships in the ontology

2.1.5 Anticipating Oral Health Inclusion in Mainstream Standards

Valerie J. Harvey Powell and W. Ted Klein

This section deals with the need to have a clear goal to include oral health in the coverage of a healthcare standard before beginning to design that standard. Failure to establish such a clear inclusive goal may risk:

- Developing inapplicable standards with regard to access control specification or,
- Developing inadequate standards with regard to attaining consistent levels of specificity across disciplines.

As standards have been prepared for the development of health information technology, the question arose as to whether dental records should be explicitly included. In the 1990s, Schleyer and Eisner (1994) envisioned "Dental Interface Objects" which would "communicate patient information between computer systems of physicians, dentists, dental specialists, and other partners in the healthcare team."

Schleyer (2004) cited the ADA House of Delegates resolution 92H-1996, calling for "the seamless availability of patient health information across health care professions, specialties and care delivery environments." (American Dental Association 1996) Schleyer felt that what was then called the National Health Information Infrastructure (NHII) could not only address "missed health care opportunities," but could also "facilitate collaboration among general dentists and specialists." Schleyer recommended an educational campaign to help dentists understand the potential benefits of NHII. He mentioned ANSI/ADA Specification No. 1000 and the dental extensions to DICOM as "essential building blocks." Schleyer felt that dentistry should "become an active participant" in the NHII. Diehl (2002) states that "cross-enterprise data integration removes the barriers that prevent timely access to accurate and professionally meaningful health information."

Farman (2002) pointed out that the DICOM (Digital Imaging and Communication in Medicine) standard, at that time, could support intraoral radiography, panoramic radiography, cephalometric radiography, CT, intraoral cameras and other modalities of interest in oral healthcare. He reports that the American Dental Association (ADA) became a member of the DICOM standards committee in 1996. In 1998 and 1999, respectively, supplements to the DICOM standard were approved covering radiography and visual light imaging used in dentistry. According to Farman, in 2000 the ADA first "suggested" and then formally recommended DICOM implementation for the communication of images in dentistry.

In order to avoid unanticipated vocabulary problems, the HL7 standard attempts to be as agnostic as possible as to vocabulary content. In fact, in the upcoming HL7 version 2.8 (under active development), all vocabulary items that are not internal HL7-only structures (like those that describe the types of technical acknowledgments, etc.) are being removed from the normative part of the standard because those who do not read the standard carefully treat the lists of 'suggested values' as the normative values that must be used. This is erroneous, and leads to under-specified vocabulary. These suggested values will be explicitly identified as values that some using HL7 have found useful, and should not be considered as mandatory for use.

In all cases when using standards, the latest version should be consulted (even if an earlier version is being implemented). Over the years, all standards include new material in later releases that are often useful for understanding best practice for using the standards, and even may provide useful hints for piecemeal extensions when an existing older version does not quite meet all the requirements, but business conditions mandate that a complete newer version cannot be fully used.

If the designers of a healthcare-related standard are not working from a goal of serving "all of healthcare," including oral health, and if the example of HL7 is not followed, there is a risk of over-constraining vocabulary by confining vocabulary to that in specific lists. An example could be a list of provider degrees or clinical credentials. Obviously if such a list (as a reference table in a relational database) contains the role designations MD, DO, DNP, and RN, but not DDS, DMD, or RDH, then dentistry would be excluded. Another kind of improper constraint could arise from misuse of a Role-Based Access Control (RBAC) matrix, where dental provider role categories are entered as not being permitted to prescribe or administer medications. These two examples are based on discovered instances involving incorrect interpretations of standards or of following outdated standards documents. Any method for specification of anatomic sites that precludes use of the anatomic site representation and identification necessary for dental care (such uniquely numbering deciduous, permanent, and supernumerary teeth) would be incapable of supporting integration of medical and dental records. At the Society for Imaging Informatics in Medicine (SIIM) conference in 2010, PACS (Picture Archiving and Communication Systems) vendors pointed out that DICOM-compliant PACS technology for veterinary practices already supported integration of medical and dental care and patient records (DICOM 2006). Another risk is not achieving the same level of specificity in the content dimension in standards for oral health as for other domains of healthcare.

2.2 Towards an Integrated Electronic Health (EHR) System: Compliance, Security and Privacy Concerns

Sushma Mishra

2.2.1 Introduction

An electronic health record (EHR) is a collection of medical information about individual patients stored in an electronic manner. It contains personally identifiable information about a patient such as social security number or medical record number, home address and health related details. An individual's personal medical information could have sensitive information about emotional problems, sexually transmitted disease, substance abuse, genetic predisposition to diseases, or sexual minority status, information potentially adversely affecting major employment opportunities or to which social stigma is attached (Cannoy and Salam 2010). Considering that an individual's personal health information is declared "privileged" by the Government, it is surprising to find that as many as 400 people may have access to one's personal medical information throughout the typical care process (Cannoy and Salam 2010). It is important to reassure the patients that their information is kept confidential for them. Such reassurance encourages patients to share all their health information, to best of their knowledge, with care providers.

The terms electronic health record (EHR) and electronic medical record (EMR) have been used synonymously in the literature; however, in 2008 the National Alliance for Health Information Technology suggested that the term EMR be used for electronic record systems that are not interoperable and that EHR be used when health information is shared electronically among multiple entities. On the other hand, the personal health record (PHR) is the electronic version of an individual's health record that the person has access to via web. Several organizations are providing the patients access to their private records or to portions of them, such as laboratory test results. In this chapter, EMR signifies separate systems used by various organizations to record health information electronically whereas EHR here refers to an integrated database of electronic health records that provides access for several entities who are sharing it. Integrating all the medical information of a person electronically for regional or nationwide use, something that is proposed in the EHR concept, has significant implications. Having a single point of access to the entire medical history of a patient bears certain challenges. Among the major widespread concerns are; where will this data reside, what would the access mechanism be and who owns the responsibility of maintaining the security and privacy standards of such records and who owns the information? Lack of interoperability is a common concern as a barrier to successful health information exchanges in an integrated health information environment.

There have been several initiatives by the government in the United States in form of regulations, guidelines and monetary incentives to expedite the process of integrating health information from disparate sources. The Health Insurance Portability and Accountability Act (HIPAA) of 1996 is a major step towards digitization of health records with clear focus on security and privacy of patients. The American Recovery and Reinvestment Act of 2009 (ARRA) provides monetary incentives to medical providers for using EHR systems rather than paper counterparts (Austin et al. 2010). Considerable effort is required to standardize the electronic systems so that interoperability issues can be dealt with effectively. The Certification Commission for Health Information Technology (CCHIT) is currently modifying its criteria to conform to the ARRA-defined requirements and is working closely with the department of Health and Human Services (HSS), the Health Information Technology (HIT) Policy Committee and the Office of the National Coordinator for Health Information Technology (ONC) to influence national EHR certification policy. On February 17, 2009, U.S. President Barack Obama signed into law HR 1, the American Recovery and Reinvestment Act, which allocates $19.2 billion dollars in funding to support the adoption and use of health information technology also known as a the "Health Information Technology for Economic and Clinical Health Act" or the "HITECH Act" (HHS.gov 2011). Impetus from federal and state government towards digitization of patient health records is aimed at avoiding errors in medical judgments from health care providers, reducing cost of healthcare delivery and improving overall care for the patient (Jha et al. 2009). Increasing popularity and adoption of (EMR) is geared towards improving quality of healthcare provided in the nation. The objective is better patient-provider communication, better communication among providers delivering care to the same patient, integration of records from different health care disciplines and subspecialties and accessibility and aggregation of records among different health care delivery sites to provide a holistic health profile for a patient. Such benefits are not without associated risk of exposure of personally identifiable information and compromise in digital health data resulting in patient anguish and possible damage to career and provider embarrassment and possible liability. It is crucial that providers utilizing EMRs address the challenges to security and privacy issues of EHR technology. Anecdotal evidence and media reports about medical security breaches suggest a rather weak preparedness on the part of the health service providers in assuring security of health data. Several security, privacy and compliance issues must be addressed within the context of creating a universal electronic health record system that provides a single point of access to patient health information.

This section explores the security, privacy and compliance challenges in EHRs and outlines some solutions to these issues. The next section explores the regulatory requirements for security and privacy of health care records primarily from HIPAA. It also discusses the guidelines for PHI for ensuring security and privacy challenges of health records. The third section lists the common challenges that we are facing in securing the information in an integrated environment. The fourth section outlines broad steps in dealing the security and privacy concerns of EHR. The final section presents the conclusion for this chapter.

2.2.2 Regulations and Guidelines

The Health Insurance Portability and Accountability Act (HIPAA) of 1996 protects the privacy of medical records of patients by preventing unauthorized disclosure and improper use of patients' protected health information (PHI). There have been Federal support and impetus for migrating to electronic medical records over the years. With considerable emphasis and monetary investment in the 1990s on the computerization of health services operations, the possibility of data manipulation and nonconsensual secondary use of personally identifiable records has tremendously increased (Baumer et. al. 2000). HIPAA declares PHI "privileged," protecting individuals from losses resulting from the fabrication of their personal data.

Businesses affected by HIPAA are directed to protect the integrity, confidentiality, and availability of the electronic PHI they collect, maintain, use, and transmit.

Three major components of HIPAA are for security and privacy of electronic records are:

2.2.2.1 The Security Rule

The security rule of HIPAA is concerned about the personal health information in electronic form. The law states that private information of individuals must be kept safe from damage of any kind. The purpose of this clause is to protect electronic patient information from alteration, destruction, loss, and accidental or intentional disclosure to unauthorized persons. HIPAA establishes behavioral standards and requires covered entities to develop practices that adhere to these behavioral standards.

The security rule requires compliance actions in the following categories:

- *Administrative safeguards*: this requires formal practices to manage security and personnel from the side of the healthcare service provider. Ensuring correct administrative safeguards entails a correct approach to governing the information security of the organization, putting correct controls in place and frequently monitoring and upgrading such controls.
- *Physical safeguards*: An important piece of the security solution of an organization lies with physical protection of the data, computers and the physical premises where it resides. This would entail creating correct physical security controls in the form of authorization controls for physical access to the computers and premises. Another important source of critical data is disposal of paper versions of the protected data or of digital media on which protected data are stored. Adequate mechanisms need to be created to deal with physical threats to data security.
- *Technical safeguards*: This category of safeguard requires creating detailed access control mechanisms to declare and monitor information access. It is also important to make sure that data in transit (moving from one point to another in the healthcare domain) is secure.
- *Organizational requirement*: This requirement assures that employees understand the serious implications maintaining the integrity and security of data that they deal with on a daily basis. The employee should have explicit business associate contract provisions so that they can affirm agreement regarding the role that is required for them.
- *Policies, procedures and documentation*: These requirements correct security policy and procedure in place to protect the data.

Meeting the security rule requirements entails coming up with a comprehensive security plan that has detailed procedures for addressing risks at several levels in the organization and that proactively addresses those risks. Examples of the planning steps include establishing security certification processes for employees and contractors, keeping employee records constantly updated to indicate the level of security appropriate to each job position, termination of role or employment, assessing the compliance of the Management Information Systems (MIS) department with the Security Rule standards and explicitly stating consequences for noncompliance with new security rules (Choi et al. 2006).

2.2.2.2 The Privacy Rule

The privacy rule of HIPAA applies to PHI in all forms, including oral, written and electronic forms. The purpose of the privacy rule is to "meet the pressing need for national standards to control the sensitive health information and to establish real penalties for the misuse or improper disclosure of this information" (Choi et al. 2006). The rules established within the privacy dimension of HIPAA, given all aspects of use of personal health records including medical records, claims, and payment information, and almost all additional information related to a patient's health care. The privacy rule protects the individual right of dictating how and when the personal information of the patient can be released. It is meant to empower an individual to play an important role in managing one's own health records. It allows patients to have a participatory approach to data management by giving them the specific right to access their medical records and request amendments, to allow or not allow access to their information in certain circumstances and be aware of the their privacy rights in this domain.

Transactions among various participants in the healthcare industries must communicate effectively and electronically patient information. Successfully meeting this requirement necessitates that the privacy and security covenants also be met.

This regulation has forced companies to revisit and reorganize their business processes. Compliance with HIPAA is not just a matter of technical products ensuring safe and secure data collection, transaction, and storage; rather, compliance is an issue of "organizational change management" (Mishra and Chin 2008). It requires instituting new structures and patterns for health care organizations to coordinate care efficiently, trust other's intentions, and responsibly maintain and protect sensitive data (Huston 2001). HIPAA influences healthcare organizations at the basic infrastructure level, thus demanding reevaluation at all levels, including the creation and implementation of technical solutions. Employing and adapting to technical solutions requires not only proper planning but also an overhaul in organizational processes (Mishra and Chin 2008). Even though more than one-third of the rules in HIPAA address administrative security requirements, many organizations focused disproportionately on technology rather than on administrative safeguards. The different types of security required by the HIPAA security rule were also not well understood by participating organizations. It is critical to establish a consistent method for linking patients with the electronic records to assure exchanging health information about the correct unique patient.

In the United States, the American Recovery and Reinvestment Act of 2009 (ARRA) provides monetary incentives to medical providers for using EHR systems rather than paper counterparts (Austin et al. 2010). In October 2009, CCHIT augmented its certification criteria with additional security criteria and provided corresponding black-box test scripts. The security criteria provide specific requirements intended to establish a minimum level of security of an EHR system. The purpose of CCHIT certification is to confirm that certified EHR systems maintain a minimum level of accuracy, reliability, security and interoperability. These characteristics are known as software quality factors (Austin et al. 2010). Regional or state-level efforts to exchange health information also will have to reconcile the differences among participants in how security policies are implemented. Organizations in ten states are working to develop and test a set of model policy requirements to bridge policy gaps for authentication and audit across these organizations.

In the case of personal health records (PHRs), which are becoming popular, security and privacy concerns have led to guidelines proposed by the government. The Office of National Coordinator for Health Information Technology (ONC) issued a "Nationwide Privacy and Security Framework for Electronic Exchange of Individually Identified Health Information" in 2008. This framework suggests eight principles for establishing a consistent approach that meets privacy and security challenges of online PHRs and electronic health information exchange. Organizations operating a PHR or Health Information Exchange (HIE) service has to follow the guidelines regardless of whether it is explicitly covered by HIPAA. These principles are expected to guide the actions of all health care-related persons and entities that participate in a network for the purpose of electronic exchange of individually identifiable health information. These principles are not intended to apply to individuals with respect to their own individually identifiable health information.

The proposed eight principles are:

- *Individual access*: Personal health information should be accessible to individuals to manage their health care. HIPAA covered entities generally make it difficult for individuals to access their personal healthcare records online (Brown 2009). This principle favors easy access to individuals for their health records.
- *Correction*: In case of a mistake in an individual's personal healthcare records, the individual should be able to correct that mistake. There should be a clear process to allow changes by the individual and to record the changes for documentation. In case of disagreement, there should be process for documenting the disagreement as well. The HIPAA privacy rule recognizes that individuals should play an important role in ensuring accuracy of their health record. Individuals have the right to have a covered entity under HIPAA to amend their PHI in a designated record set. In case a correction is made, the covered entity is entitled to inform its business associates and others who are known to have their PHI that the record was amended.
- *Openness and Transparency*: Healthcare providers should aim for complete openness and transparency to the individuals about policies, procedures and technologies employed to collect and disseminate individually identifiable information. The information should be provided in easily understandable format to the individual providing details about who accesses the information, how is it transmitted, how is it used and what control the individual has of it.

- *System Complexity*: With the health information technologies evolving into increasingly complex systems, with better access to health information, larger storage capacity and interoperability across networks, it is important that the individuals, who information is stored in these systems, trust the technologies and the care providers to keep their information safe. Openness and transparency is thus essential in establishing this trust through adequate information provided to the individuals about how the system is being used. Health information organizations (HIOs) and entities that participate in HIOs should provide clear notice of their policies and procedures regarding how they use and disclose individuals' identifiable health information and how they will protect the privacy of this information.
- *Individual Choice*: Individuals should have the control over deciding what specific part of the personally identifiable information should be disclosed and to whom. The individual choice principle of the Privacy and Security Framework emphasizes that the opportunity and ability of an individual to make choices with respect to the electronic exchange of their individually identifiable health information is an important aspect of building trust (hhs.gov 2011). The Privacy and Security Framework (PSF) also recommends that the options available for choices should depend on the nature of information being exchanged and the purpose of the exchange. The privacy rule empowers the individuals to participate actively in managing their own information.
- *Collection, Use and Disclosure Limitations*: health information about individuals should be collected, used and disclosed as required by the policies and procedures. The privacy rule generally requires covered entities to take reasonable steps to limit the use or disclosure of PHI to the minimum necessary to accomplish the intended purpose. This principle also suggests that for routine or recurring requests and disclosures, covered entities must implement reasonable policies and procedures (which may be standard protocols) to limit information disclosures or requests. It also suggests that a covered entity should limit the business associate's uses and disclosures of for PHI to be consistent with its own policies and procedures. The business associate may not have the similar stringent policies about the use of PHI, hence the restriction.
- *Data Quality and Integrity*: There should be reasonable care taken to ensure that data being collected and transmitted is complete, accurate and timely. It is also important to ensure that it has not been altered or destroyed in an unauthorized manner.
- *Safeguards Principle*: there should be reasonable assurance that administrative, technical and physical safeguards are provided to ensure confidentiality, integrity and availability of data. It is important to protect the personally identifiable data from inappropriate access, use or disclosure. The Safeguards Principle in the Privacy and Security Framework emphasizes that trust in electronic health information exchange can only be achieved if reasonable administrative, technical, and physical safeguards are in place.
- *Privacy Rule*: the HIPAA privacy rule supports the Safeguards Principle by requiring covered entities to implement appropriate administrative, technical, and physical safeguards to protect the privacy of protected health information (hhs.gov).

2.2.2.3 Accountability

All the guidelines should be followed and implementation should be verified through auditing, monitoring and other procedural and technical processes.

The Accountability Principle in the Privacy and Security Framework emphasizes that guidelines should be followed and all the activities and mechanisms in accordance with HIPAA compliance should be reported. This principle is important to build trust in electronic exchange of individually identifiable information. The privacy rule in HIPAA provides the foundation for accountability within an electronic health-information-exchange environment. It requires covered entities to comply with administrative requirements and extend such obligations to business associates. This rule also establishes mechanisms for addressing non-compliance with privacy standards through covered entity's voluntary compliance, a resolution agreement and corrective action plan or imposing civil penalties (hhs.gov).

The Certification Commission for Healthcare Information Technology (CCHIT) is an independent, voluntary, private-sector initiative that has been designated by the Department of Health and Human Services (HHS) as a recognized certification body for electronic health records (EHRs) and their networks (Brown 2009). CCHIT has modified its criteria to certify PHRs. It is likely that CCHIT certification will become the commonly accepted requirement for PHRs as well (Brown 2009).

2.2.3 Challenges with Integrated Electronic Health Records

The U.S. health care system faces multiple challenges such as increasing cost and inconsistent quality. It is perceived that the electronic health records have the potential to improve the efficiency and effectiveness of health care providers. The American Recovery and Reinvestment Act of 2009 makes national, integrated health information systems a priority. Even though there is a broad consensus on benefits of such an integrated system, health care providers have been slow to adopt it. A recent study on adoption of electronic health records suggests that only 17% of U.S. physicians use either a minimally functional or comprehensive electronic-records systems (Jha et al. 2009). Integration efforts pose serious challenges to organizations in terms of technical preparedness as well as organizational willingness. Employing and adapting to technical solutions requires not only proper planning but also an overhaul in organizational processes. Some of the areas identified as major challenges for integration of electronic medical records are:

2.2.3.1 Getting Patient Consent

There is confusion about the "correct" way of obtaining patient permission to disclose personal health information. There are several reasons to determine prevalent practice (Dimitropoulos and Rizk 2009):

- A lack of understanding about HIPAA requirements to get patient permission for certain disclosures. Organizations have interpreted and executed this requirement differently.
- A set of different state laws that lack clear guidance on when to seek permission and when not to seek permission.
- Ethical and moral obligation to get the permission before sharing any information.
- Organizational policies require getting permission as an added security layer to their security practices.

There is also confusion about the terms used for obtaining patients' permission. This is due to use of different terms in HIPAA privacy rule for different purposes (Dimitropoulos and Rizk 2009). Adding to the confusion is the variance in state laws of terms such as *consent, authorization* and *release*, to describe a patient's written permission to disclose health information.

2.2.3.2 Ensuring Privacy and Security of Patient Information

HIPAA requires a certain level of preparedness from organizations implementing the security and privacy rules of this legislation. Various organizations' interpretations of HIPAA requirements to secure information and protect privacy vary significantly adding to the confusion about how integrated health information should be treated. There is a general lack of understanding about privacy rule implications to allow disclosure of health information for treatment, payment and health care operations. Also, the state laws add to confusion with reference to when the rule is being applied or how is it being applied.

The primary causes of variation identified in security policies were attributable to a general misunderstanding about appropriate security practices, including what is technically available and what provisions can be applied more broadly (Dimitropoulos and Rizk 2009). Some organizations get concerned when they do not find the participating organization to be dealing with security requirements effectively. The security rule addresses administrative, physical and technical security. Even though more than one-third of the rule addresses administrative security requirements, many organizations focused disproportionately on technology rather than on administrative safeguards (Dimitropoulos and Rizk 2009). An over-emphasis on technical safeguards is unable to protect the organization from insider threats to security which is significantly more common compared to vulnerabilities originating outside an organization.

2.2.3.3 Data Access Mechanisms and Authorization Techniques

There is a need to develop standard authentication and authorization protocols to be implemented with electronic systems holding health data. Organizations require a fair amount of trust on other participating members to share their records with a reasonable assurance that the other party is keeping the information secure. In an integrated environment, data should flow seamlessly from one system to another resulting in several access points across the systems. Considering the critical nature of the data in such systems, our existing access control models must be used innovatively.

2.2.3.4 Linking Data to a Unique Person

If organizations intend to share data across databases to realize the vision of one record per patient, there has to be predefined agreed upon ways of linking the databases such that records are accurately identified. If the correct record for a patient is not identified, that might lead to serious clinical and privacy threats. It is important because different organizations involved in providing care to a patient use locally assigned patient identifiers which lose meaning outside the organizational boundaries. Correctly identifying patients and providers not only is critical in the delivery of high quality care and for electronic HIE, but also is a fundamental issue in other information security domains, such as authentication and authorization (Dimitropoulos and Rizk 2009).

Even though we have seen a lot of progress in adoption of EMR in the recent years, a lot needs to be achieved. Most of the providers are not realizing the full benefits from EMR since they shy away from using all its capabilities. The use of EMR technology improves efficiency and safety but the way it is being used currently restricts it to the data that is fed in the system or data in the linked systems. The information has to be entered manually and there is no easy access to the historical records of a specific patient.

2.2.3.5 Data Storage and Handling

HIPAA requires healthcare providers to be more stringent with storing and handling of patient data, in the system well as during transmission of the information to other systems. Transmission of information from one system to another requires use of encryption techniques. Benaloh et al. (2009) argue for using encryption control measures for patient health records. The approach calls for patient enabled encryption keys such that the patient participates in their own security management of the data.

2.2.3.6 Disaster Recovery Preparation

Disasters, natural or man-made, could prove catastrophic to the information held in systems. With a greater emphasis on storing the patient information electronically, comes an increased responsibility to plan for disaster recovery techniques for such systems. The systems also require enhanced interoperability to deal with data from various sources.

The challenges in complying with regulatory requirements lie in the ever changing nature of technology and the associated security vulnerabilities. It is important to continuously assess, evaluate and address these challenges proactively. As the EMR is implemented in provider practices, a full-risk assessment of the administrative, technical and physical safeguards must be addressed. Each HIPAA security rule specification should be addressed and procedures should be put in place to minimize risk

2.2.4 Addressing These Challenges

Security violations in electronic health records, such as unauthorized access or unauthorized alteration of individual information could lead to potential problems for all the involved parties. Though the concept of EHR is appealing to improve effectiveness of processing of health care data, but electronic health data need caution while designing and deploying the system. The proportion of damage in EHR compromise would be significantly higher than that in a paper-based system (Goldschmidt 2005). To encourage healthcare service consumers and providers to use electronic health records, it is crucial to instill confidence that the electronic health information is well protected and that consumers' privacy is assured (Liu et al. 2007). The traceability of data in a computer system also has to be considered an asset in controlling information or containing damage from an unauthorized access. This does not happen with paper records; unauthorized information access is not tracked *or* monitored. This does not mean there should not be concern about attempts to gain access to electronic medical records for unauthorized or criminal purposes. Some of the common solutions to the integration of electronic health records are provided below:

2.2.4.1 Common Agreement on Patient Consent for Disclosure

The development of a common approach to obtaining and managing patient consent for disclosure is critical. There are several state laws that have more stringent standards for security and privacy than HIPAA, which does not preclude state laws being enforced. Due to differing expectations statewide, organizations cannot come up with a standard privacy requirement that can satisfy all the security needs for participating organization in HIEs. Several options are being considered by state and federal bodies to come up with satisfactory solutions for interstate sharing of information.

2.2.4.2 Harmonizing State Privacy Laws

It is important to harmonize state privacy laws to enable a nationally integrated HIE. This has to be a coordinated effort among states to help prevent the codification of policies that could make nationwide electronic HIE impossible. There are several ongoing initiatives in this direction.

2.2.4.3 Standard Access Control and Authorization Policies

More work is required to establish how security and privacy policies will be implemented among participants. There has to be an agreement by the involved parties not only on the content of such policies but also a consensus on implementation and adoption approaches as well. The access control models should be based on a "need to know" basis (Kurtz 2003). It better to provide access based on the role of the participant in the organization than a blanket access power to persons or organizations. The care providers should access only the records that they are providing care for.

2.2.4.4 Inter-Organizational Agreements (IOAs)

There has to be clearly defined inter-organizational agreements between organizations sharing the data in electronic health record systems. These agreements provide the basis of trust in the relationship between participating organizations. There is an ongoing effort on getting consensus form the partners on creating a legal agreement in case of any breach of trust. The IOA Collaborative has developed a core set of privacy and security provisions and plans to pilot-test two model agreements for interstate electronic HIEs – one agreement for a public health setting and the other for exchange among private entities (Dimitropoulos and Rizk 2009).

2.2.4.5 Educating the Consumer and the Provider

Electronic HIEs can be a new concept to consumers nationwide and thus require a widespread effort to educate the consumer about the pros and cons of such a collaborative effort. Such an effort will engage consumers in the discussion about security of the records and will make them an informed participant in this ongoing effort. One of the key findings in the assessment of variation was that many health care providers misunderstand the capabilities and benefits of electronic HIEs and have concerns about the security of electronic health record (EHR) systems (Dimitropoulos and Rizk 2009). The efforts are directed towards disseminating consistent educational information to providers about the benefits of EHRs and electronic HIE, with a focus on privacy and security, to help encourage their participation in electronic HIE.

2.2.4.6 Standardization and Interoperability

In order to make patient information shareable across several healthcare providers, it is important to standardize the system and EMR specifications. The aim of this sharing of information should be a single record for a patient the provides complete medical history compiling information from all the primary care physicians, surgeons, dentists, pharmacies or any other healthcare provider the patient has visited. This concept of total integration leads to development of the electronic healthcare record (EHR). As challenging as it might be, EHR truly is far behind in its implementation, except in certain environments, such as the Department of Veterans Affairs.

2.2.4.7 Audit Controls and Monitoring

Continuous audit control and monitoring should be provided to ensure the integrity of data. Auditing system logs provide insights into for data access on "need to know'" basis and developing such audit trails would be beneficial in the long run. Random and directed review of the audit trail should be accomplished regularly to test compliance with confidentiality policies. It is crucial to review the feeder systems for audit trail capabilities, as these could be vulnerable without proper information security and auditing capabilities.

2.2.4.8 Clear Policies, Procedures and Controls

Policies, controls and procedures of accessing data should be clearly defined. These policies should be communicated very well to the users through regular training and education. Regular backup of the database must be established to include the capability to reload the database in case of disaster.

2.2.4.9 Disaster Recovery Plan

Design of the disaster recovery plan should be carried out to assure minimum risk of systems downtime and data loss in case of a calamity. Disaster recovery plans are crucial for data recovery process especially in the health care domain. Eventually, all of the records of the patients will be in electronic form and loss of access to this data could jeopardize patient care. Care should be taken to provide the correct services for the risk involved. Backup copies of data with fail-over capabilities are important to maintain. There should be stringent mechanisms in place to ensure continued operation and data integrity in case of a disaster (Kurtz 2003).

2.2.4.10 Physical Security of the Information

Physical protection of important information in form of printers, disposal of copies in paper or digital form and computers on which the data resides should be ensured.

2.2.4.11 Integrating Dental Records with EHR

There has been little effort in integrating the dental records into the EHR, with the primary exception of certain U.S. Federal EHR technologies. According to Groen and Powell (2010), "While patient interaction with PHR systems is still very limited, the National Dental EDI Council (NDEDIC) has recognized their importance and begun to focus on ensuring the participation of dental insurance stakeholders in the development of PHR systems." Further, according to Groen and Powell, "UHIN (the Utah Health Information Network) is an example of a state health information network that supports the dental community and is focused on helping to reduce costs for dental practices. Dental claims, payments, reports and x-rays can be transferred electronically through UHIN."

2.2.5 Conclusion

The Health Insurance Portability and Accountability Act (HIPAA) of 1996 suggests that the privacy, security and electronic transaction standards for maintaining the patient information for all healthcare providers. HIPAA targets two goals (Choi et al. 2006): insurance flexibility (electronic record can be easily accessed and transferred thus would prevent refusal of coverage due to change of jobs) and administrative ease (reducing healthcare cost due to standardizing the transactions). Hence, electronic data interchange is an important element in assisting the organizations to meet with high patient load and enhance business partner relationships in healthcare organizations. HIPAA seeks to validate and assist with the inevitability of electronic data transactions, while also addressing privacy and security issues that may stem from converting to the use of potentially vulnerable electronic transactions. The main challenge ahead is to continue work toward a common set of privacy and security policies and practices that respect local preferences in each state yet facilitate nationwide electronic HIE. For the success of integrated electronic health record technology, it is crucial to create a broad base of support from various stakeholders and develop consensus-based polices that could be broadly adopted and shared. This section explores various issues and concerns in creating EHR and discusses several possible ways of meeting such challenges.

2.3 Physicians' Dental Data Needs and Oral Healthcare Providers' Medical Data Needs: The Clinical Rationale

Shin-Mey Rose Yin Geist and Valerie J. Harvey Powell

2.3.1 Physicians' Needs for Dental Records

Physicians require dental records:

- For diagnosing and assessing systemic diseases and health status of their patients
- For coordination and collaboration of healthcare
- For research purposes
- For forensic purposes

More than 200 systemic diseases can present oral symptoms and/or signs. Dental records prepared by an alert dentist provide invaluable information for early diagnosis and monitoring the progress of these diseases. Conditions most common or highly relevant to oral health with respect to systemic disease are presented in this section. Please also see Appendix C for pertinent literature on individual categories of diseases and conditions (C-1 through C-36) where medical-dental collaboration is valuable for patient care or research.

2.3.2 Diabetes Mellitus

Diabetes mellitus (DM), along with its complications, is one of the most complex and difficult diseases for healthcare professionals to manage worldwide. Over the last decade, there has been a rapid rise in the incidence and prevalence of DM due to global changes in lifestyle. It was projected that by 2030, there will be an estimated 366 million patients with diabetes in the world. In the United States, currently at least 25.8 million children and adults – 8.3% of the population – have diabetes. Among them, 18.8 million are diagnosed and 7.0 million are undiagnosed (American Diabetes Association 2011a).

Managing complications of diabetes such as heart disease and stroke, hypertension, retinopathy, chronic kidney disease, neuropathy, and lower-limb amputations demands a high expenditure of healthcare resources. The *total cost of diabetes* in the United States in 2007 was estimated at $218 billion. The costs of diagnosed diabetes care are estimated at $174 billion. The costs of undiagnosed diabetes, prediabetes, and gestational diabetes amount to an additional $44 billion (American Diabetes Association 2011b). Early diagnosis and treatment of diabetes will prevent or reduce complications and can save tremendous health care costs and improve quality of life. Dental records reporting periodontal disease hold promise for the diagnosis of diabetes. The association of diabetes and periodontal disease has been well established; diabetic individuals have a high prevalence of periodontitis. Many patients with severe periodontitis have been referred for diabetes evaluation and subsequently diagnosed with diabetes. Recently it was found that periodontitis could be an independent predictor for diabetes incidence. Physicians will find the benefit of patients' dental record of periodontitis and its progression helpful in diagnosing diabetes and monitoring the progression of the disease (Demmer et al. 2008; Choi et al. 2011).

2.3.3 Xerostomia, Candidiasis, and Frequent Dental Infections

Xerostomia, candidiasis and frequent dental infections are common in patients with poorly controlled diabetes (Soysa et al. 2006; Borges et al. 2010; Khovidhunkit 2009;

Ueta 1993). These records can also be helpful in diagnosing diabetes as well as providing physicians with a picture of the patient's DM status.

There are indications that collaborative and coordinated dental care can reduce the expenditure in health care resource for diabetes. Due to immunity impairment, diabetes patients have higher risk for infection and infection complications; timely elimination of the chronic odontogenic infections can prevent costly severe head and neck infection and even septicemia (Calvet et al. 2001; Rajagopalan 2005; Huang et al. 2005; Rao et al. 2010). Evidence has shown, although with some controversy, that periodontal treatment improves glycemic control in diabetes (Taylor et al. 2008; Taylor 2003; Grossi 2001; Jones et al. 2006; Janket et al. 2005). Research on periodontal disease and increased risk for CVD in diabetes yields interesting results that periodontal bacteria are associated with coronary disease (Desvarieux et al. 2005; Janket et al. 2008). Although the direct cause and effect relationship is not yet fully established, such research has raised general awareness of the importance of oral health. Many dental offices monitor A1c level of diabetes patients, provide glucose checks, and a tobacco cessation program to collaborate and coordinate diabetes patients' healthcare. These provisions have shown a positive result (Geist et al. 2011).

2.3.4 Chronic Kidney Disease

Chronic Kidney Disease (CKD) is a major burden to the healthcare system. CKD is an irreversible and progressive disease for which diabetes and hypertension are major risk factors. There are 26 million people in the United States with this disease. CKD usually progresses to kidney failure (usually called End Stage Renal Disease or ESRD). Once patients reach this stage, they need costly renal replacement therapy, either dialysis or a kidney transplant. Since 1972, the Medicare national insurance program for ESRD has paid 80% of the costs of renal replacement therapy including dialysis and transplantation for approximately 90% of patients in the United States (National Kidney Foundation 2002, 2009). In 2007, 527,283 US residents received treatment covered by this program and the total cost was $35.32 billion in public and private expenditures (National Kidney and Urologic Disease Information Clearinghouse 2010). There are 158,739 US patients living with a functioning kidney transplant in 2007. Every healthcare effort should be made to reduce mortality and morbidity due to kidney failure, improve the quality of life of patients and reduce the attendant healthcare expenditures. Oral health care providers and nephrologists are encouraged to communicate often to provide good oral health and to reduce dental infection and its complications. Patients should have a coordinated oral health care program before and after kidney transplant to prevent dental infection and immunosuppressant-induced oral health problems (National Institute of Dental and Craniofacial Research 2011).

2.3.5 HIV Infection and AIDS (HIV/AIDS)

HIV/AIDS is another global epidemic. By the end of 2007, there were 33 million people in the world living with HIV infection (WHO 2010). In the United States, CDC estimates that more than one million people are living with HIV (Centers for Disease Control and Prevention 2010a). The cost of lifetime medical care for HIV infected individuals each year is estimated to be $20 billion (Centers for Disease Control and Prevention 2010b).

No other systemic diseases have as high a significance in oral health as HIV/AIDS. Early on in this epidemic, many studies demonstrated a wide variety of oral lesions in individuals with HIV/AIDS. These lesions, from infections to neoplasms, are common; studies have shown that about 40–50% of HIV positive persons have oral fungal, bacterial or viral infections, often occurring early in the course of the disease (Petersen 2004). Manifestations of these infections have been used in diagnosing HIV infection and subsequent disease progression to AIDS (Greenspan 1987; van der Waal et al. 1991; Coogan et al. 2005). The presence of oral candidiasis, oral hairy leukoplakia or Kaposi's sarcoma strongly suggests HIV infection. After the inception of Highly Active Anti-Retroviral Therapy (HAART), these oral lesions often changed in frequency and severity to a certain degree; however, they are still valuable in monitoring disease process and treatment failure, especially in circumstances where viral load or CD4 counts are not easily or frequently accessible (Ramirez-Amador et al. 2007; Hodgson et al. 2006). With HAART, many oral lesions related to the HAART medications' adverse effects can affect patients' quality of life (Hodgson et al. 2006) and need to be treated collaboratively with physicians and other healthcare providers. In summary, dentists' knowledge of oral lesions and the advantages of the accessibility of oral manifestations in dental care can contribute valuable information in early disease diagnosis, progression and/or treatment failure, to the physicians who care for persons with HIV infection.

2.3.6 Hemophilia

It is estimated that 20,000 people in the United States have hemophilia. It is a rare disease, but its treatments are expensive and demand extensive coordination. Individuals with hemophilia are encouraged to enroll in the federal government sponsored hemophilia treatment centers (HTCs). More than 100 federally funded HTCs are located throughout the United States. Many HTCs are located at major university medical and research centers so all the treatment that a patient needs will be coordinated easily to increase effectiveness, and to reduce complications and costs. The hemophilia teams at these centers include nurse coordinators, hematologists (adult or pediatric), social workers, physical therapists, orthopedists, dentists and nutritionists. A CDC study showed that people who used an HTC were 40% less likely to die of a hemophilia-related complication compared to those who did not receive care at a treatment center. It also demonstrated that people who used a treatment center were 40% less likely to be hospitalized for bleeding complications (Centers for Disease Control and Prevention 2011). Individuals with hemophilia are encouraged to maintain optimal oral health. Their oral health records are an important source of information for coordinated care, especially for surgical dental procedures such as wisdom teeth extractions. Recent recommendations specify that only a hematologist may prescribe factor concentrates to avoid complications, minimize costs and optimize the treatment outcome.

2.3.7 Autoimmune Diseases

The NIH estimates that up to 23.5 million Americans have an autoimmune disease (AD). Depending on the classification system, there are 80–100 different autoimmune diseases. Many of them affect multiple organs and different parts of the body (systemic autoimmune diseases), giving affected individuals a variety of symptoms and signs (NIH National Institute of Allergy and Infectious Diseases 2005). This problem makes diagnosis difficult. Particularly when an individual, affected by different autoimmune diseases, exhibits an overlapping array of symptoms and signs. The most common systemic autoimmune disorders are SLE, rheumatoid arthritis and Sjögren syndrome, and most of the time they occur in the same individual. Diagnosis and treatment can be challenging and require a multidisciplinary approach. These diseases often have oral manifestations in the early stage and many times the oral lesions provide important clues in establishing early diagnosis.

2.3.8 Sjögren Syndrome

Sjögren syndrome (SS) is one of the most common systemic autoimmune diseases. It can cause dysfunction of the exocrine glands and of other organs such as the kidneys, gastrointestinal system, blood vessels, lungs, liver, pancreas and the central nervous system. The characteristic symptoms are dry mouth and dry eyes due to the reduction of flow of salivary and lachrymal glands, but patients may also experience extreme fatigue and joint pain and have a 20 times higher risk of developing lymphoma compared to the general population (Zintzaras et al. 2005). Currently it is estimated that four million Americans are affected by this debilitating disease (Sjögren's Syndrome Foundation 2009). Of these, about 50% exhibit primary Sjögren syndrome. The other 50% of cases are secondary Sjögren syndrome, which involves the presence of other systemic autoimmune disorders such as rheumatoid arthritis, lupus or scleroderma. Diagnosis of Sjögren syndrome can be challenging. The average time between first symptoms and diagnosis is 10 years, while patients are already suffering from physical, psychological and social disabilities.

The early sign of dry mouth may not be perceived by the affected individuals because it takes 40–50% of salivary function loss to feel dry (Dawes 1987). However, the oral manifestations, mainly oral candidiasis and dental decay at the root surface and incisal edge, serve as signs of oral dryness. Some individuals may experience frequent oral traumatic ulcers due to lack of lubrication of food. These clinical signs along with easy access for a lower lip minor salivary gland biopsy may contribute valuable information in establishing a diagnosis in an early stage.

2.3.9 Systemic Lupus Erythematous (SLE)

SLE is another common systemic autoimmune disorder. SLE affects many organs and systems in the body, producing widely variable symptoms. Oral lesions occur in about 40% of the patients, and include involvement in Sjögren syndrome. SLE can appear as thinning of the oral mucosa (erythema) with ulcers and white radiating lines at the border of the areas of redness. This observation is called lichenoid mucositis and assists in establishing the diagnosis.

2.3.10 Cancer

Coordination and collaborative care is crucial before, during and after cancer therapy. It is especially important in chemotherapy and radiation therapy. Most chemotherapeutic agents used in cancer treatment interrupt cell metabolism, inhibit cell division and cause biological cell death of rapidly proliferating cancer cells. They also kill normal cells that divide frequently, such as bone marrow cells, mucosal cells in the digestive tract (including the oral cavity), and hair follicle cells. These results in the most common side effects of chemotherapy: bone marrow suppression, immunosuppression, mucositis and hair loss. Mucositis and increased risk for infection due to immunosuppression are major concerns. Although these side effects are mainly reversible, when they happen during therapy they can be too severe for the therapy to continue. They may delay or interrupt cancer therapy and decrease its effectiveness. For example, latent dental infection can become active due to immunosuppression, resulting in severe and sometimes lethal head and neck infections such as Ludwig angina. Before patients start chemotherapy, it is essential that they have a comprehensive oral examination. All infection sources must be removed to prevent inter-treatment dental infections.

For patients diagnosed with leukemia or lymphoma, pre-chemotherapy tooth extraction may be prohibitive due to the myelosuppression and immunosuppression of the disease itself. However, palliative measures can be taken to reduce or avoid chemotherapy complications.

Advanced medical technology has recently made hematologic stem cell transplant (HCT) – once the last resort treatment of blood cell malignancies such as leukemia and many solid tumors – a widely used and potentially curative procedure. This new procedure, in addition to traditional bone marrow transplant (BMT), has made oral health care a vital part of HCT management before, during and after the course of therapy. Pre- and post-transplant immunosuppressant treatment may cause short-term or long-term oral complications. These complications include mucositis, infections, oral bleeding, graft-versus-host disease, salivary changes and dry mouth, taste alterations, secondary malignancies in oral cavity, and jaw bone necrosis. Vigilant oral care can reduce mortality and morbidity, increase the success rate of engraftment and improve the quality of life of the recipients (Epstein et al. 2009).

2.3.11 Chronic Graft-Versus-Host Disease (CGVHD)

HCT, BMT, and kidney and other organ transplant recipients are expected to have degrees of graft-versus-host disease (GVHD) in the months to years following the transplant. GVHD is a condition in which alloreactive donor T cells recognize host tissue antigens as foreign and mount an immune response against the host tissue similar to systemic autoimmune diseases. Acute GVHD is usually managed by the transplant team while the patient is still in the medical center. However, more than 50% of patients develop chronic GVHD, which usually appears within 6–12 months of transplantation. Oral manifestations may be the initial or only signs of this reaction. Dental records of these oral lesions, which can be ulcerative or erythematous, and can include reticular lichenoid mucositis and frequent mucocele formation, can help in the diagnosis of cGVHD in the community health care setting. Patients may quickly be referred back to the original medical center if necessary.

2.3.12 Bisphosphonate-Associated Osteonecrosis

Since 2003, a new disease entity, bisphosphonate-associated osteonecrosis (BON), has emerged in cancer patients who have received intravenous nitrogen-containing bisphosphonates (Geist et al. 2005). This form of bisphosphonate has been used in treating bone cancer such as multiple myeloma and solid tumors that are known to metastasize to bone such as prostate cancer, breast cancer, and lung cancer. It is used to reduce or prevent skeletal events. The disease mechanism is not fully understood, but current evidence indicates that BON almost exclusively involves the jawbone and is most prevalent in patients who have received intravenous nitrogen-containing bisphosphonates such as pamidronate and zoledronic acid for cancer therapy. In most cases, necrosis of the jawbones appeared after dental surgical procedures such as tooth extractions. Patients with a history of intravenous nitrogen-containing bisphosphonate therapy are advised to avoid invasive dental procedures, and oral healthcare providers are warned to take precautions in treating such patients. The oral healthcare community urges oncologists to refer patients for oral health care before initiating IV bisphosphonate use to avoid future surgical dental procedures that may increase the risk of bisphosphonate-associated jawbone necrosis (Migliorati et al. 2011).

2.3.13 Head and Neck Cancer

Oral healthcare providers have a long history of collaboration with surgeons, oncologists, otolaryngologists and other specialists in managing head and neck cancer patients. This is probably due to the common treatment area of the oral cavity. It is probably more so in Taiwan, where there is a high prevalence of nasopharyngeal carcinoma (NPC). NPC is a common form of head and neck cancer among Southern Chinese and the treatment is almost exclusively high dose external irradiation with a minimal dosage of 65 Gy. In order to encourage compliance, increase the survival rate and improve the quality of life of the survivors, complications of radiation therapy must be managed collaboratively among the radiation oncologist, ENT specialists, dentists, dental specialists and other health professionals. In the early 1970s, tumor boards were established in major hospitals where NPC and other head and neck cancer patients were treated. It was in these tumor board conferences that the involved specialists contributed their expertise to help define the treatment plan for individual patients and resolve issues of complication. Because of the involvement of oral healthcare providers and ENT specialists, the most severe complication of radiation therapy, osteoradionecrosis, has been greatly reduced (Hahn 1983; Geist et al. 1993; Chen et al. 2000). Today, oral health care of head and neck cancer patients before, during, and after radiation therapy has become the standard of care for head and neck cancer treatment worldwide (Vissink et al. 2003; National Cancer Institute 2011).

Due to the complexity of cancer patient management and the multidisciplinary care involved, a teamwork approach should be adopted in every health care system where any type of cancer patient is treated. Oral health care providers should be included in the team. Some hospitals do not have an oral health care component for their cancer management team. This omission can be detrimental to their patients' overall health during cancer therapy. Hospitals should be encouraged to maintain if not expand oral health care to incorporate emerging techniques and medicine to improve the outcome of cancer treatment (Parzuchowski JS et al, 2011). Hospitals should be encouraged to maintain, if not expand oral health care to incorporate emerging techniques and medicine to improve the outcome of cancer treatment.

Before patients start radiation or chemotherapy, it is essential that they have a comprehensive oral examination. All infection sources must be removed to prevent inter- and post-treatment dental infections. These infections may delay or interrupt cancer therapy and decrease its effectiveness. Before IV bisphosphonate use, patients should have appropriate dental treatment to avoid future surgical dental procedures which may increase the risk of bisphosphonate-associated jawbone necrosis.

2.3.14 Gardner Syndrome

Gardner syndrome is an inherited disease complex with multiple abnormalities that may involve the skin, retina, skeleton and teeth. One of the components of the syndrome is familial colorectal polyposis. These polyps have a high rate of malignant transformation into invasive adenocarcinoma. Studies have shown that by age 30, about 50% of patients with Gardner syndrome will develop colorectal carcinoma. It is crucial to diagnose this syndrome in early life so preventive removal of the polyps can be done early. Multiple osteomas of the mandible and multiple supernumerary teeth are common findings. Dental records of these lesions can contribute to early diagnosis and prevent malignancy in patients with this syndrome.

2.3.15 Oral Healthcare Providers' Medical Data Needs

With advances in medical and dental sciences and technology, many dental patients present with multiple medical conditions that may require modifications in dental management. It is essential to have patients' relevant medical information accurately stated and updated in the record so a risk and benefit assessment can be done for every dental treatment, and that certain precautions be taken, to deliver dental care safely and efficiently. A patient's self reported health history is not always reliable (Pakhomov et al. 2008; Leikauf et al. 2009). For example, a patient may not report the status of COPD, which precludes supine positioning during long periodontal procedures. A patient may not report clearly and precisely about his or her cancer status and cancer treatment plan to permit the dentist to decide which dental treatment procedure takes priority. In general, a patient's medical record should be included in his or her health record because dental care is delivered to a whole person. However, for practical purposes, information with high relevancy needs to be sought. This includes medical data needed for assessing the risk of:

- Office emergencies
- Post-surgery bleeding
- Post-treatment infection
- Certain other conditions

In addition to the above, when coordinating the preparation of patients for HCT, BMT, or other organ transplant, for chemotherapy and/or radiation therapy, and for implantation of various devices, relevant medical data is also needed.

2.4 Standardized/Structured Messages Facilitate Efficient Information Sharing and Benefit Patient Care

Shin-Mey Rose Yin Geist

Due to the medical advances and evolution of medical subspecialties, large portions of the population, especially those with chronic medical conditions, often receive healthcare from multiple specialties. Care coordination by sharing patients' health information among different specialties becomes essential for quality of care to maximize the resources of the healthcare system. The key to care coordination is communication, which takes the form of consultation or referral.

Consultation or referral is a process involving three steps:

- *Initiation of the process*: confirming relevant patient information, providing reasons for the consultation or referral, and requesting specific information.
- *Responding*: The response to this consultation provides direct answers to the request.
- *Interpretation*: The final step of this process is interpretation of the response and making clinical decisions. When these three steps are carried out adequately and in a timely manner, the process can be efficient, benefiting patients and reducing costs for the healthcare system. Each step has its own challenges of knowledge, time, manpower, and sometimes, financial demand.

It has been widely recognized that communication among healthcare providers regarding consultation/referral can be time consuming, labor intense, and many times, futile. It is a major source of inefficiency and a quality issue in the healthcare system (Geist et al. 2008; O'Malley et al. 2011).

This section will focus on the knowledge part of the consultation-referral, addresses the importance of standardized-structured communications and indicates how these can greatly streamline the consultation/referral process.

Knowing what information to request or answer in the consultation/referral is the key to efficient communication. The information should be relevant and current, meaning problem-focused information and the current understanding of the disease and paradigm of management. This relevant information can be organized into a concise standardized/structured communication message (Geist et al. 2008).

Resources for standardized/structured communication messages are derived from standards of care and clinical practice guidelines in prevention, detection, evaluation and treatment of various diseases.

Many health organizations either regularly update their clinical practice guidelines or develop new guidelines for managing patients with various diseases. The Institute of Medicine defines guidelines as "systematically developed statements to assist practitioner and patient decisions about appropriate health care for specific clinical circumstances" (Field et al. 1990). Health care organizations also develop and update scientific statements, scientific advisories and position statements. These publications serve as tools to increase healthcare professionals' knowledge and awareness of effective, state-of-the art science related to the causes, prevention, detection or management of specific diseases, or to provide rapid, clear and consistent statements of the organization's position on scientific issues. Published periodically every 5–6 years, depending on the scientific evidence that has emerged, these publications reflect major paradigm shifts in the understanding of disease behavior and management.

The American Diabetes Association (ADA) publishes their clinical practice guidelines as clinical practice recommendations, which consist of position statements on various topics related to diabetes. These statements are reviewed annually and updated as needed. *Standards of Medical Care in Diabetes* is one of these position statements and is published every January (American Diabetes Association 2011). The American Heart Association publishes guidelines on various topics on cardiovascular diseases such as prevention of endocarditis (Wilson et al. 2007), myocardial infarction management (ACC/AHA 2008) and many others.

These clinical practice guidelines or scientific statements, being current, evidence-based, widely recognized and deeply influential, not only provide assistance in clinical decision making. They also establish the parameters of interdisciplinary conversation and have a major impact on consultation concerns and consultant responses. In essence, they provide the common ground for communication and the structure of the consultation questions.

By compliance with standards of care or clinical practice guidelines, many interdisciplinary communications can be brief and to the point to avoid redundancy and confusion.

An example would be the primary care provider (in this case a dentist) requesting a specialist (in this case a cardiologist) to provide a pre- surgical cardiovascular risk assessment for a patient who reported history of heart attack 3 months ago. Communication can be standardized and structured by following the current ACC/AHA 2007 Guidelines on Perioperative Cardiovascular Evaluation and Care for Noncardiac Surgery (Fleischer et al. 2007). These current guidelines provide an algorithm to direct the clinician to reach a clinical decision. The dentist needs to request verification of the date of the heart attack, the extent of the infarct as well as residual LV function, and the severity of coronary artery disease. Once this information is obtained from the cardiologist, the dentist should be able to reach a clinical decision on when and how to provide dental care by using the algorithm (see Fig. 2.13).

Routinely requesting a formal pre-surgical cardiovascular risk assessment can cause unnecessary delay and cost of healthcare resource.

2.4.1 Other Examples of Clinical Practice Guidelines That Influence Interdisciplinary Consultations

2.4.1.1 Hypertension

Hypertension is one of the most ancient diseases and is a major global health issue. The history of hypertension has shown that in the 1930s (Moser 2006), high blood pressure was considered a natural process and should be left alone. In the 1940s, hypertension was diagnosed only when blood pressure was greater than 180/110. Until the 1950s, elevated blood pressure was still considered necessary for the adequate perfusion of vital organs. Over the next half-century, the definition, prevention, diagnosis and treatment of hypertension have gone through tremendous changes. The changes in concepts and management are well reflected in the national guidelines: the Joint National Committee on Prevention, Detection, Evaluation and Treatment of High Blood Pressure (JNC) Reports. These reports are published as clinical practice guidelines by a committee that is sponsored by the National Heart, Lung and Blood Institute (NHLBI), a branch of the National Institutes of Health of the US Department of Health and Human Services. From the first JNC report in 1976 to the current 7th JNC report published in 2003

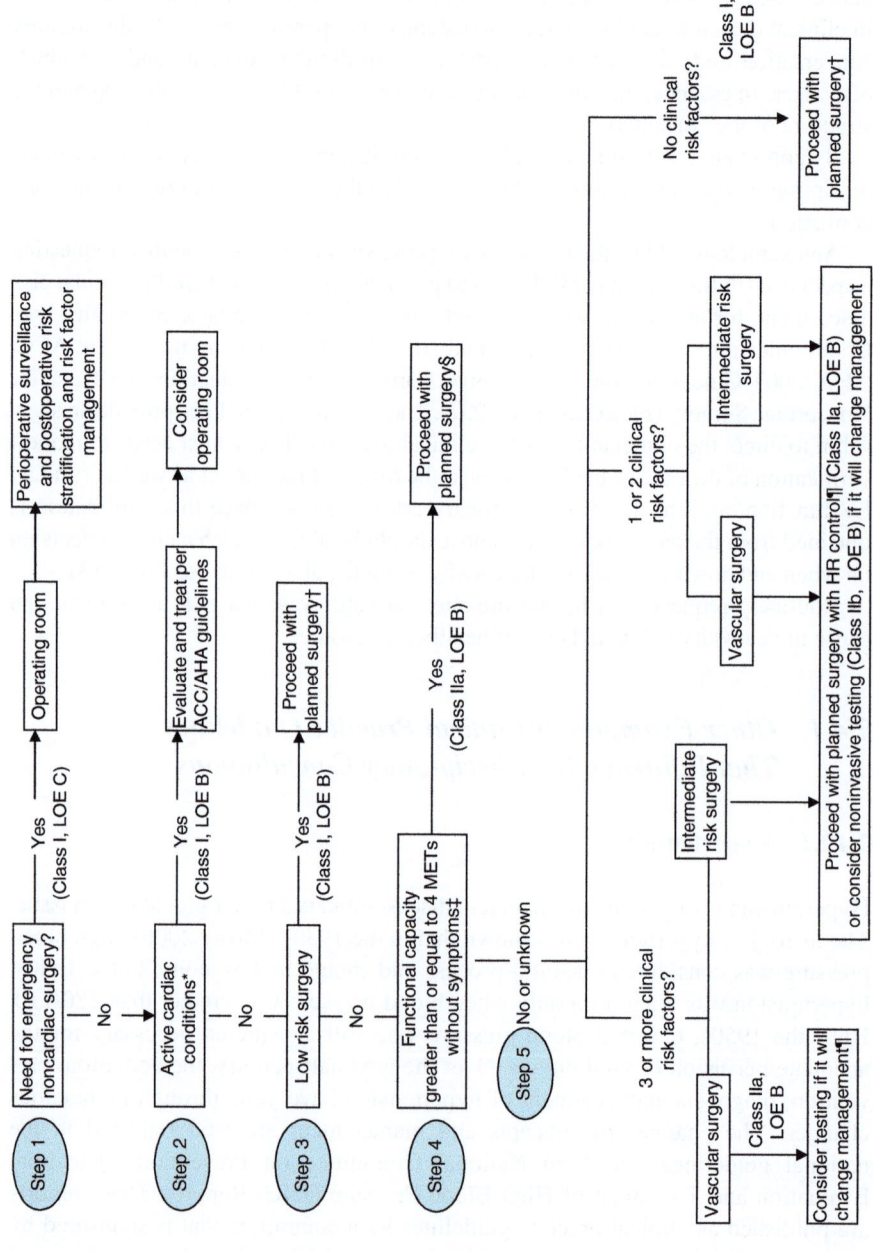

(Lenfant 2003), committees have been formed every 4–6 years to issue new sets of guidelines. They update the management of hypertensive patients based on the scientific understanding of the physiology, epidemiology, pathology and availability of pharmaceutical therapeutic agents. The guidelines guide physicians, other health care providers, patients and the public on new definitions, classifications, treatment rationales and options, and management of hypertension and its complications. In the first JNC report, no specific action was recommended unless the diastolic pressure was ≥105 mmHg. There were no recommendations for the staging of hypertension based on systolic pressure. There were fewer than 30 drugs available to treat hypertension at that time. In the 7th JNC report (Lenfant 2003), normal blood pressure for adults 18 years and older was defined as <120/80 mmHg. Prehypertension was defined for individuals whose blood pressure falls between 120/80 and 140/90 mmHg. Individuals with prehypertension who also have diabetes or kidney disease should be considered candidates for appropriate drug therapy if a trial of lifestyle modification fails to reduce their BP to 130/80 mmHg or less. JNC seven suggests that all people with hypertension (BP ≥140/90 mmHg) be treated. The treatment goal for individuals with hypertension and no other compelling conditions is <140/90 mmHg. Based on recent evidence, the 7th JNC emphasizes the importance of systolic blood pressure as a major risk factor for CVDs. There were more than 100 antihypertension drugs available at the time of publication of the 7th report of JNC.

All these changes have had a major impact on interdisciplinary communication. Dentists know when to refer patients for hypertension evaluation and treatment. Dentists also know how to manage dental patients with hypertension without sending unwarranted consultations to request permission from physicians to treat dental patients who have hypertension.

2.4.1.2 Heart Murmurs and Antibiotic Prophylaxis for Prevention of Infective Endocarditis

Heart murmurs are abnormal sounds either heard during the heart cycle, by stethoscope or detected on an echocardiogram. A heart murmur may have no pathological significance or may be an important clue to the presence of valvular or other structural heart abnormalities. A murmur that has no pathological significance is often referred to as an innocent, functional or physiologic murmur. Innocent murmurs are

---

Fig. 2.13 Cardiac evaluation and care algorithm for noncardiac surgery based on active clinical conditions, known cardiovascular disease or cardiac risk factors for patients 50 years of age or greater (Fleisher et al. 2007). (Reprinted with permission Circulation. 2007;116:e418–e500 ©2007 American Heart Association, Inc.)

Fig. 2.14 Cardiac conditions associated with the highest risk of adverse outcome from endocarditis for which prophylaxis with dental procedures is reasonable (Wilson et al. 2007)

Prosthetic cardiac valve or prosthetic material used for cardiac valve repair
Previous IE
Congenital heart disease (CHD)*
Unrepaired cyanotic CHD, including palliative shunts and conduits
Completely repaired congenital heart defect with prosthetic material or device, whether placed by surgery or by catheter intervention, during the first 6 months after the procedure†
Repaired CHD with residual defects at the site or adjacent to the site of a prosthetic patch or prosthetic device (which inhibit endothelialization)
Cardiac transplantation recipients who develop cardiac valvulopathy

*Except for the conditions listed above, antibiotic prophylaxis is no longer recommended for any other form of CHD.
†Prophylaxis is reasonable because endothelialization of prosthetic material occurs within 6 months after the procedure.

common in children and are quite harmless. Other causes of innocent heart murmur are pregnancy, fever, thyrotoxicosis (a condition resulting from an overactive thyroid gland) or anemia.

2.4.1.3 Pathologic Heart Murmurs (Organic Heart Murmurs) that Are Caused by a Variety of Valvular Defects

Prior to the current American Heart Association (AHA) guidelines regarding the prevention of infective endocarditis (IE), an organic heart murmur had great clinical significance. This was because previous AHA guidelines on antibiotic prophylaxis (AP) for IE prevention recommended AP for many heart conditions; the list was long and complex. An organic heart murmur was often used as a surrogate marker to identify conditions for which AP was recommended because almost all heart conditions recommended previously for AP were associated with an organic (pathologic) heart murmur. An organic heart murmur thus had great clinical significance (Dajani et al. 1997; Bonow et al. 2006). When a patient reported a heart murmur without further information regarding its nature (organic or innocent), its clinical significance was somewhat ambiguous. Clarification of the nature of the heart murmur was a major reason for medical consultations and contributed to inefficiencies in health care (Geist et al. 2008; Lessard et al. 2005).

The AHA 2007 guidelines on AP for (IE) prevention (Wilson et al. 2007) excluded many of the conditions associated with organic heart murmur from the list of conditions that are reasonable for AP, such as aortic stenosis and mitral valve prolapse (MVP) with regurgitation and about a dozen other heart conditions. The new guidelines defined a clear and short list of heart conditions for which AP is reasonable, thus making the pursuit of the nature of a heart murmur an insignificant clinical issue in this aspect (Fig. 2.14).

- Prosthetic cardiac valve or prosthetic material used for cardiac valve repair
- Previous IE

- Congenital heart disease (CHD)[12]
  - Unrepaired cyanotic CHD, including palliative shunts and conduits
  - Completely repaired congenital heart defect with prosthetic material or device, whether placed by surgery or by catheter intervention, during the first 6 months after the procedure[13]
  - Repaired CHD with residual defects at the site or adjacent to the site of a prosthetic patch or prosthetic device (which inhibit endothelialization)
- Cardiac transplantation recipients who develop cardiac valvulopathy

With these changes, the reasons for and requested information in consultations have drastically reduced and the increased clarity has improved the efficiency in communication. Dentists simply need to confirm with cardiologists if their patients have any of the heart conditions associated with the highest risk of adverse outcome from endocarditis for which prophylaxis with dental procedures is reasonable. (See Appendix A for a standard/structured consultation form)

2.4.1.4 Diabetes

The American Diabetes Association (ADA) publishes standards of medical care in *Diabetes* every January. The standards contain current treatment and possible complications, and therefore serve as tools for risk and benefit assessment for all health care providers who manage patients with diabetes (American Diabetes Association 2011).

The ADA's clinical recommendations are closely linked to other major diabetes care organizations such as World Health Organization (WHO) and the International Diabetes Federation (IDF). These recommendations provide a standardized message, such as patient's target A1c level and risk for hypoglycemia, microvascular and macrovascular complications risk and management, insulin-resistance-risk-control and many other diabetes issues. When an oral healthcare provider consults with a physician regarding dental care for a patient who has diabetes, questions of current A1c level and A1c target should be routinely asked.

2.4.1.5 Coronary Artery Stent

Coronary angioplasty, also called percutaneous coronary intervention (PCI), is a procedure designed to open clogged coronary heart arteries. More than 70% of the PCI include the placement of stent(s) in the artery to prop it open. In 2006, there were 652,000 PCI procedures with stents, of which approximately 76% were drug-eluting stents and 24% bare-metal stents. Individuals with coronary stent(s) are recommended to take dual antiplatelet therapy: thienopyridines (clopidogrel or

---

[12]Except for the conditions listed above, antibiotic prophylaxis is no longer recommended for any other form of CHD.

[13]Prophylaxis is reasonable because endothelialization of prosthetic material occurs within 6 months after the procedure.

ticlopidine) in combination with aspirin to reduce the incidence of major adverse cardiac events and stent thrombosis.

In 2007, the American Heart Association, American College of Cardiology, Society for Cardiovascular Angiography and Interventions, American College of Surgeons, and American Dental Association jointly published a Science Advisory: Prevention of Premature Discontinuation of Dual Antiplatelet Therapy in Patients with Coronary Artery Stents (Grines et al. 2007). It is recommended that individuals with bare-metal stents should stay on the dual antiplatelet therapy for 3 months, individuals with drug-eluting stents for 12 months. There should be coordination of care between the patient's cardiologist and other healthcare providers who perform invasive or surgical procedures and are concerned about perioperative and postoperative bleeding. These healthcare providers must be made aware of the potentially catastrophic risk of premature discontinuation of thienopyridine therapy. Dental practitioners are strongly discouraged from manipulating patients' antiplatelet therapy. The advisory stated that there is little or no indication for interruption of antiplatelet drugs for dental procedures. When concerned about prolonged bleeding during or after invasive dental procedures, dental practitioners should either postpone the procedure or consider using local hemostasis measures. The same issue was also addressed in the American College of Chest Physicians practice guidelines on the perioperative management of antithrombotic therapy (Douketis et al. 2008).

These advisory and current guidelines provide relevant information for dental practitioners before even initiating the consultation to ask about discontinuance or alteration of the antiplatelet regimen.

2.4.1.6 Chronic Kidney Disease

Prior to 2002, different terms were used to describe chronic kidney disease: diminished renal reserve, renal insufficiency, renal failure and end-stage renal disease (ESRD). Severity of kidney malfunction was measured with abstract criteria such as percentage of nephrons' function loss. These non-specific terms and vague disease stage criteria made interdisciplinary and even intradisciplinary communication difficult, with negative consequences to patients' care.

In 2002 The National Kidney Foundation's (NKF-USA) Kidney Disease Outcomes Quality Initiative (KDOQI) published a guideline on chronic kidney disease (CKD), in which a new definition of chronic kidney malfunction and criteria for staging the severity of the malfunction were introduced (Kidney Disease Outcome Quality Initiative, 2002). The term Chronic Kidney Disease (CKD) was proposed for a spectrum of function loss based on the level of glomerular filtration rate (GFR). In 2005, KDIGO (Kidney Disease: Improving Global Outcomes), an independent non-profit organization under the administration of NKF, endorsed this definition and staging system (Levey et al. 2005). From that point on, global communication regarding chronic kidney disease was improved. Nevertheless, the definition and staging system are not perfect; while they have attained global acceptance, there are also controversies. The main concern was the over- and misdiagnosis of CKD and possible overuse of specialty resources. The position KDOQI and KDIGO is that current definition/staging of CKD is simple and easy to apply (Eckardt et al. 2009). It raises awareness of CKD and improves the prognosis, in the long run benefiting patients and reducing the costs of the healthcare system. In response to these controversies, KDIGO has convened a workgroup to develop global clinical practice guidelines for the definition, classification/staging and prognosis of CKD. The consensus has been reached to keep the current definition for CKD with the addition of clinical diagnosis and albuminuria staging, to modify the classification system (Levey et al. 2010). The future guidelines will facilitate improved interdisciplinary communication even more.

2.4.1.7 Renal Dialysis

Individuals undergoing long-term renal dialysis (hemodialysis (HD)) have a dialysis access which can be an arteriovenous (AV) fistula or a synthetic graft. Patients undergoing renal dialysis (peritoneal dialysis (PD)) have a PD catheter dialysis access. The access serves as a life line to the patient because it provides access for blood going through the dialysis machine and returning to the body. Infection of the access can be a serious complication; emergent access must be made and new long-term access has to be made. Due to the invalid focal infection theory, patients with hemodialysis access had been given antibiotic prophylaxis for any invasive medical or dental procedure causing transient bacteremia to prevent access infection. New evidence indicates that the majority of hemodialysis access infections are most often caused by staphylococci, Gram-negative bacteria, or other microorganisms in association with surgery when the access was placed, or resulting from wound or other active infections. There is no convincing evidence that microorganisms associated with transient bacteremia from dental procedures cause infection of these access. In 2003, the AHA published a scientific statement on nonvalvular cardiovascular device-related infections. The statement does not recommend antibiotic prophylaxis after HD access placement for patients who undergo routine dental, respiratory, gastrointestinal, or genitourologic procedures causing transient bacteremia. Prophylaxis is only recommended for patients when they undergo incision and drainage of infection at other sites or replacement of a hemodialysis access (Baddour et al. 2003).

2.4.2 Permanent Pacemaker and Implantable Cardioverter-Defibrillator (Cardiovascular Implantable Electronic Device)

Because of the focal infection theory, patients with pacemakers and implanted defibrillators had been given antibiotic prophylaxis for any invasive medical or dental procedure causing transient bacteremia to prevent infection of the devices. According to the AHA's 2003 statement on nonvalvular cardiovascular device-related infections, individuals with pacemakers and defibrillators only need antibiotic prophylaxis when undergoing incision and drainage of an abscess or replacement of pacemaker or defibrillator (Baddour et al. 2003). Based on new evidence, in 2010 the American Heart Association published a scientific statement to update guidelines on permanent pacemaker (PPM) and implantable cardioverter-defibrillator

(ICD) infections and their management. The statement does not recommend antibiotic prophylaxis for dental or other invasive procedures not directly related to device manipulation to prevent CIED infection (Baddour et al. 2010).

2.4.3 Patients Who Are Taking Oral Anticoagulants

Warfarin is a synthetic vitamin K antagonist. It has been used as an oral anticoagulant since the 1950s for the primary and secondary prevention of venous thromboembolism, for the prevention of systemic embolism in patients with prosthetic heart valves or atrial fibrillation, for the primary prevention of acute myocardial infarction in high-risk individuals, for the prevention of stroke, recurrent infarction or death in patients with acute myocardial infarction. Although Warfarin is effective, this medication is both challenging to clinicians and patients. The anticoagulation status of the patient must be closely monitored by a laboratory test – the international normalized ratio (INR) – to keep the patient in a narrow therapeutic range without causing a bleeding problem. Many kinds of food are rich in vitamin K; consumption of too much vitamin K-rich food will cancel the antocoagulant effect of Warfarin. Patients on Warfarin must follow dietary instructions. Many medications also interact with Warfarin. Many clinicians, including dentists who provide surgical procedures to patients taking this medication, often face the dilemma of continuing or discontinuing warfarin therapy or adjusting the dosage for fear of prolonged bleeding after surgery. These issues were addressed in the American College of Chest Physicians' Evidence-Based Clinical Practice Guidelines (8th Edition) in the Perioperative Management of Antithrombotic Therapy section (Douketis et al. 2008). The guideline developers recommend continuance of Warfarin therapy around the time of dental procedures and co-adminstration of an oral prohemostatic agent to control local bleeding.

Dabigatran is an alternative to Warfarin. It provides an anticoagulant effect similar to warfarin but does not need INR monitoring. Dabigatran is a direct thrombin inhibitor and is not a vitamin K antagonist. Dabigatran has been approved for use in Europe, Britain, and Canada since 2008 to prevent blot coagulation. In October 2010, the drug was approved by the U.S. Food and Drug Administration for prevention of stroke in patients with non-valvular atrial fibrillation. Its use is recommended by the American College of Cardiology Foundation/American Heart Association as a Class I recommendation (Wann et al. 2011).

2.4.4 Patients Who Are Taking Antiplatelets

Consultation requests to physicians asking if a patient's antiplatelet regimen should be altered for dental surgery is one of the unwarranted reasons for consultation (Geist et al. 2008), and are often done because of fear of post operative bleeding. However, stopping a patient's antiplatelet therapy can carry a risk for fatal thrombosis. This issue was addressed in the section of coronary artery stents.

2.4.5 Bleeding Time (BT) and Platelet Function Assay-100 (PFA-100)

In assessing perioperative excessive bleeding, clinicians often request BT or PFA-100. The College of American Pathologists (CAP) and the American Society of Clinical Pathologists (ASCP) published a position statement in 1998 stating that BT cannot reliably identify individuals who have recently ingested aspirin or who have a drug-induced platelet defect. It concluded, "in the absence of a bleeding history, BT does not predict the risk of bleeding associated with surgery" (Peterson et al. 1998). Currently, no laboratory tests are predictive of surgical bleeding in patients taking antiplatelets.

PFA-100 is a sensitive test for drug effects; however, its value in prediction of surgical bleeding is not established. Patient history is the most cost-effective screening tool in predicting surgical bleeding.

The current American College of Chest Physicians Evidence-Based Clinical Practice Guidelines on the Perioperative Management of Antithrombotic Therapy recommend against the routine use of platelet function assays to monitor the antithrombotic effect of aspirin or clopidogrel in patients who are receiving antiplatelet drugs (Douketis et al. 2008).

In summary, the evidence-based clinical practice guidelines, scientific statements, advisory statements and position statements from various specialty organizations provide parameters for interdisciplinary communication.

2.4.6 Cancer Patient Management

National Cancer Institute of the U.S. Institutes of Health has developed and maintains a comprehensive online database of the most current, credible, and accurate information regarding cancer patient management. This database is also called Physician Data Query (PDQ). The PDQ contains peer-reviewed summaries on cancer treatment, screening, prevention, genetics, complementary and alternative medicine and supportive care. It also includes a registry of cancer clinical trials from around the world, and directories of physicians, professionals who provide genetics services, and organizations that provide cancer care. The PDQ is provided in professional and patient versions to facilitate communication among healthcare providers and between patients and their care providers (National Cancer Institute 2010).

Oral complications of chemotherapy and head/neck radiation can be quite significant. The PDQ contains the current standard information for head and neck radiation therapy, including dosage, delivery methods, prevention and management of oral mucositis, infections, taste alterations, salivary dysfunction, dental decay, truisms and risk levels of osteoradionecrosis. It also addresses prevention and management of the oral complications of various cancers and hematopoietic stem cell transplantation (National Cancer Institute 2011).

These information resources will serve as a risk/benefit assessment tool and will provide common language for communication.

2.4.7 Limitations of Structured Communication

Today, it is every healthcare provider's responsibility to update his/her knowledge in practice guidelines in order to practice team-based care. Communication is a dynamic process, and the content of the communication varies as the disease pattern changes and treatment advances. The strength of standard/structured communication can sometimes become a limitation to a clinician who is not abreast with current knowledge. A standard/structured consultation form may need to be updated often and may restrict free information flow.

However, limitations always can be overcome by continuing education that is designed to bring all parties of healthcare providers up to date. Various medical healthcare specialist organizations and oral healthcare organizations should work together to share each other's expertise and advocacy so patients will benefit from integrated and coordinated health services. The health system will benefit from cost reduction with collaboration in care and unwarranted consultations and laboratory tests.

Adaptation of an electronic health record system will reduce the administrative burden of time and the tasks of generating new consultation forms and transmitting consultation requests and responses.

2.5 Designing and Implementing Efficient Structured Communication Among a Patient's Medical and Dental Providers

Shin-Mey Rose Yin Geist

For efficiency of information sharing, confidentiality of patient information, record keeping and legal purposes, interdisciplinary communication takes the form of consultation and referral so that it can be well documented and easy to retrieve. The process of consultation/referral involves request, response and interpretation to reach a clinical decision. Each step of the process has its challenges. The biggest one is the content of the request and response. Once the content of the consultation/referral form is standardized by applying knowledge of current clinical practice guidelines and/or scientific statements, the requests and responses can be organized into a concise and structured communication message to improve the quality of the consultation/referral and consequently the efficiency of patient care (Geist et al. 2008).

Principles of designing efficient structured communication among a patient's medical and dental providers consist of:

- *Request Forms*: Designing a straightforward request form with standard questions based on current standards of care or clinical practice guidelines, and
- *Answer Lists*: Providing a standard answer list in the response for the consultant to check.

Fig. 2.15 Oncology consult form for cancer patient regarding part or future bisphosphonate therapy

Referral:
Mr. / Ms. _____ will need chemotherapy / radiation therapy for _____ cancer. Please assess his / her dental needs and prepare his / her oral cavity for the therapy to minimize the discomfort and the risk for oral infection and other complications during and after the therapy.

Chemotherapy / radiation therapy will be initiated on _____, 20 _____
Chemotherapy agent(s) include:
_____

The areas of the radiation will be
_____

The total radiation dosage will be
_____

The radiation delivery mechanism will be
_____

For example, a primary care provider (in this case a dentist) requests a specialist (in this case a cardiologist) to provide information for cardiovascular risk assessment for a patient with a reported history of myocardial infarction (MI) who needs two teeth extracted under local anesthesia. Instead of asking the cardiologist about the patient's risk from dental treatment, the oral healthcare provider should ask specific questions regarding the date, extent, and treatment for the MI, and outcome of that treatment; in other words, the patient's current cardiac status. Once the information is received, the oral healthcare provider will plug the information into the algorithm provided in the ACC/AHA 2007 guidelines on perioperative cardiovascular evaluation, care for noncardiac surgery (Fleisher et al. 2007), and take necessary precautions for indicated treatment.

For a dental patient who is reported to have diabetes mellitus, oral healthcare providers should issue a standardized/structured consultation requesting the most recent HbA1c level and glycemic control target; see the consultation form Appendix A.

When an oral healthcare provider considers giving a dental patient antibiotic prophylaxis (AP) to prevent infective endocarditis (IE), he or she should provide the cardiologist with a list of heart conditions for which AP is reasonable. This should take the form of a checklist which should be clear, concise and efficient. The list of conditions is based on the American Heart Association's 2007 evidence-based practice guidelines on IE prevention (Wilson et al. 2007) and is a well recognized as common ground for communication. See the consultation form Appendix B.

When a consultation is to be sent to a cancer patient's oncologist, it can be designed as follows (Fig. 2.15):

On the other hand, when an oncologist refers a cancer patient to an oral healthcare provider to prepare the oral cavity for radiation therapy or chemotherapy, the same strategy can be used to design the referral as follows (Fig. 2.16):

When a hemophilia patient or patients with other bleeding disorders need dental care, the hematologist can refer patient to an oral healthcare provider by offering preparation of patient to coordinate the dental care, or the oral healthcare provider

Request:	from Dental Provider:	Date:

Mr./Ms. _____ reports a history of _____ cancer. Comprehensive oral examination reveals that he/she has a dental diagnosis of _____ and needs _____ treatment. Please provide the following information to facilitate the dental treatment of Mr./Ms. _____

Response:	from Medical Provider:	Date:

Current cancer status of Mr./Ms. _____
Was Mr./Ms. _____ given IV bisphosphonates? YES ____ NO ____
Is Mr./Ms. _____ currently taking IV bisphosphonate? YES ____ NO ____
Is IV bisphosphonate therapy planned for the future? YES ____ NO ____

Fig. 2.16 Oral health referral form for cancer patient needing chemotherapy or radiation therapy

can request the hematologist to prepare the patient for the dental care. This is an example of mutual respect of each other's expertise and collaboration to improve the efficiency of patient care.

When there are no clear clinical practice guidelines to follow, and there is a conflict in opinion regarding treatment, a clear statement should be made either in the request or in the response. For example, currently there are controversies regarding antibiotic prophylaxis (AP) for dental treatment of patients with artificial joints. The purpose of the consultation in this case is to inform the orthopedic surgeon that since there is no clear evidence indicating a benefit from this practice the oral healthcare provider would leave the decision regarding AP to the orthopedic surgeon. If the surgeon believes that it would be beneficial to the patient then he or she should prescribe the antibiotics of choice and take the responsibility for administering the medication. See the Appendix A for an example consultation.

2.5.1 Transmission Methods

How to transmit and receive standardized/structured consultation or referral in a timely fashion is another challenge. In designing an efficient way to meet this challenge, one must examine the pitfalls of the traditional consultation and referral transmission mechanism.

2.5.2 Illegibility

Traditional consultation letters are written on blank forms, with the dentist's or physician's often illegible writing. See Appendix D. This can be a major barrier to communication among healthcare workers. See Appendix E for a barely legible consultation request. This problem would be prevented by key-in electronic communications.

2.5.3 Demands on Time and Manpower

The traditional paper-based handwritten consultation is a time consuming and labor intense process. The patient usually carries it to the physician and brings it back to the oral healthcare provider. Sometimes it is mailed to the patient or the physician and returned by mail. It is paper forms are often lost during the process. In recent years, many hospitals and clinics have adapted electronic health record systems (EHR). Consultation requests are transmitted to the consultants through facsimile then scanned and stored in the EHR, and the returned responses are received and stored in the same manner. This has shortened the transmission time and improved record keeping, but it demands extra manpower to track the facsimile and do the scanning. A recent study has shown that nurse care managers or non-physician staff members contribute positively in the process of communication (O'Malley et al. 2011). However, there are times when the consultation requests can only be answered by physicians, such as when comments on laboratory results or treatment decisions are required. In such cases, the nurses care manager or non-physician staff must track down the physician for the response, which is not always easy to accomplish in a timely manner.

2.5.4 Implementation Through Health Information Technology (HIT)

Today, electronic health records (EHRs) are common in medical and dental practice. Although not all systems are compatible with each other by default or by choice to protect patient's confidentiality, each system has the capacity to electronically generate, transmit and store the standardized/structured consultation/referral.

Some major healthcare corporations have already yielded positive results in electronic consultation/referral because their systems are used by large numbers of participants of primary care providers and specialists (Chen et al. 2011; Stoves et al. 2010). This may not be feasible for small, individual practices. One easy solution: an electronically generated consultation request can be sent through email to a consultant, who can directly answer and return the request form electronically. The consultation can then be stored in the patient's electronic health record. This direct communication between the primary care health care provider and specialist eliminates the need to involve additional personnel who can delay a response and leads to the possible breach of confidentiality.

In conclusion, although the time has not yet arrived for all healthcare providers to have universal access to their patients' medical and dental electronic records, HIT can definitely improve the efficiency of the consultation/referral process and consequently the patient care.

2.6 Matching Patients to Achieve Unique Patient Identification

Monica Chaudhari

The medical and dental insurances and care systems that have evolved separately with little integration are now exploring a joint outcomes assessment approach to confirm and quantify the link between systemic and oral by measuring the two-way impact on clinical, economic, and humanistic outcomes, such as patient health-related quality of life.

One such joint outcomes research was conducted using the linked data from both Washington Dental Service (WDS) and Group Health Cooperative (GH). WDS is a founding member of the Delta Dental Plans Association delivering dental care to more than two million people through employer-sponsored programs. GH is a nonprofit health care system that coordinates care and coverage to more than half a million residents of Washington state and Idaho. Secondary enrollment data from WDS and GH, clinical (laboratory, pharmacy and diagnosis) data from GH and claims data from WDS were used on enrollees continuously and dually insured between 2002 and 2006.

The inception of this research project pivoted on a strategy devised to identify the same subjects between WDS and GH, i.e. to uniquely identify individuals. This strategy has been discussed at length by Theis et al. (2010). The ability to successfully match individuals' records in non-related databases entailed identifying a number of overlapping variables with personal information, their information richness and the accuracy with which they are recorded in individual databases. Generally, the challenge in uniquely matching a patient across different databases is that across healthcare entities, data standards may differ, personal identifiers may be coded differently and data update and retention rules may be applied differently. Incorrectly specified information from keying-in-errors may add to these challenges resulting in higher non-match rates with larger datasets. On the other hand, too few overlapping variables may increase the likelihood of duplicate matches resulting in misclassification bias. (Blakely and Salmond 2002).

To optimize matching, two approaches, deterministic and probabilistic, are usually used for record linkage based on the reliability of the overlapping identifiers. While deterministic linkage requires exact match on one or more identifiers used iteratively to link and verify the linkage, probabilistic matching uses information from many variables and allows for disagreement by assigning weights to all possible record pairs. When reliable identifiers are available, deterministic approaches are usually preferred because they achieve acceptable results, are less cumbersome and require less development time than probabilistic matching. (Liu 1999; Gill et al. 1993; Roos and Wajda 1991) Because of the enormity of data with half a million subscribers to be matched, we conducted an initial test to assess the performance of deterministic linkage approach in a sub-sample.

We first explored the linkage utility of personal identifiers within respective databases by examining them for missing or invalid values and their consistency over time. The GH database was inspected for the time period 2004–2005. The variables in GH database with the greatest number of unique values, and thus potentially the most discriminating, were social security number (SSN), telephone number, last name, first name, and date of birth. However, significant year-to-year variability in telephone number, city and zip code made these variables less suitable for deterministic linkage.

The SSN, while collected, was not used as the principal personal identifier in either of the databases and was found missing for nearly 100% of dependents of the WDS subscribers. Unlike GH that retained a unique patient identifier for each individual across all enrollment-disenrollment cycles, a new unique identifier was assigned at WDS when an enrollee changed employer groups. This caused duplication of records with multiple identifiers for the same individual, also termed as 'weak warm body mapping'. This term is coined due to the implications it bears on tying (mapping) the histories of an individual (a warm body) that are captured by the system under different identifiers over different periods.

Figure 2.17 illustrates the differences between the GH and WDS approaches to coded patient identifiers within their respective systems.

- The figure is intended to reflect broadly the difference between the two systems and is not representative of the true processes (Fig. 2.17).

To avoid problems emanating from weak warm body mapping and the frequent absence of dependents' SSN, we inspected WDS records for subscribers and dependents separately for the entire study period 2002–2006. The issue of weak warm body mapping was resolved by ensuring existence of a unique identifier within WDS database for both dependants and subscribers on a combination of personal identifiers like subscribers' member-id (most of the times, it was subscribers' SSN also shared by their dependents), last name, first name and birth date.

All subscribers had unique SSN but there were few who had more than one SSN on the unique combination of last name, first name and birth date if it was not missing or on the combination of last name and first name if birth date was missing. Such subscribers were not included in the study. We also made sure that all the subscribers included in the study had a single unique identifier in the database on the above combination. The dependents of only the selected subscribers who had single unique identifier in the database for the combination of their first name, last name and subscriber's member-id were included in the study. This ensured reliable traceability of their dental history and benefits within WDS database. See Fig. 2.18 for the decision flow used to manage the weak warm body mapping.

To test our confidence in the four linkage variables, SSN, last name, first name and birth date, we then performed four deterministic linkages with four employer groups dually insured by GH and WDS, restricting to adults born between January 1, 1932, and December 31, 1961 and enrolled in 2004 or 2006. To improve matching precision, the Group Health and WDS datasets were then standardized by removing duplicates and names were cleaned (e.g. removing prefixes, suffices, punctuation). Subsequently, as shown in Table 2.11, the linkage showed 96% or higher exact matches of the minimum of the total unique identifiers from WDS and GH respectively with matches on just SSN, SSN + last name, SSN + birth date, last name + first name + birth date. This also suggested that insurance data are homogeneous; employer groups send identical administrative data to both dental and health care insurers.

Content with the high degree of matching on combinations of the four linkage variables, we finally developed the entire linked dataset for our research study,

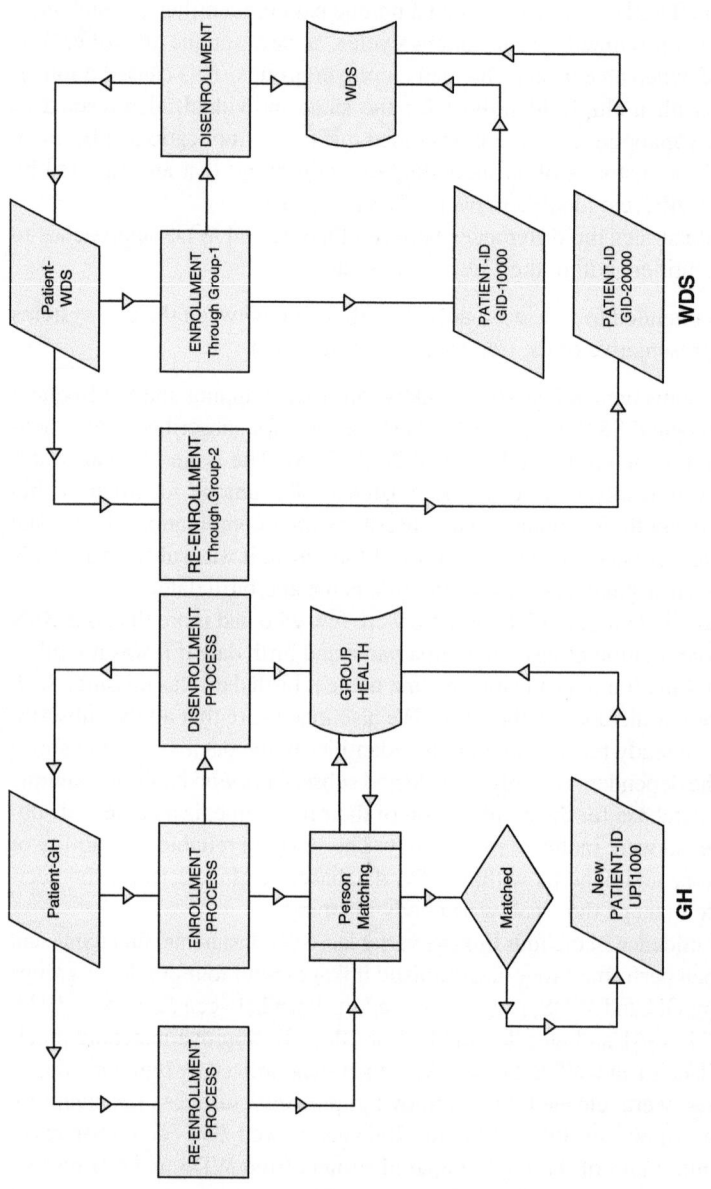

Fig. 2.17 GH and WDS approaches to coded patient identifiers

2 HIT Considerations: Informatics and Technology Needs and Considerations

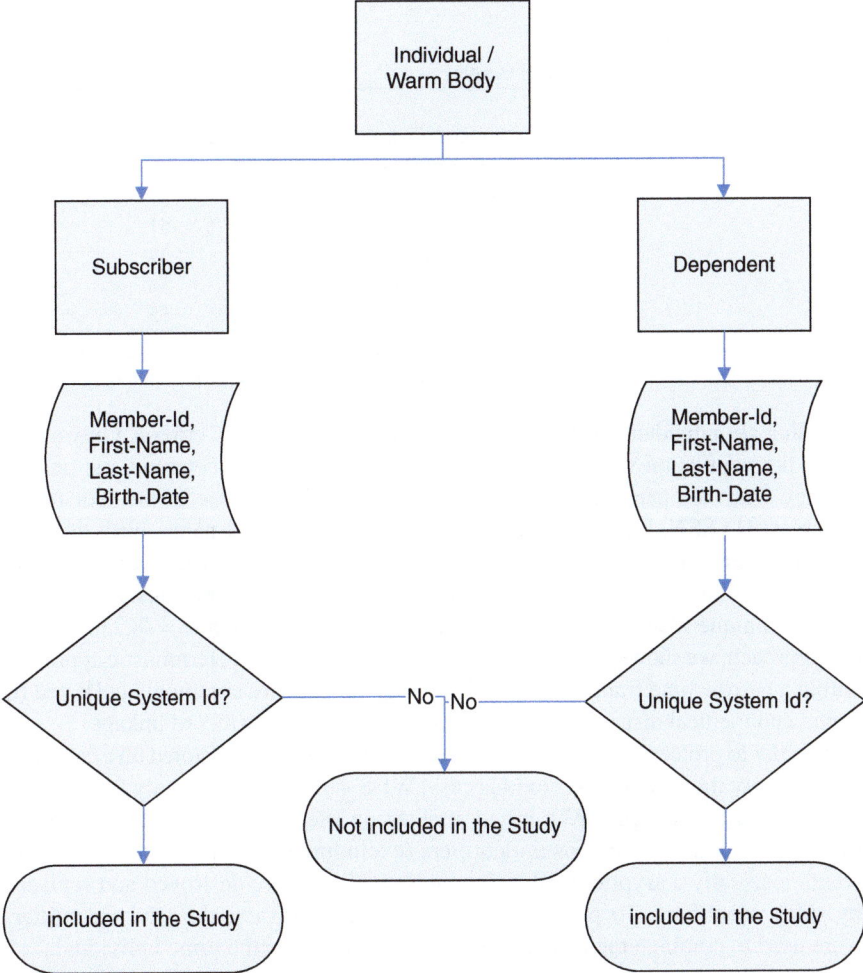

Fig. 2.18 Weak warm body decision flow

Table 2.11 Test match-merges of WDS data to four GH plans with known WDS dental coverage

Data elements examined	Number of unique matches (% agreement with WDS)
Social security number[a]	97.7
Social security number + last name[a]	96.9
Social security number + birth date[a]	97.3
Last name + first name + birth date[a]	96.0

[a]Duplicates on each of the four combinations were deleted from both datasets

Table 2.12 Linkage results of WDS data to GH data among persons aged 40–74 with 5-year continuous enrollment

Exact merge	% of individuals linked in agreement with GH
SSN	41
SSN + last name + first name + birth date	36
n – 1 deterministic merge	
SSN + last name + first name	37
Last name + first name + birth date	51
SSN + first name + birth date	37
SSN + last name + birth date	38
Total of the n – 1 deterministic merge	**55**

*Duplicate social security numbers, last names, first names or birth dates were deleted from each merge group in both datasets.

including all individuals from WDS and GH who met the study criteria. Only a subset of the population would be successfully linked. An $n-1$ deterministic linkage strategy was then performed on four sets of merges with three of the four merge variables: (1) SSN, last name, first name; (2) last name, first name, birth date; (3) SSN, first name, birth date; and (4) SSN, last name, birth date. We grouped the four $n-1$ deterministic merges into one dataset and removed all duplicates using Group Health's unique identifier to obtain our final linked population (n=78,230). Using this approach, we showed (Table 2.12) that a relatively simple deterministic approach, within a narrow time frame and with demographic variables commonly collected by dental and medical insurance carriers, results in high-quality record linkage.

In order to protect confidentiality, all personal identifiers were stored on a computer file that only the GH analyst could access. WDS sent SSNs separately from names and birth dates through a Web-based application (Secure File Transfer). Once the linkage was complete, personal identifiers (excluding the unique system identifier which is usually a cryptic number for each enrollee) were destroyed and replaced by study identifiers. To protect confidentiality and privacy, the study identifiers were used to combine medical and dental information on the same individuals.

Now that we had a validated method to identify uniquely the same individual across the GH and WDS databases, we were able to examine the actual joint outcomes research question, i.e. what is the nature and degree of association between periodontal disease and diabetes.

2.7 Improved Electronic Healthcare Technologies (EHT) Through the Harmonization of Application Design and Clinician Needs

Mureen Allen

2.7.1 Introduction

There is general excitement as the healthcare industry lumbers slowly but surely to full electronic integration of healthcare systems. In 2004, President Bush decreed that every American should have an electronic health record by 2014, since then the clock has been ticking. Many public-private collaborations since 2004 have been formed to accelerate the adoption and use of electronic health records. Until the funded mandate of the American Recovery and Reinvestment Act (ARRA) to adopt and use electronic health records the momentum of adoption by healthcare providers has been relatively slow.

The electronic health record (EHR) is only one component of what is essential for electronic integration. There are many other components essential for a fully integrated healthcare system including, but not limited to, laboratory information systems (LISs), medication management systems, registry systems, patient health records (PHRs), and biometric devices, etc., which collectively represent electronic health technologies (EHTs). It is imperative that attention be paid to these technologies to increase their acceptance and use by healthcare providers.

For many years the adoption of electronic health technologies, especially EHRs, has been woefully lacking. There are a number of factors that will drive the adoption and successful use of these technologies including, (1) whether they seamlessly integrate with the clinical workflow to support context-specific delivery of care, (2) their relative ease of use and (3) the completeness of the data. If EHTs support all three of these criteria then resistance to their adoption will decline precipitously.

2.7.2 Context-Specific Delivery of Information to Improve Care

At this point, you might be wondering why should the developers of EHTs pay attention to the clinical workflow or much less try to integrate seamlessly into the workflow. The answer is unmet information needs. There are a number of studies (Covdell et al. 1985) indicating that during healthcare encounters, providers often have information needs that go unmet. These needs exist even when healthcare providers interact with EHTs.(Allen et al. 2003) Healthcare providers typically rely on the information at hand (memory, reference textbooks, journals, and colleagues) to help make decisions about a specific aspect of a patient's care. The difficulty with relying on these is that memory can be faulty or limited, reference textbooks often do not contain the latest treatment protocols, journals are too numerous and too detailed, and colleagues are often unreliable. Clearly, a better method is needed. This is where EHTs can play an important role. EHTs are capable of providing the knowledge to support the provider in the decision-making process. EHTs should seamlessly supplement the information requirements of the health care provider in a timely, context-specific manner. In addition, EHTs should be capable of reusing data entered in the health record to drive context-specific care. To facilitate this capability EHTs need to take into account the clinical workflow, the ability to capture structured and codified data from all aspects of documentation and the ability to collate and reuse data once they are stored in the electronic record.

Information captured through structured, codified data facilitates the ability to deliver context-specific information at the point of care, including links to guidelines or protocols, clinical decision support, performance measurement, the measurement of individual patient and population management.

The factors essential for context-specific information retrieval are discussed below and an example of each is provided. For each of the examples the context is indicated by **bold** text and the resultant information and action based on the context is indicated by underline text:

(a) **Who requires the information**? EHTs should understand that information needs of users might vary. Within the clinical context the EHT should anticipate the needs of a medical student, resident, or specialist.

> **Example 1**
>
> Dr. Jones, an **oncologist**, is reviewing Mrs. Black's electronic medical record. Mrs. Black, a **40 year old female with leukemia, has failed standard treatment**. As he prepares to update the treatment section of her record, he sees an alert entitled treatment options. As he opens the alert, he sees a list of treatment studies, a list of published references about failed leukemia treatment and finally a number of experimental treatment protocols that are available for Mrs. Black, including a clinical trial for patients who have already received and failed standard therapy.
>
> Dr. Jones reviews the various recommended treatment options and determines the best options for Mrs. Black. On Mrs. Black's arrival Dr. Jones, review the treatment options with her.
>
> In this example, the doctor has access to a clinical decision support tool that tracts treatment protocols.

(b) **What does the user want**? Context-specific information needs will vary from one user to the next. A medical student might need information to help him learn a topic whereas a specialist might need cutting edge information to help manage a difficult patient. A nurse's needs might be different from that of a physician.

> **Example 2**
>
> Mr. Smith is a **50 year old diabetic**, who was just **admitted to the hospital** for **treatment of a leg ulcer**. **Nurse** White starts to review Mr. Smith's record, including the treatment sections, where she sees the clinical protocol for diabetic leg ulcers. There are a number of standing orders relevant to Mr. Smith care including wound cultures, blood tests etc.
>
> In this example, the nurse has access to an electronic clinical protocol, which will guide how she cares for the patient.

(c) **Who does the user need information about**? Health needs about individuals vary. The context-specific information needs about a 50 year old woman is different from that of a 20 year old woman. Specifically, context-specific needs will vary based on the socio-economic status, ethnicity, age, or gender of the patient.

> **Example 3**
> Dr. Jackson, **a dentist**, is meeting with **a new patient** Mr. Brown who **has diabetes, and hypertension**, both of which are **apparently well-controlled**. As Dr. Jackson reviews Mr. Brown's electronic record, she notices the clinical data available from his previous providers. She notices, based on his record, that Mr. Brown is overdue for a routine dental prophylaxis. In addition, Dr. Jackson notices that recently Mr. Brown's **blood glucose readings** on his home monitor are **higher than usual**. Dr. Jackson suspects, based on Mr. Brown's signs and symptoms that he has gingivitis, which she confirms on examination.
>
> In this example, the user has all the relevant information to make critical decisions relevant to the patient's condition.

(d) **Where is the user when he has the information needed**? The needs of the user in emergency room will differ from the user in the ambulatory center.

> **Example 4**
> Mrs. Anderson is in the **emergency room** complaining of **shortness of breath and mild indigestion. She is 45**, and **slightly overweight. The emergency room physician** taking care of her, pulls up her ambulatory healthcare record, he notes that apart from **mild heartburn and smoking** Mrs. Anderson has no other history. The ER physician enters his clinical findings into Mrs. Anderson's record and as he begins to enter her diagnosis, he reviews a list of potential diagnoses. As he reviews this list, he notices that one of the potential diagnoses is a heart attack. He quickly orders a blood test that confirms that Mrs. Anderson is having a heart problem and she is admitted. Afterwards, he reviews the recommendation and learns that women usually present with atypical symptoms when compared to men.
>
> In this example, the system takes into context the user and the location and determines the appropriate potential diagnoses.

To date, current systems are not capable of using context-specific information to drive workflow. However, developers and researchers are beginning to add intelligent electronic health technology incrementally.

2.7.3 Usability

The usability of an interface is of critical importance for the accurate use of any application. Healthcare technologies have their own specific set of usability issues. A good user interface (UI) enhances the users' experience. It is well known that user satisfaction with an application is often driven by the friendliness and intuitiveness of the UI. Measurable benefits that stem from a good UI include workflow efficiency and data accuracy. Logically, the effects of a bad UI are the opposite of the good UI, namely, user dissatisfaction, workflow inefficiency and data inaccuracies. Users typically will not interact with applications with non-intuitive interfaces.

A bad UI may even be dangerous. Poor usability has the potential to introduce a set of errors that affect the patient's health. Issues include selecting incorrect medications from a pick list, ordering the incorrect dose of a medication, etc. (Horsky et al. 2005; Koppel et al. 2005). Because of the possibility of a disastrous error caused by the UI, there is a need to study formally the user interface of EHTs to determine how they affect the clinical workflow and more importantly how they influence care. Ultimately, there is a need to develop standardized user interfaces that have been proven to mitigate the risk for errors attributable to the UI (Armijo et al. 2009).

> **Example 5**
> Dr. Bailey is a busy dentist. He pulls up his patient's electronic medical record, and notices that that his patient, James, is a 5 year old male, weighing 50 lbs. who is complaining of a toothache. After his examination Dr. Bailey concludes that James has an early dental infection and using his electronic prescribing system decides to prescribe Augmentin. As he enters the order, Dr. Bailey scrolls through the drop-down menu of all antibiotics including many variants of Augmentin. There is no context associated with the list of Augmentin so Dr. Bailey selects the first antibiotic on the list and sends the prescription electronically to the pharmacy. At the pharmacy, when James' mother goes to pick up the prescription the pharmacist is concerned. The pharmacist confirms that the prescription is for a child and calls the doctor's office. It seems that in his haste, Dr. Bailey selected the incorrect medication strength.
>
> In this example, the design of the user interface results in an error on the part of the user.

With EHTs, it is now possible to present a large volume of information all at the same time. This places an additional cognitive burden on the user to determine what is relevant or worse to ignore information that is irrelevant and potentially harmful. If EHTs are to be successful, they need to present information to the user in such a manner to minimize the cognitive burden on the user.

2 HIT Considerations: Informatics and Technology Needs and Considerations

> **Example 6**
>
> Dr. Hendricks examines Mrs. Boxer and diagnoses a dental abscess. Dr. Hendricks determines that he best course of action is to incision and drain the abscess. Prior to the procedure, he reviews Mrs. Boxer's electronic record and notes her list of active medical conditions and her history of mitral valve prolapse. He reviews the list of past medical conditions and determines that he can proceed with the procedure. Just prior to the incision and drainage, the patient, seeing the scalpel in Dr. Hendricks' hand tells the doctor that she developed a heart infection after a previous surgery. Dr. Hendricks stops and reviews every part of Mrs. Boxer's electronic record. After some time, Dr. Hendricks finds the relevant information in the medical summaries. The medical summary in question was in a folder buried in the electronic record with 20 other summaries and the contents were not indexed for search.
>
> In this example, the user is forced to review the entire document in the medical record to find the relevant information. There is not a simple method available to facilitate retrieval of all the relevant information.

The design of an EHT can contribute to user error. All information stored in an EHT should be indexed, catalogued and searchable. EHTs that require the user to search consistently and proactively all components of the EHT to find all relevant information will lead to potentially life-threatening errors. Obscure data buried within an EHT can lead to the user not having all the relevant information readily available. However, giving the user a simple method of searching all the content in the EHT ensures that he finds the relevant information.

Ultimately, usability is a critical component of EHTs. It is not sufficient, for healthcare providers to have technologies in their offices for documentation, it is imperative that these technologies take into consideration how healthcare providers process information, how they look for information. In addition, these technologies should have failsafe mechanisms to prevent errors of omission and commission.

To encourage the development of safe EHTs there needs to be a better understanding of the technologies, how these can lead to user errors and how such errors can be mitigated. There is a need for studies to identify the best practices with respect to the development of the user interface of EHTs. The results of these studies should be codified as recommendations and guidelines that all EHT are required to adhere to minimize the likelihood of errors.

2.7.4 The Totality of the Data

The success or failure of EHTs will depend on the totality of the data available to the healthcare provider. Clinical decisions are driven by the availability of data at the point of care. Data are generated each time a patient interacts with the healthcare system and even today, as we transition to EHTs, the data are still siloed and often not accessible across the healthcare system. For the healthcare system to be effective, data available electronically in one system should be available to other systems. The test result for a patient should be available to all of the treating healthcare providers (with the appropriate authority and consent) and not just the ordering physician. Essentially all available data should be accessible to the healthcare provider at the time of decision-making.

The aggregation of a patient's data from multiple disparate sources is crucial. Whether forming a centralized database or using a record locator system to find the patient records on distributed systems, it is critical that at the time the healthcare provider needs to make a decision about a patient, he can view all the data available for that patient.

Example 7
Mr. Brown pays a visit to Dr. Smith for the first time. He has a Personal Health Record which supports codified data. Before he arrived at the office, Mr. Brown was able to download a copy of his records and send a structured copy to the doctor's office so that the data can be imported into the Dr. Smith's medical record. In the office, Dr. Smith reviews and accepts the data from Mr. Brown's PHR. Based on this new information Dr. Smith receives an alert that shows deficits in Mr. Brown's care including persistent hypertension and elevated blood glucose. In addition, Dr. Brown sees a list of best practices for Mr. Smith many with which have been complied. For those measures and alerts that have not been complied with Dr. Smith has the ability to order the necessary tests and/or medications.

In this example, the completeness of the data from the PHR enabled Dr. Smith to provide very personalized care.

Example 8
Mrs. Jones is in the dentist's office for a toothache. As Dr. Roberts asks her about her medical history, Mrs. Jones knows that she has a low blood count but she cannot remember how low. Fortunately, Dr. Roberts has an electronic dental record, which is connected to a health information network that receives data from other healthcare providers, laboratories and pharmacies. As he does a quick check of her laboratory records, he realizes that she has a very low platelet count that could potentially lead to life-threatening bleeding if he attempts an invasive procedure in the office.

In this example, the critical piece of data was available only because the dentist had access to the medical lab tests from another provider.

2.8 Electronic Decision Support in Medicine and Dentistry

Miguel Humberto Torres-Urquidy

2.8.1 Medicine and Dentistry: Differences in Electronic Decision Support

One of the constant themes throughout this book is the idea that systemic health and oral health are connected and that despite the historical separation of the medicine and dentistry, both professions can benefit from increased use of health IT and informatics. In some cases, the designs and developments that influence medicine are equally applicable to dentistry, like enterprise master patient index. Unfortunately, electronic Clinical Decision Support (CDS) has developed differently for medicine and dentistry. In this chapter, we examine how this occurred, review some of the differences, speculate on why CDS is less robust in dentistry and explore ways to improve CDS in dentistry.

2.8.1.1 Historical Drivers of CDS Divergence

In the early days of health IT, computer technology was limited only to large medical institutions that could afford computer technology. The cost of the hardware, software, maintenance and support were distributed across a large number of providers, administrators, etc. In contrast, dentists usually worked in small solo or group practice and in isolation from other dentists. The same cost for health IT was born by a much smaller number of people. Thus, it is not surprising the dentists were unable incorporate computer technology early. The one dental institution that could afford Health IT was a Dental School. However, these entities saw little or no benefit in acquiring computer technology, nor did they have the manpower to develop such systems.

2.8.1.2 Clinical Drivers of CDS Divergence

CDS systems in medicine, especially in hospitals, thrive on the integration with the electronic patient record. The CDS process takes into consideration all the patient data already in the system and produces warning, alerts and other automatic analysis.
Some of the early seminal works on medical CDS include:

- Musen et al. (Shortliffe et al. 2001) described several classic examples CDS systems in medicine. Musen mentioned that although early prototypes were developed in the sixties, full fledged applications did not start appearing until a decade later.
- The Leeds Abdominal Pain System developed by F.T. deDombal, using Bayes theorem, was developed to help in the identification of acute abdominal pain

including appendicitis, diverticulitis, a perforated ulcer, etc. The Leeds system (Shortliffe et al. 2001), used sensitivity, specificity and disease prevalence data of signs and symptoms to calculate the probability of the possible explanations.
- In 1976, Shortliffe and colleagues developed MYCIN which focused on the management of patients with infection through the prescription of antibiotics. MYCIN used as knowledge a set of production rules commonly used in the field of Artificial Intelligence.
- Years later in 1985, a system devoted to the identification of possible diagnoses was developed by Randy Miller and colleagues at the University of Pittsburgh. They developed the Quick Medical Reference (QMR) (Bankowitz et al. 1989). QMR represented medical knowledge by using "disease profiles," which in turn were a synthesis of information collected "from review of the published literature and expert opinion. Disease profiles consisted of a list of all history, physical, and laboratory data reported to occur in the given disease." As well, each finding would have a sensitivity level and a positive predictive value.

Although these and other systems were not fully adopted, they provided the foundation under which current expert systems work in hospitals.

In dentistry, White (1996) and more recently Mendonça (2004) conducted a review of the state of CDS in dentistry which, like medical CDS, has been available for several years (Walker 1967). These systems can be found in subspecialties such as dental emergencies, orofacial pain, oral medicine, oral radiology, orthodontics, pulpal diagnosis and removable prosthodontics. Examples include:

- The Diagnostic Aid Resource Tool (DART) for oral medicine. This software contains a diagnostic module which through a "statistical data-base manager" retrieves diseases matching the possible patient diagnoses.
- ORAD (White 1989) provides decision support in the interpretation of radiographic lesions. ORAD requests information through 16 questions which then are analyzed using Bayesian methods. ORAD is capable of diagnosing up to 140 possible diseases and is currently available on the Internet.
- Invisalign provides decision support with orthodontic cephalometric analyses and treatment planning procedures (Melkos 2005). Currently it is possibly the most commonly used decision support system in dentistry.
- OralCDx (Sciubba 1999) assists in the identification of precancerous lesions using oral brush biopsies. OralCDx utilizes a neural network-based image processing system to detect oral epithelium cancerous or precancerous cells.
- Both Invisalign and OralCDx, provide decision support over the distance and operate more like a lab test than the traditional decision support.

In medicine, the driving force behind CDS has been the challenge of dealing with uncertainty when diagnosing disease and delivering treatment. The diagnostic space in medicine requires physicians to consider a large number of possibilities. Further, in medicine, diagnosis is a very important and distinct process. A diagnostic session includes the selection of diagnostic procedures followed by an interpretation of the results. Thus, the medical profession has invested more resources in creating tools that would assist in reducing uncertainty.

In dentistry decision making is intrinsically linked to the definition of a diagnosis-treatment complex. Uncertainty is not as strong a component of the diagnostic reasoning as in medicine. For example, the diagnosis of common dental problems (caries, missing teeth, periodontal problems) is a simple determination of present or not. Most of the diagnostic information usually is obtained at initial examination through direct observation or using immediate, at hand methodologies. Emphasis on treatment instead of diagnosis is enforced by the fact that dentists are not reimbursed for diagnoses. They are paid for treatment. Further, in order to obtain third party payments, a diagnosis is not a necessary element of the paperwork, only the treatment. Hence dentists are trained to focus more on treatment planning than on diagnosis in Dental School.

2.8.2 Why Electronic Decision Support Is Less Common in Dentistry than in Medicine?

There are several reasons why this seems to be the case. In this section, we focus in three possible explanations of why CDS is less common in dentistry.

2.8.2.1 Our Level of Understanding of the Way We Diagnose Patients

Since the 1950s, there have been several efforts in medicine to define and formalize the underlying cognitive processes occurring when humans search and identify diagnosis. Ledley and Lusted (1959) dissected how physicians use "complex reasoning" and provided systematization to the intangible processes that occur in the physicians' mind. Ledley et al. introduced the mathematical concepts of symbolic logic; probability and value theory which have helped us operationalize diagnostic reasoning. Subsequent efforts in medicine built on this key paper and created a large array of decision support tools from as early as the sixties (Warner et al. 1964). Thus, the amount of effort invested by the medical profession in understanding these processes is far larger than in dentistry. There are Divisions in medical schools, professional associations and dedicated journals in the area medical decision-making that contrast with the lack of the same in dentistry.

In dentistry, several efforts have been made to understand the way dentists reach diagnoses especially for caries (Crespo et al. 2004; Bader and Shugars 1997). However, our understanding is limited since diagnostic information is not routinely recorded in dental records (Bader and Shugars 1997b). Both groups identified that dentists use cognitive structures called "illness scripts" and that "these scripts develop from continuous exposure to patients." Bader points out; dentists follow a pattern recognition process that is inextricably linked to treatment decisions instead of a pure diagnostic approach.

2.8.2.2 Application Areas

Physicians have to deal with significant uncertainty and sometimes pursue treatment without a clear diagnosis (Sox 1988). Physicians define a preliminary diagnosis and initiate treatment expecting a specific response in order to define subsequent actions, while taking into consideration incoming additional diagnostic information. Physicians also have to decide between a large array of diagnostic tests that vary in terms between not only a large array of diagnostic tests that vary in terms not only of availability and cost but also risk and between specificity. Thus, medicine can greatly benefit from the use of decision support tools that ameliorate uncertainty at the diagnostic level.

On the other hand, Abbey observes, "the dentist is often more challenged by deriving the treatment plan than by deciphering the diagnosis" (Weed 1991). Abbey continues by saying that in medicine the varieties in clinical presentation of systemic diseases with "superimposed signs and symptoms" require physicians to select a different array of diagnostic aids that subsequently help in reaching a diagnosis. In dentistry, the possible signs and symptoms are confined to the head and neck region. Additionally, dentists routinely use a limited number of diagnostic aids compared to medicine (although new dental diagnostic aids have appeared in recent years). "Dental radiography is mostly morphological rather than quantitative," Abbey continues. Also, dentists rely heavily on personal capabilities including his/her senses and information obtained directly from patients. Use of laboratory data is limited.

2.8.2.3 The Way Knowledge Is Represented and the Inference Mechanisms

According to both White and Mendonça, several knowledge representation mechanisms include algorithmic systems that use "logical classification methods." One advantage of these systems is that they do not require large datasets however, they lack flexibility and if a change needs to be made, these systems would struggle to meet this requirement. Usually well understood diagnostic processes would fit this category well; in the case of dentistry, we have examples of decision support systems that use this principle in oral pathology (Rubin 1994). In the case of statistical systems, ORAD is a classical example where using a Bayesian method it analyzes the responses from 16 questions and provides a diagnosis from 140 possible lesions. In the area of rule based systems in dentistry, we found a system called RHINOS which provides differential diagnoses for headache and facial pain. Finally, there is a dental system that uses neural networks for prediction of location and relationship between past and present dental conditions (Okuda et al. 1997).

As we have shown, the application of different inference mechanisms is common in dentistry. However, most of these systems usually appear as prototypes in academic units and are not present in dental offices. The inability to migrate CDS to the dental office is for one or more of the following reasons:

- Traditional dental practice, in a day to day basis, does not require CDS (the clinician is good enough to make satisfactory decisions);
- There are no external factors that would increase the need for better decision making, for example evaluation of treatment quality or the necessity of always present treatment alternatives;
- The status quo of computer technology prevents the implementation of CDS and
- A combination of some or all of these.

2.8.3 What Needs to Be Done in Order to Increase the Adoption of Electronic Decision Support in Dentistry?

Current dental software lacks the proper human interface that could facilitate an easy integration in regular dental practice. This problem needs to be solved before any subsequent steps can be taken into incorporating other functionality such as CDS into dental practice. As mentioned before, current successful decision support systems do are not integrated with in office software. Preliminary studies point toward that direction (Thyvalikakath, personal communication). Other areas need further study:

2.8.3.1 Health and the Use of Diagnostic Information

The profession needs to step toward an "Oral physician" model, moving away from being "denturists" (a focus on diagnosis and science rather than dental procedures) and being more involved in the systemic aspects of the patient health. Population age is project to increase and thus the longevity of our patients. As a direct consequence of an aging population, chronic diseases are going to be more common, thus, dental practitioners should be able to proactively deal with patients with complex medical histories. For example, a dentist as an oral physician can increase their role as early detectors of patient systemic problems and intervening in modifying health related habits.

2.8.3.2 Education

Dental education programs should incorporate the concept of using informatics tools to facilitate the diagnosis and treatment planning. Currently, dental education does not consider the use of information technology to facilitate these steps in clinical practice.

2.8.3.3 Justification

Developers should correctly identify the needs of dentists and justify the implementation of CDS. We should avoid the approach of having a hammer looking for a nail as has been common amongst our medical counter parts. As described before there are intrinsic differences between medicine and dentistry, thus developers need to identify where decision support would maximize the effectiveness of the practicing dental professional. Proponents of higher accountability, guidelines and evidence based practice would agree that decision support could foster these areas in dentistry; however, it is important to identify what are the specific areas in which dentistry would really benefit from the tool.

2.8.3.4 Workflow

A key element in decision support is the ability of systems to provide the information when is needed and that it does not interrupt other critical or more important activities. It is necessary to understand the dental office as a healthcare delivery system and not as a "one-size fits all" customer when developing software applications.

2.8.3.5 Professional Environment and Interactions with the Rest of the Health Care Delivery System

The complexity of certain medical treatments will increase in the middle term because of advancements in other areas, such as genetics. This will require dentists to interact in new ways with fellow healthcare professionals thus creating a need to join a multidisciplinary health delivery system. The dentist will have to coordinate his/her actions at new levels of complexity. Additionally, evidence-based dentistry, quality, pay per performance and other elements that are common in the other areas of health care will start influencing the way we interact with patients, thus will be necessary the implementation of decision support tools.

2.9 Early CDS Application for Dentistry – Medical History for Dentist

Franklin M. Din

2.9.1 Background

Back in the early 2000s, this editor decided to produce a Clinical Decision Support application that was relevant to Dentistry. This contribution will discuss the challenges faced during the development of the application and show the results of the choices that were dictated by those challenges.

The first determination I made during the design of the application was to define what constitutes Clinical Decision Support (CDS). This is not a trivial question. Most people tend to view CDS as something that is implemented in real time at the immediate point of care in response to a clinical event. An example is an alert that pops up to warn a provider about a drug-drug interaction immediately upon the submission of a drug order, based on the patient's current condition, current drug regimen and the latest drug monographs. This view, while valid is also too limiting. CDS at its foundation is an application that helps a provider make a decision by analyzing all relevant factors. The idea of immediacy is not part of the definition. So, I approached my CDS application as an aide to help a dentist during the diagnosis and treatment planning phases rather than an aid to help during the immediacy of care.

Next, I had to decide on what domain to address. I determined that the biggest gap in the integration of medical and dental data is the dentist's understanding of how systemic medical conditions affect, influence and direct dental care and oral health. Hence, I decided that the greatest impact of CDS in dentistry is to help guide dentist about the interrelationship of systemic and oral concerns and to deliver this functionality at the medical history review/diagnostic/treatment planning phase of the dental workflow. In the real world of dentistry, this happens at the time of the initial oral visit

The next decision was to determine which IT platform, what programming language, what database application to use. I chose to write the application in Visual Basic 6.0. At the time, it was the only programming language I knew. The platform I chose was a PC running on Microsoft Windows. Not only is this the dominant platform in the world, but this was also my computer's setup. I chose MS Access as the database since I had the program as part of my MS Office package and I had extensive experience creating and writing subroutines for MS Access applications. So these decisions were not the result of a massive cost benefit analysis but rather a chose imposed by what I had available and what I already knew.

As I began development of the CDS application for the PC, I started using a PALM IIIc handheld which I really liked. The PALM platform was the first truly usable handheld device. Much like a iPhone™ and Android™ phones the PALM IIIc allowed the user to download and install apps that were developed by third party developers and offered for purchase at app sites (Handango and Palm Gear were the two biggest web based app stores at that time). I decided that if I could, I would like to develop a version of this CDS application for the PALM. I thought that providing a mobile CDS app was a good way to introduce CDS with a minimal investment. With the PC version, the user was tied to a PC. The CDS was only usable if the dentist had a computer in the operatory. With the PALM, the CDS was available anywhere the dentist was.

Unfortunately, I was not skilled enough of a programmer to write directly to the PALM platform. However, I was fortunate enough to discover a company called AppForge which produced a software application the allowed a developer to write a

Fig. 2.19 PALM IIIc image

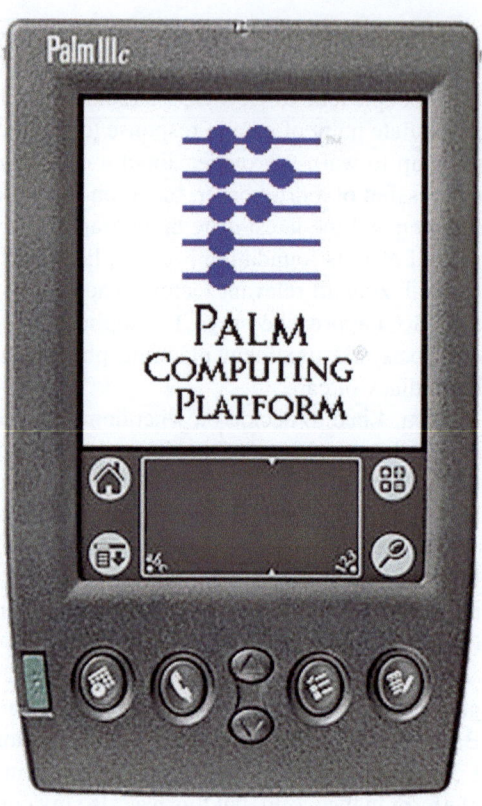

program in Visual Basic 6.0 in the VB Development environment, and then compile the code to run on PALM handhelds running on PALM OS 3.5. I purchased this software and developed a PALM version.

So, I ended up writing two versions of the Medical History for Dentist CDS application:

- A PC version using MS Access as the database
- A PALM III version to be used in any PALM handheld running the PALM 3.5–4.1 operating system. (Fig. 2.19)

Both the PC and PALM versions were designed to be standalone application since I did not have time, resources or permission to attempt integration with existing electronic record systems. The use of MS Access enabled the option of adding my application to an Electronic Dental Record (EDR) application in the future. The API and database connectivity are well understood in MS Access. So my MHD application could be added as a module in which the MHD is activated via event triggers in the EDR.

The PALM version was developed to provide mobility. At the time clinical records were still largely paper. This PALM version will allow the user to search for information manually to inform his treatment plan.

2.9.2 PALM Version

2.9.2.1 Hardware Considerations

The design of the PALM application was a significant challenge. The PALM IIIc, the primary hardware platform, (Fig. 2.19) has limited capabilities by today's standards. The relevant specs on the PALM IIIc are as follows:

- Operating System – PALM OS 3.5
- CPU Clock – 20 MHz
- CPU – 32 bit Motorola DragonBall EZ MC68EZ328
- CPU Core – Motorola 68000
- Maximum data set for processing – 68 K
- RAM (total device memory) – 8 Meg EDO RAM
- ROM – 2 Meg
- Display Type – Color Reflective TFT, 8 bit/pixel
- Display Resolution – 160×160 pixels
- Pixel density – 68.4 pixel/in.
- Display size – 2.34×2.34 in.

For those experienced in programming, the specs clearly demonstrate significant programming challenges. Each is described below:

2.9.2.2 Display

- The 8 bit color depth limits the range of colors that can be displayed to 256 colors. Therefore, very colorful applications with gradations and shadows are not possible.
- Pixel density (dot pitch) of 68.4 pixel/in. results in curves that are not completely smooth. In fact, many curved lines show distinct pixilation. Thus, images and figures tend to be simple.
- The 160 pixel wide screen, the dot pitch of 68.4, plus the built in default font size limits the amount of information that can be written in a single line. For longer text, especially text in tables, this means a lot of scrolling.

2.9.2.3 Memory

- The total memory for the included base applications and all third party applications is 8 Meg. This includes any data required to run the application. This was especially difficult for the MHD application since all the data regarding medical and dental conditions is included in the 8 Megs.
- The "chunks" of data and code to process and display the data is limited to 64 K blocks. If more than 64 K is needed, the code must be restructure so that any single module/subroutine/data load does not exceed 68 K.
- The 8 Meg total and 64 K blocks mean that memory management is paramount to the successful development of applications for the PALM III. Programming

with these limitations is more like the early days of programming for the PC in the early 1980s as opposed to programming modern applications.

2.9.2.4 CPU

- The CPU speed of 20 Mhz is very slow compared to modern CPUs. Programs written for the PALM III needed to avoid intensive calculations. Workarounds, like breaking a calculation into simpler components needed to be incorporated into the programming code.

2.9.2.5 Foundation Software Considerations

The CDS application was programmed to run on PALM handhelds or PALM compatible hardware running PALM OS 3.5. However, rather than program directly for PALM OS 3.5, I used a third party application, AppForge, that promised a write once and compile too many mobile platform functionality. At the time, Symbian and Microsoft Pocket PC were competing OS and hardware. The AppForge application compiled the VB code to run through a translator program installed on the PALM device, AppForge's Booster 3.5 (Fig. 2.20), which executed the application.

2.9.2.6 The Application

Once the application and the AppForge Booster are installed, the MHD application icon appears in the main screen. See Fig. 2.21.

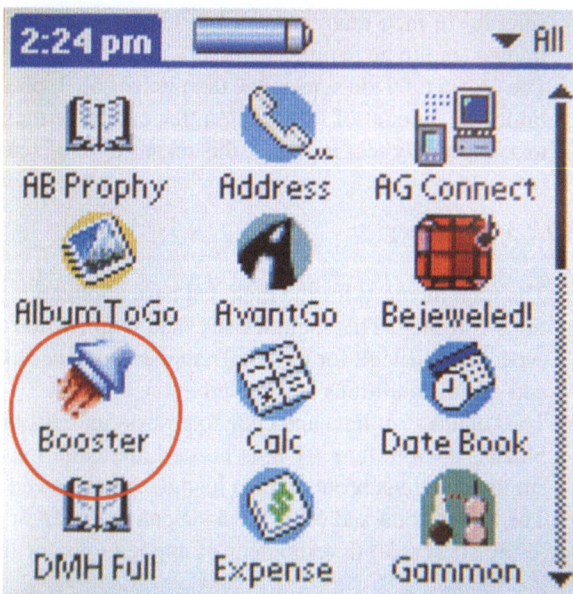

Fig. 2.20 PALM screenshot for booster icon

2 HIT Considerations: Informatics and Technology Needs and Considerations

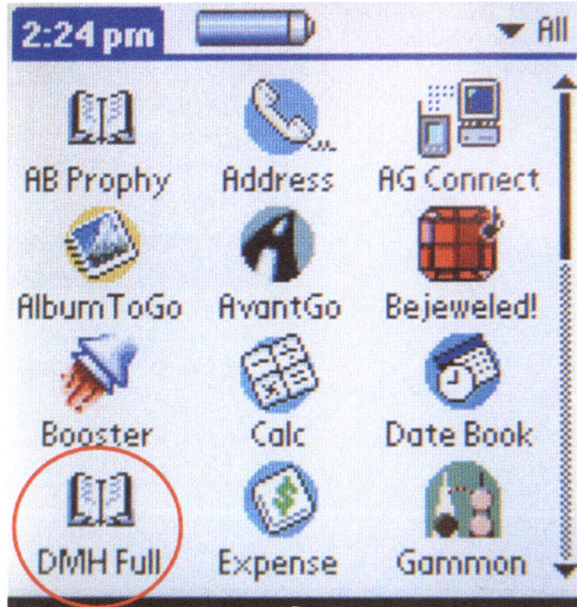

Fig. 2.21 PALM screenshot for medical history for dentists application icon

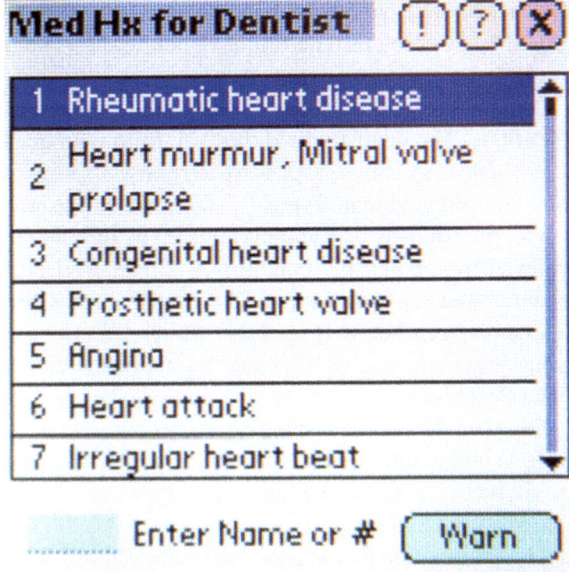

Fig. 2.22 PALM screenshot for medical history for dentists application

By tapping on the icon, the application opens to the main screen, Fig. 2.22 below.

The application is designed to have the user select the medical condition and then display the relevant dental alert/precautions. It was designed this way to fit the typical data gathering workflow. All dentists are required to conduct a medical history review of their patients. The dentist captures this information by listing a set of

Fig. 2.23 PALM screenshot for thyroid problem selection

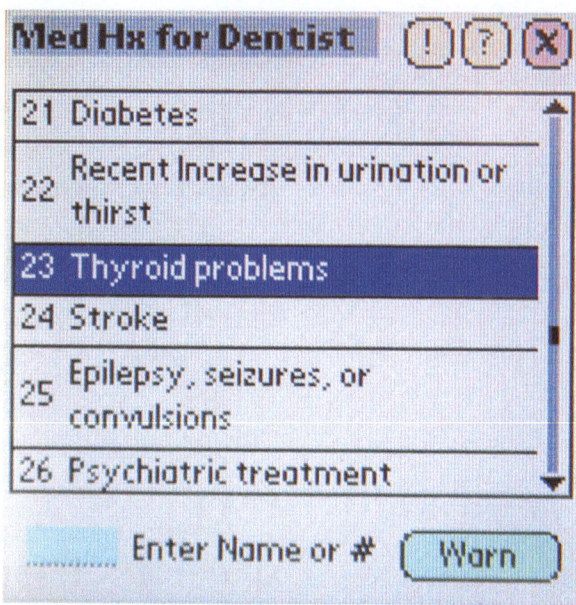

general medical conditions that are known to have relevance to dental care. In the screenshot above, you can see the first seven conditions all relate to a specific category of heart problem. The Fig. 2.23 below shows some additional medical conditions that impact dental care.

In the paper world, a patient would indicate that he/she had one or more of these conditions. The dentist would then ask follow-up questions to obtain more detail. For instance, in above, a positive response to item 23 indicates that the patient has a thyroid problem. Typically, the next question is to find out if the problem is hyperthyroidism or hypothyroidism. In this application, the same process is achieved by tapping the condition, "23. Thyroid problems." This highlights the selection and makes it active. The user then taps the "warn" button. This leads to a new screen below (Fig. 2.24) which offers two choices, hyperthyroidism or hypothyroidism. The user would tap one of the choices in order to highlight and select the choice.

Based on the patient response, the user taps one of the choices. The "!M" code in the last column indicate that there is more information to follow. When the user taps one of the two choices, the screen automatically changes to produce more information. See Fig. 2.25 below.

The information that is presented comes in two flavors.
- Basic information on the condition
- Specific warning/precaution

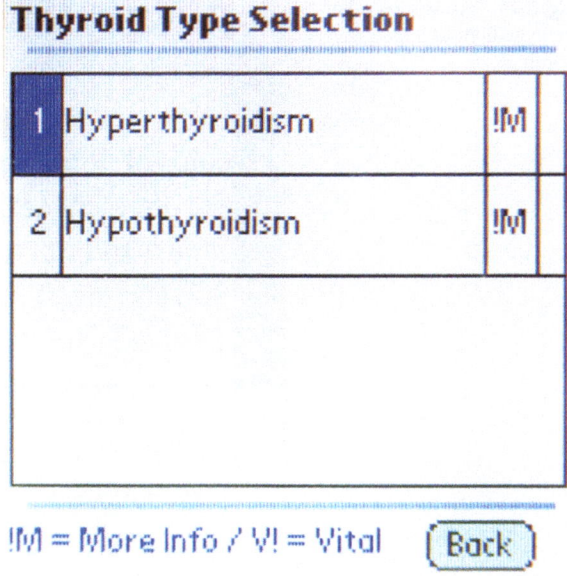

Fig. 2.24 PALM screenshot for thyroid problem sub-type selection

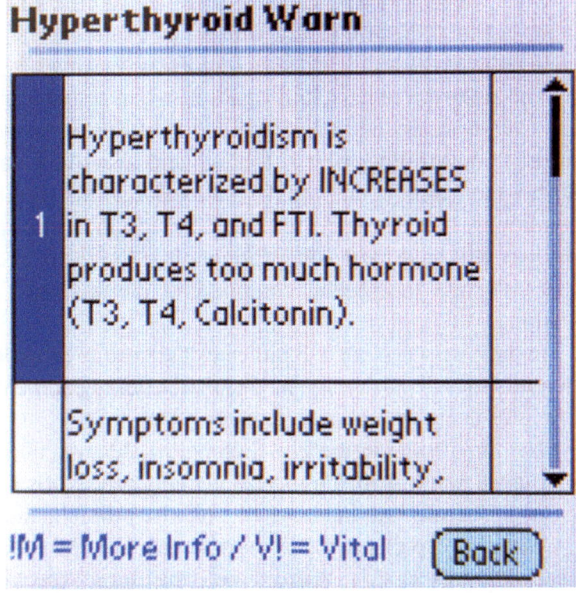

Fig. 2.25 PALM screenshot for hyperthyroid general warning

Fig. 2.26 PALM screenshot for hyperthyroid important warning

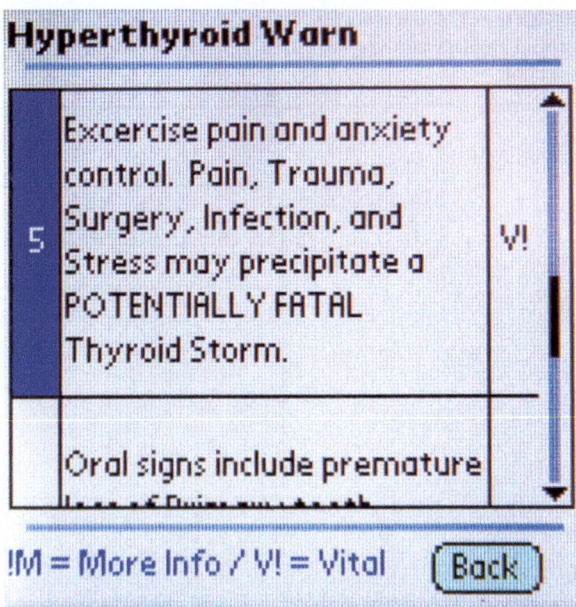

In the screenshot above you will see an example of basic information in the first item. In Fig. 2.26 below, you will see an example of a specific warning. The "V!" code indicates that this is a very important warning.

The inclusion of basic information and an actual warning/precaution is purposeful. CDS is supposed to leverage IT to improve a provider's decision making. One of the things IT does best is to store and to retrieve vast amounts of information. Rather than assume that the dentist recalls all the significant details about medical conditions, I chose to provide that information in this application. This insures that the user will have the basic information of the medical condition. It also allows the user to relate the medial condition to the warning … to see the logic in the warning.

In the case where a CDS indicates the need to provide a medication, the application provides details on the medication. Looking at the main screen again, item 4 in Fig. 2.27 deals with prosthetic heart valves.

The third bullet in the Fig. 2.28 below, "Prosthetic Heart Valve Warn" window, see screen below, indicates both a warning/precaution ("V!") and more information ("!M"). The warning indicates "… require prophylactic antibiotics."

When we tap this item, the next screen, Fig. 2.29, below provides details on the necessary prescription. You will note that item 2 specifies the protocol for children along with the notation for more information.

When you tap item 2, you will see a template for the prescription, Fig. 2.30. Note that the top line is a formula for calculating the correct dose for a child (highlighted in yellow).

2   HIT Considerations: Informatics and Technology Needs and Considerations

Fig. 2.27 PALM screenshot for prosthetic health valve selection

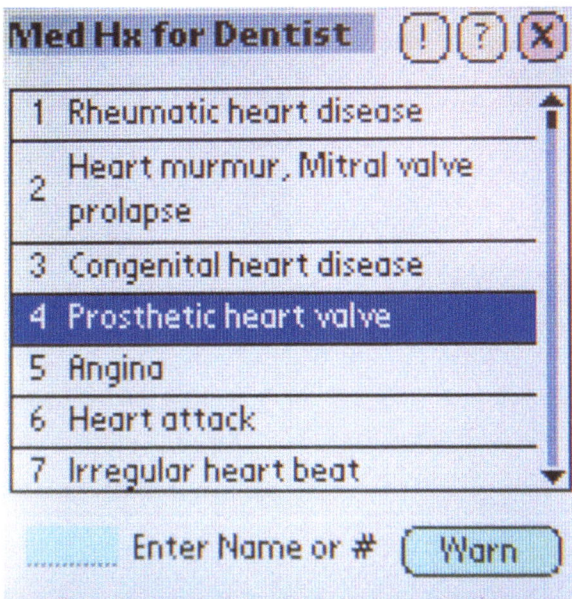

Fig. 2.28 PALM screenshot for prosthetic health valve warning

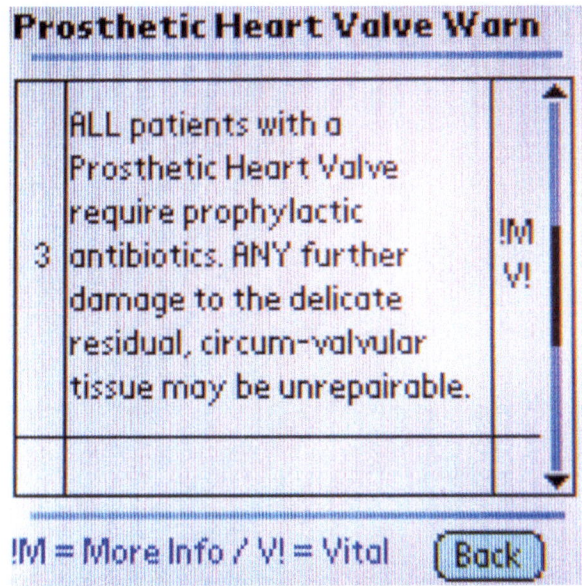

You will also note that there is a button to show an alternative prescription. In this alternate prescription, Fig. 2.31, you will see a button for an alternate prescription. Tapping this button produces the original prescription in Fig. 2.30. You can switch back and forth as needed using the "Alt Rx" button.

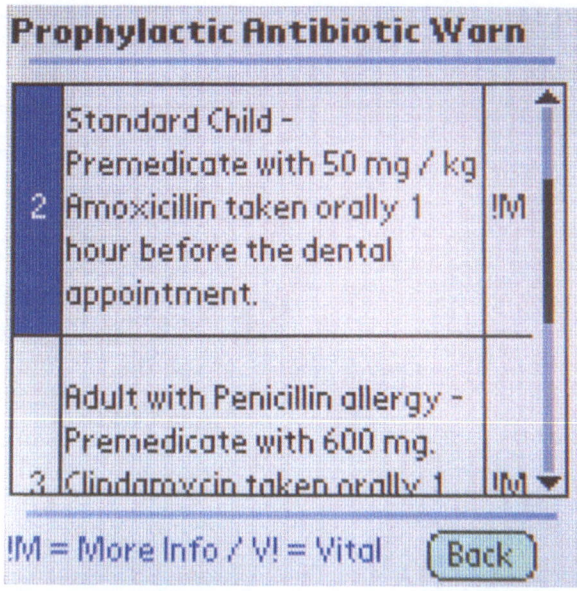

Fig. 2.29 PALM screenshot for prophylactic antibiotic warning

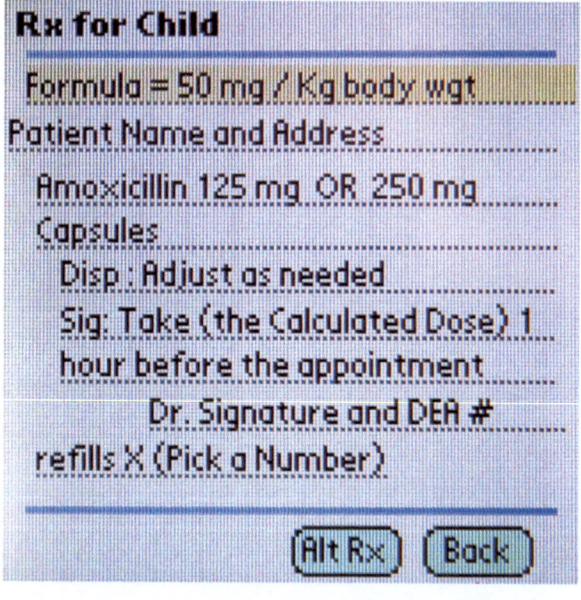

Fig. 2.30 PALM screenshot for prophylactic antibiotic dosing for child

Because the use of prophylactic antibiotics is important to dentists, I also created an adjunct CDS application, AB Prophylaxis, focused on the when to use prophylactic antibiotics. As with the full CDS application, this application includes both the basic information and the actual warning/precaution. The main screen in Fig. 2.32 below shows the basic regimens.

Fig. 2.31 PALM screenshot for prophylactic antibiotic alternative dosing for child

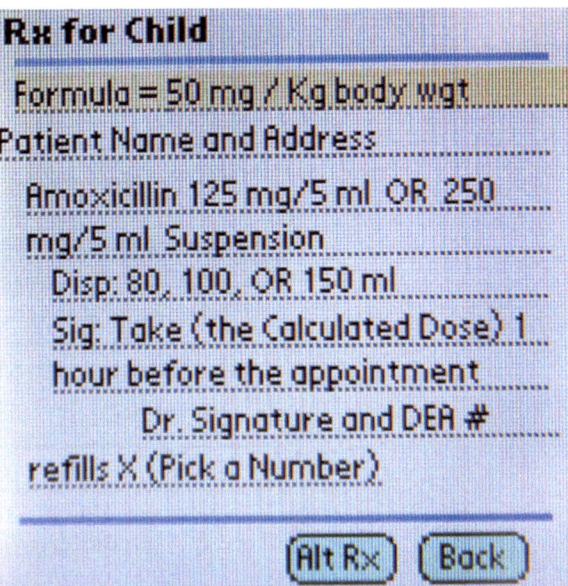

Fig. 2.32 PALM screenshot for prophylactic antibiotic dosing options selection

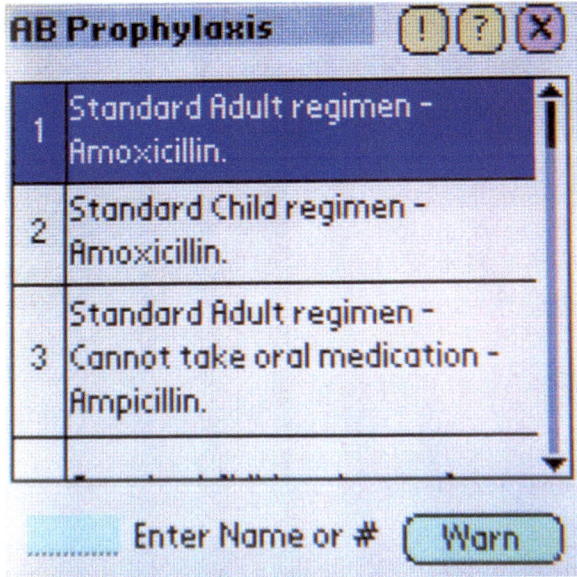

The AB Prophylaxis application restructures the information in the MHD to make it simpler to find information. For instance, Fig. 2.33 below provides a link to identify "high risk patients." In the full MHD application, this information is scattered throughout the application.

Fig. 2.33 PALM screenshot for high risk patient selection

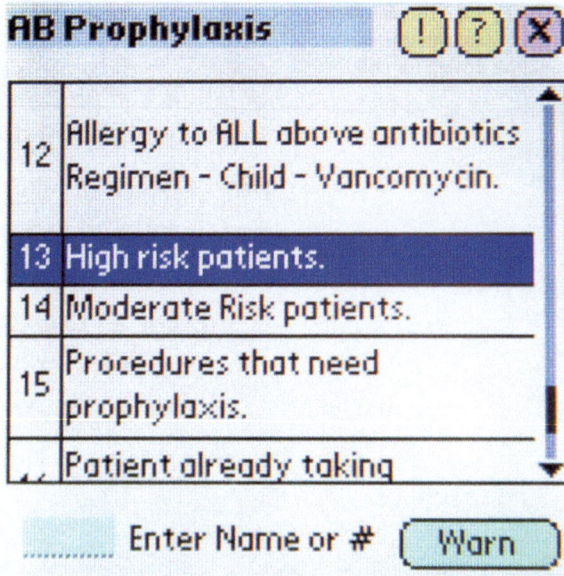

Fig. 2.34 PALM screenshot for high risk patient warning

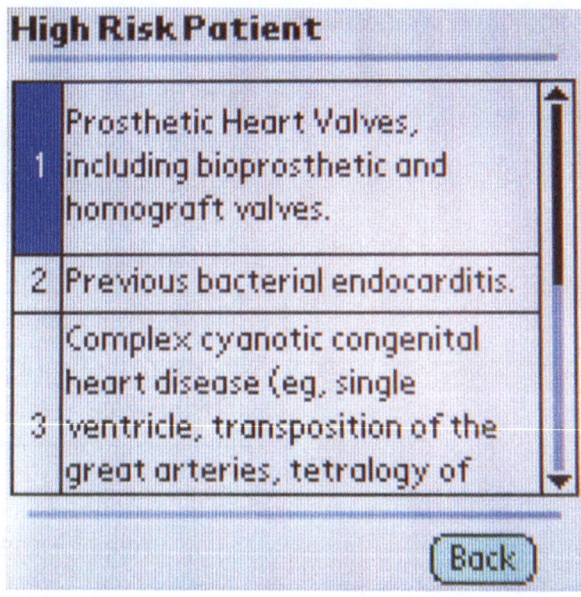

By selecting "13, High Risk Patient" and tapping the "Warn" button, the new screen, Fig. 2.34, shows the conditions that qualify as high risk patient.

The use of the two applications is one of the workarounds dictated by the limitation of the PALM IIIc and similar platform. To include both sets of functions in a single application using complex queries and virtual data objects would be very difficult to accomplish.

2.9.3 PC Version

While there is a separate PC/MS Access database version of the MHD application, the information delivered is the same as the PALM application. The differences are:

- The PC database version has prettier screens and the application can be incorporated into an EDR through the MS Access programming interface.
- The PC version allows the user to print the medical history and the associated CDS warning/precautions and background information. This allows the user to make this CDS process part of the official patient record.

2.9.4 Summary

This was an early attempt to create a usable CDS application for Dentistry. It addresses the need to integrate medical and dental information in order to improve patient care. Newer attempts at dental CDS can benefit from an understanding of this early iteration.

References

ADA Foundation Streamlines. Enhances association charitable activities. J Am Dent Assoc. 2003;134(4):424.

Centers for Disease Control and Prevention (2010a) HIV in the United States, CDC fact sheet. http://www.cdc.gov/hiv/resources/factsheets/us.htm [Accessed 18 June 2011]

Centers for Disease Control and Prevention (2010b) Projecting Possible Future Courses of the HIV Epidemic in the United States http://www.cdc.gov/hiv/resources/factsheets/us-epi-future-courses.htm [Accessed 18 June 2011]

Centers for Disease Control and Prevention (2011) Hemophilia, Data and Statistics. http://www.cdc.gov/ncbddd/hemophilia/data.html [Accessed 18 June 2011]

Fleisher LA, Beckman JA, Brown K, Calkins H, Chaikof EL, Fleischmann KE, Freeman WK, Froehlich JB (2007) ACC/AHA 2007 Guidelines on Perioperative Cardiovascular Evaluation and Care for Noncardiac Surgery : A Report of the American College of Cardiology/American Heart Association Task Force on Practice Guidelines (Writing Committee to Revise the 2002 Guidelines on Perioperative Cardiovascular Evaluation for Noncardiac Surgery). Circulation 116:e418 e500. doi: 10.1161/CIRCULATIONAHA.107.185699

Hammond WE, Cimino JJ. Standards in biomedical informatics. In: Shorliffe EH, Cimino JJ, editors. Biomedical informatics: computer applications in healthcare and biomedicine. New York: Springer; 2006.

Howerton Jr WB, Mora MA. Advancements in digital imaging: what is new and on the horizon? J Am Dent Assoc. 2008;139(Suppl):20S–4.

Jernigan DB, Davies J, Sim A. Data standards in public health informatics. In: O'Carroll PW, Yasnoff WA, Ward ME, Ripp LH, Martin EL, editors. Public health informatics and information systems. New York: Springer; 2010. p. 213–38.

Jones JA, Miller DR, Wehler CJ, et al (2006) Does periodontal care improve glycemic control? The Department of Veterans Affairs Dental Diabetes Study. J Clin Periodontol 34(1):46–52.

National Institute of Dental and Craniofacial Research (2011) Dental Management of the Organ Transplant Patient. NIH Publication No. 11-6270, http://www.nidcr.nih.gov/OralHealth/Topics/OrganTransplantationOralHealth/OrganTransplantProf.htm [Accessed 18 June 2011]

National Kidney and Urologic Disease Information Clearinghouse (2010) Kidney and Urologic Diseases Statistics for the United States, http://kidney.niddk.nih.gov/kudiseases/pubs/kustats/ [Accessed 18 June 2011]

Newell, A (1982) "The knowledge level." Artificial Intelligence 18, 1, 87–127

Parzuchowski JS, Jordon J, Burgess L,. Witsell M, Sobol L, Rontal M., Balaraman S, Ignatius R, Venuturumilli P, Krauss D, Chen P, Fontanesi J, Akervall J (2011) Lead-time from diagnosis to start of radiation shortened by 44% for head and neck cancer when patients go through a multidisciplinary clinic. Journal of Clinical Oncology, 2011 ASCO Annual Meeting Proceedings (Post-Meeting Edition) 29,15_suppl (May 20), 2011: e16627 [Accessed 18 June 2011]

Powell MA. Money in Mesopotamia. J Econ Soc Hist Orient. 1996;39(3):224–42

Smith B (1998) The Basic Tools of Formal Ontology. In Formal Ontology in Information Systems from Nicola Guarino (ed.), Amsterdam, Oxford, Tokyo, Washington, DC: IOS Press (Frontiers in Artificial Intelligence and Applications), pp. 19–28

Staad S, Studer R (2009). Handbook on Ontologies. Springer; 2nd ed. Berlin, Heidelberg

Wilson W, Taubert KA, Gewitz M, et al (2007) Council on Scientific Affairs of the American Dental Association as related to dentistry. Prevention of Infective Endocarditis: Guidelines From the American Heart Association: A Guideline From the American Heart Association Rheumatic Fever, Endocarditis, and Kawasaki Disease Committee, Council on Cardiovascular Disease in the Young, and the Council on Clinical Cardiology, Council on Cardiovascular Surgery and Anesthesia, and the Quality of Care and Outcomes Research Interdisciplinary Working Group. Endorsed by American Academy of Pediatrics, Infectious Diseases Society of America, International Society of Chemotherapy for Infection and Cancer, Pediatric Infectious Diseases Society. Circulation 116,1736–1754. doi: 10.1161/CIRCULATIONAHA.106.183095

Knowledge Representation and Ontologies

Ai J, Smith B, Wong DT. Saliva ontology: an ontology-based framework for a Salivaomics Knowledge Base. BMC Bioinformatics. 2010;11:302.

American Dental Association. Current dental terminology. Chicago: American Dental Association; 1991.

Baader F, Horrocks I, Sattler U. Description logics. In: Handbook on ontologies. Berlin/Heidelberg/ New York: Springer; 2004. p. 3–28.

Bertaud-Gounot V, Richard F, Le Moing C, Duvauferrier R. Ontology of dental emergencies for diagnostic classification. Cape Town: Medinfo; 2010.

Campbell KE, Oliver DE, Spackman KA, Shortliffe EH. Representing thoughts, words, and things in the UMLS. J Am Med Inform Assoc. 1998;5(5):421–31.

Canadian Dental Association. Uniform system of codes and list of services. Ottawa: CDA; 2001.

Falkman G, Gustafsson M, Jontell M, Torgersson O. SOMWeb: a semantic web-based system for supporting collaboration of distributed medical communities of practice. J Med Internet Res. 2008;10(3):e25.

Gangemi A, Guarino N, Masolo C, Oltramari A, Schneider L. Sweetening ontologies with DOLCE. In: Gómez-Pérez A, Benjamins VR, editors. Knowledge engineering and knowledge management. Ontologies and the semantic web, 13th international conference. EKAW 2002. Siguenza: Springer; 1–4 Oct 2002. p. 166–81.

Gasevic D, Djuric D, Devedzic V. Model driven architecture and ontology development. 1st ed. Berlin/Heidelberg: Springer; 2006.

Grenon P, Smith B, Goldberg L. Biodynamic ontology: applying BFO in the biomedical domain. In: Pisanelli DM, editor. Ontologies in medicine. Amsterdam: IOS Press; 2004. p. 20–38.

Gruber TR. A translation approach to portable ontology specifications. Knowl Acquis. 1993;5(2):199–220.

Guarino N. In: Guarino N, editor. Formal ontology in information systems. Proceedings of the first international conference (FOIS'98). Trento: IOS Press; 1998. p. 3–15.

Leake JL. Diagnostic codes in dentistry–definition, utility and developments to date. J Can Dent Assoc. 2002;68(7):403–6.

Long JJ, Goldberg L. Diagnostic criteria of Sjögren's syndrome: a study in knowledge transfer. ADEA/AADR/CADR meeting & exhibition, Orlando, Mar 2006. p. 1461.

Musen M. Generation of model-based knowledge-acquisition tools for clinical-trial advice systems. Stanford: Stanford University; 1988.

Noy N, Tudorache T, Nyulas C, Musen M. The ontology life cycle: integrated tools for editing, publishing, peer review, and evolution of ontologies. AMIA Annu Symp Proc. 2010;2010:552–6.

Ogden DK, Richards IA. The meaning of meaning: a study of the influence of language upon thought and of the science of symbolism. New York: Harcourt Brace; 1930, 1923.

Rubin DL, Shah NH, Noy NF. Biomedical ontologies: a functional perspective. Brief Bioinform. 2008;9(1):75–90.

Sandholm T. The philosophy of the grid: ontology theory – from aristotle to self-managed it resources. Report No.: Technical Report TRITA-NA-0532. Stockholm: Royal Institute of Technology; 2005.

Smith B, Brochhausen M. Establishing and harmonizing ontologies in an interdisciplinary Health Care and Clinical Research Environment. Health Technol Inform. 2008;134:219–34.

Torres-Urquidy MH, Schleyer T. Formal conceptualization of dental diagnoses: status report. In: Okada M, Smith B, editors. Proceedings of the second interdisciplinary ontology meeting, Tokyo, Feb–Mar 2009, p. 17–23.

Wächter T, Schroeder M. Semi-automated ontology generation within OBO-edit. Bioinformatics. 2010;26(12):i88–96.

World Health Organization. Application of the international classification of diseases to dentistry and stomatology ICD-DA, vol. 3. Geneva: World Health Organization; 1994.

World Wide Web Consortium (W3C). OWL web ontology language overview. 2011. http://www.w3.org/TR/owl-features/. [Accessed 30 May 2011]

Anticipating Oral Health Inclusion in Mainstream Standards

American Dental Association. Council on dental practice: supplemental record 1 – seamless electronic patient record. Supplement to annual reports and resolutions. Chicago: American Dental Association; 1996. p. 282–3.

DICOM (2006) DICOM correction item CP-643, add veterinary identification tags. ftp://medical.nema.org/MEDICAL/Dicom/Final/cp643_ft.pdf.

Diehl M. What data integration means to the practicing dentist. Dent Clin N Am. 2002;46: 606–15.

Farman AG. Use and implication of the DICOM standard in dentistry. Dent Clin N Am. 2002;46: 565–73.

Schleyer TKL. Should dentistry be part of the national health information infrastructure? J Am Dent Assoc. 2004;135(12):1687–95.

Schleyer T, Eisner J. The computer-based oral health record: an essential tool for cross-provider quality management. CDA J. 1994;22:57–64.

Towards an Integrated Electronic Health (EHR) System: Compliance, Security and Privacy Concerns

Austin A, Smith B, Williams L. Towards improved security criteria for certification of electronic health record systems. Proceedings of SEHC'10. Cape Town; 3–4 May 2010.

Baumer DL, Earp JB, Payton FC. Privacy of medical records: IT implications of HIPAA. ACM Comput Soc 2000;30(4):40–7.

Benaloh J, Chase M, Horvitz E, Lauter K. Patient controlled encryption: ensuring privacy of electronic medical records. CCSW'09. Chicago; 13 Nov 2009.

Brown B. Improving the privacy and security of personal health records. J Health Care Compliance. 2009.

Cannoy S, Salam A. A framework for healthcare information assurance policy and compliance. Comm ACM. 2010;53(3):126–31.

Choi Y, Caption K, Krause J, Streeper M. Challenges associated with privacy in health care industry: implementation of HIPAA and the security rules. J Med Syst. 2006;30(1):57–64.

Dimitropoulos L, Rizk S. A state-based approach to privacy and security for interoperable health information exchange. Health Aff (Millwood). 2009;28(2):428–34.

Goldschmidt PG. HIT and MIS: implications of health information technology and medical information systems. Commun ACM 2005;48(10):69–74.

Groen P, and Powell VJH. Electronic dental records (EDR): 'open source' and commercial-off-the shelf (COTS) solutions. Virtual Medical Worlds. 2010. At http://www.hoise.com/vmw/10/articles/vmw/LV-VM-08-10-5.html. 23 Aug 2010.

Hhs.gov. Nationwide privacy and security framework for electronic exchange of individually identified health information. 2008. www.hhs.gov/healthit/documents/NationwidePS_Framework.pdf. Retrieved on 23 Feb 2011.

Hhs.gov. 2009. http://www.hhs.gov/ocr/privacy/hipaa/administrative/enforcementrule/hitechenforcementifr.html. Retrieved on 23 Feb 2011.

Huston T. Security issues for implementation of e-medical records. Comm ACM. 2001;44(9). doi:10.1145/383694.383712.

Jha AK, DesRoches CM, Campbell EG, Donelan K, Rao SR, Ferris TG, Shields A, Rosenbaum S, Blumenthal D. Use of electronic health records in U.S. hospitals. N Engl J Med 2009;360:1628–38.

Kurtz G. EMR confidentiality and information security. J Health Inf Manag 2003;17(3):41–8.

Liu V, May L, Caelli W, Croll P. A sustainable approach to security and privacy in health information systems. Proceedings of 18th Australasian conference on information systems security & privacy in health IS. Toowoomba; 5–7 Dec 2007.

Mishra S, Chin AG. Assessing the impact of governmental regulations on the IT industry: a neoinstitutional theory perspective, in Ramesh Subramanian, editor. Computer Security Privacy Politics. 2008:36–53.

References for Physicians' Dental Data Needs and Oral Healthcare Providers' Medical Data Needs: The Clinical Rationale, Standardized/Structured Messages Facilitate Efficient Information Sharing and Benefit Patient Care, and Designing and Implementing Efficient Structured Communication Among a Patient's Medical and Dental Providers

ACC/AHA. Performance measures for adults with ST-elevation and Non–ST-elevation myocardial infarction. A report of the American College of Cardiology/American Heart Association task force on performance measures (writing committee to develop performance measures for ST-elevation and non–ST-elevation myocardial infarction). Circulation. 2008;118:2596–648.

American Diabetes Association. Standards of medical care in diabetes – 2011. Diabetes Care. 2011;34 Suppl 1:S11–61.

American Diabetes Association. Cost of diabetes, diabetes statistics. 2011b. http://www.diabetes.org/diabetes-basics/diabetes-statistics/.

Baddour Larry M, Bettmann Michael A, Bolger Ann F, et al. Nonvalvular cardiovascular device-related infections AHA scientific statement- 2003. Circulation. 2003;108:2015.

Baddour Larry M, Epstein Andrew E, Erickson Christopher C, et al. Update on cardiovascular implantable electronic device infections and their management a scientific statement from the American Heart Association 2010, endorsed by the Heart Rhythm Society. Circulation. 2010;121:458–77.

Bonow RO, Carabello BA, Kanu C, et al. ACC/AHA 2006 guidelines for the management of patients with valvular heart disease: a report of the American College of Cardiology/American Heart Association task force on practice guidelines (writing committee to revise the 1998 guidelines for the management of patients with valvular heart disease): developed in collaboration with the society of cardiovascular anesthesiologists: endorsed by the society for cardiovascular angiography and interventions and the society of thoracic surgeons. Circulation. 2006;114(5):e84–231.

Borges BC, Fulco GM, Souza AJ, de Lima KC. Xerostomia and hyposalivation: a preliminary report of their prevalence and associated factors in Brazilian elderly diabetic patients. Oral Health Prev Dent. 2010;8(2):153–8.

Calvet HM, Yoshikawa TT. Infections in diabetes. Infect Dis Clin North Am. 2001;15(2):407–21, viii. Review.

Chen AH, Yee Jr HF. Improving primary care-specialty care communication: lessons from San Francisco's safety net: comment on "referral and consultation communication between primary care and specialist physicians". Arch Intern Med. 2011;171(1):65–7.

Chen YP, Tsang NM, Tseng CK, Lin SY. Causes of interruption of radiotherapy in nasopharyngeal carcinoma patients in Taiwan. Jpn J Clin Oncol. 2000;30(5):230–4.

Choi YH, McKeown RE, Mayer-Davis EJ, Liese AD, Song KB, Merchant AT. Association between periodontitis and impaired fasting glucose and diabetes. Diabetes Care. 2011;34(2):381–6. Epub 2011 Jan 7.

CDC information. Hemophilia. http://www.cdc.gov/ncbddd/hemophilia/data.html.

CDC fact sheet. HIV in the United States. http://www.cdc.gov/hiv/resources/factsheets/us.htm.

Coogan MM, Greenspan J, Challacombe SJ. Oral lesions in infection with human immunodeficiency virus. Bull World Health Organ. 2005;83(9):700–6. Epub 2005 Sep 30.

Dajani AS, Taubert KA, Wilson W, et al. Prevention of bacterial endocarditis. Recommendations by the American Heart Association. Circulation. 1997;96(1):358–66.

Dawes C. Physiological factors affecting salivary flow rate, oral sugar clearance, and the sensation of dry mouth in man. J Dent Res. 1987;66 Spec No:648–53.

Demmer RT, Jacobs Jr DR, Desvarieux M. Periodontal disease and incident type 2 diabetes: results from the first national health and nutrition examination survey and its epidemiologic follow-up study. Diabetes Care. 2008;31(7):1373–9. Epub 2008 Apr 4.

Dental management of the organ transplant patient. http://www.nidcr.nih.gov/OralHealth/Topics/OrganTransplantationOralHealth/OrganTransplantProf.htm.

Desvarieux M, Demmer RT, Rundek T, et al. Periodontal microbiota and carotid intima-media thickness: the oral infections and vascular disease epidemiology study (INVEST). Circulation. 2005;111(5):576–82.

Diabetes Care. Association between periodontitis and impaired fasting glucose and diabetes. Diabetes Care. 2011;34(2):381–6. Epub 2011 Jan 7.

Douketis JD, Berger PB, Dunn AS, et al. The perioperative management of antithrombotic therapy: American college of chest physicians evidence-based clinical practice guidelines (8th edition). Chest. 2008;133(6 Suppl):299S–339.

Eckardt KU, Berns JS, Rocco MV, Kasiske BL. Definition and classification of CKD: the debate should be about patient prognosis–a position statement from KDOQI and KDIGO. Am J Kidney Dis. 2009;53(6):915–20.

Epstein JB, Raber-Drulacher JE, Wilkins A, Chavarria MG, Myint H. Advances in hematologic stem cell transplant: an update for oral health care providers. Oral Surg Oral Med Oral Pathol Oral Radiol Endod. 2009;107(3):301–12.

Field MJ, Lohr KN, editors. Clinical practice guidelines: directions for a new program, institute of medicine. Washington, D.C.: National Academy Press; 1990. p. 38.

Fleisher LA, Beckman JA, Brown KA, et al. ACC/AHA 2007 guidelines on perioperative cardiovascular evaluation and care for noncardiac surgery: a report of the American College of Cardiology/American Heart Association task force on practice guidelines (writing committee to revise the 2002 guidelines on perioperative cardiovascular evaluation for noncardiac surgery) developed in collaboration with the American society of echocardiography, American Society of Nuclear Cardiology, Heart Rhythm Society, Society of Cardiovascular Anesthesiologists, Society for Cardiovascular Angiography and Interventions, Society for Vascular Medicine and Biology, and Society for Vascular Surgery. J Am Coll Cardiol. 2007;50(17):e159–241.

Fleisher LA, Beckman JA, Brown KA, et al. 2009 ACCF/AHA focused update on perioperative beta blockade incorporated into the ACC/AHA 2007 guidelines on perioperative cardiovascular evaluation and care for noncardiac surgery: a report of the American College of Cardiology Foundation/American Heart Association task force on practice guidelines. Circulation. 2009;120(21):e169–276.

Geist JR, Chen FH. Nasopharyngeal carcinoma. Computed tomographic imaging of four cases. Oral Surg Oral Med Oral Pathol. 1993;75(6):759–66.

Geist SM, Geist JR. Improvement in medical consultation responses with a structured request form. J Dent Educ. 2008;72(5):553–61.

Geist RY, Geist JR, Jaw AM. Osteonecrosis related to bisphosphonates: a new concern for dentistry. J Mich Dent Assoc. 2005;87(11):40–2.

Geist SR, Geist JR, Sordyl CM, LeBow J. Benefits of casual random blood glucose assessment of diabetic dental patients in an urban dental school clinic. J Dent Educ. 2011;75:212–3.

Greenspan D, Greenspan JS. Oral mucosal manifestations of AIDS? Dermatol Clin. 1987;5(4):733–7.

Grines CL, Bonow RO, Casey Jr DE, et al. Prevention of premature discontinuation of dual antiplatelet therapy in patients with coronary artery stents: a science advisory from the American Heart Association, American College of Cardiology, Society for cardiovascular angiography and interventions, American College of Surgeons, and American Dental Association, with representation from the American College of Physicians. Circulation. 2007;115(6):813–8.

Grossi SG. Treatment of periodontal disease and control of diabetes: an assessment of the evidence and need for future research. Ann Periodontol. 2001;6(1):138–45. Review.

Guest editorial: Dr. Poul Erik Petersen, Chief. WHO Oral Health Programme. Strengthening the prevention of HIV/AIDS-related oral disease: a global approach. Community Dent Oral Epidemiol. 2004;32:399–401. http://www.who.int/oral_health/publications/cdoe0432/en/.

Hahn LJ. Osteoradionecrosis of the mandible: clinical observation and treatment in 45 cases. Taiwan Yi Xue Hui Za Zhi. 1983;82(3):451–60.

Hodgson TA, Greenspan D, Greenspan JS. Oral lesions of HIV disease and HAART in industrialized countries. Adv Dent Res. 2006;19:57–62.

Huang TT, Tseng FY, Liu TC, et al. Deep neck infection in diabetic patients: comparison of clinical picture and outcomes with nondiabetic patients. Otolaryngol Head Neck Surg. 2005;132(6):943–7.

Janket SJ, Wightman A, Baird AE, et al. Does periodontal treatment improve glycemic control in diabetic patients? A meta-analysis of intervention studies. J Dent Res. 2005;84(12):1154–9.

Janket SJ, Jones JA, Meurman JH. Oral infection, hyperglycemia, and endothelial dysfunction. Oral Surg Oral Med Oral Pathol Oral Radiol Endod. 2008;105(2):173. Epub 2007 Oct 1. Review.

Jones JA, Miller DR, Wehler CJ, et al. Does periodontal care improve glycemic control? The department of veterans affairs dental diabetes study. J Clin Periodontol. 2007;34(1):46–52. Epub 2006 Nov 24.

Khovidhunkit SO, Suwantuntula T, Thaweboon S, et al. Xerostomia, hyposalivation, and oral microbiota in type 2 diabetic patients: a preliminary study. J Med Assoc Thai. 2009;92(9):1220–8.

Kidney and Urologic Diseases Statistics for the United States. http://kidney.niddk.nih.gov/kudiseases/pubs/kustats/.

Kidney Disease Outcome Quality Initiative. K/DOQI clinical practice guidelines for chronic kidney disease: evaluation, classification, and stratification. Am J Kidney Dis. 2002;39: S1–246.

Leikauf J, Federman AD. Comparisons of self-reported and chart-identified chronic diseases in inner-city seniors. J Am Geriatr Soc. 2009;57(7):1219–25. Epub 2009 May 21.

Lenfant C, Chobanian AV, Jones DW, et al. Seventh report of the joint national committee on the prevention, detection, evaluation, and treatment of high blood pressure (JNC 7): resetting the hypertension sails. Hypertension. 2003;41(6):1178–9.

Lessard E, Glick M, Ahmed S, Saric M. The patient with a heart murmur: evaluation, assessment and dental considerations. J Am Dent Assoc. 2005;136:347–56.

Levey Andrew S, de Jong Paul E, Coresh Josef, et al. The definition, classification and prognosis of chronic kidney disease: a KDIGO controversies conference report. Kidney Int. 2011;80(1):17–28. http://www.kidney-international.org.

Levey AS, Eckardt KU, Tsukamoto Y, et al. Definition and classification of chronic kidney disease: a position statement from kidney disease: improving global outcomes (KDIGO). Kidney Int. 2005;67:2089–100.

Migliorati CA, Epstein JB, Abt E, Berenson JR. Osteonecrosis of the jaw and bisphosphonates in cancer: a narrative review. Nat Rev Endocrinol. 2011;7(1):34–42. Epub 2010.

Moser M. Historical perspectives on the management of hypertension. J Clin Hypertens. 2006;8(8 suppl 2):15–20.

National Cancer Institute. PDQ (physician data query). Bethesda: National Institutes of Health; 1990. Available at: http://www.cancer.gov/cancertopics/pdq/cancerdatabase.

National Cancer Institute. Oral complications of chemotherapy and head/neck radiation PDQ. Bethesda: National Institutes of Health; 2010. Available at: http://www.cancer.gov/cancertopics/pdq/supportivecare/oralcomplications/HealthProfessional.

National Cancer Institute. PDQ® oral complications of chemotherapy and head/neck radiation. Bethesda: National Cancer Institute. Available at: http://cancer.gov/cancertopics/pdq/supportivecare/oralcomplications/HealthProfessional. Date last modified 24 Mar 2011. [Accessed 8 May 2011]

National Kidney Foundation. KDOQI clinical practice guidelines for chronic kidney disease: evaluation, classification, and stratification part 3. Chronic kidney disease as a public health problem. Am J Kidney Dis. 2002;39(2 Suppl 1):S1–266. http://www.kidney.org/professionals/kdoqi/guidelines_ckd/p3_pubhealth.htm.

National Kidney Foundation. Insurance Choice for medicare ESRD Patients. 2009. www.kidney.org/…/INSURANCE_CHOICE_MEDICARE_ESRD-MSP_new.pdf.

NIH National Institute of Allergy and Infectious Diseases. The autoimmune diseases coordination. Committee Rep Congr: Prog Autoimmune Dis Res. 2005. http://www.niaid.nih.gov/topics/autoimmune/Documents/adccfinal.pdf.

O'Malley AS, Reschovsky JD. Referral and consultation communication between primary care and specialist physicians. Arch Intern Med. 2011;171(1):56–65.

Pakhomov SV, Jacobsen SJ, Chute CG, Roger VL. Agreement between patient-reported symptoms and their documentation in the medical record. Am J Manag Care. 2008;14(8):530–9.

Peterson P, Hayes TE, Arkin CF, et al. The preoperative bleeding time test lacks clinical benefit: College of American Pathologists' and American Society of Clinical Pathologists' position article. Arch Surg. 1998;133(2):134–9.

Prevalence of diabetes in the United States. data from the 2011 National Diabetes Fact Sheet. http://www.cdc.gov/diabetes/pubs/pdf/ndfs_2011.pdf. Released 26 Jan 2011.

Projecting possible future courses of the HIV epidemic in the United States. http://www.cdc.gov/hiv/resources/factsheets/us-epi-future-courses.htm.

Rajagopalan S. Serious infections in elderly patients with diabetes mellitus. Clin Infect Dis. 2005;40(7):990–6. Epub 2005 Feb 24. Review.

Ramírez-Amador V, Ponce-de-León S, Anaya-Saavedra G, Crabtree Ramírez B, Sierra-Madero J. Oral lesions as clinical markers of highly active antiretroviral therapy failure: a nested case–control study in Mexico city. Clin Infect Dis. 2007;45(7):925–32. Epub 2007 Aug 23.

Rao DD, Desai A, Kulkarni RD. Comparison of maxillofacial space infection in diabetic and non-diabetic patients. Oral Surg Oral Med Oral Pathol Oral Radiol Endod. 2010;110(4):e7–12. Epub 2010 Jul 24.

Sjögren's Syndrome Foundation. 2009. http://www.sjogrens.org/home/about-sjogrens-syndrome.

Soysa NS, Samaranayake LP, Ellepola AN. Diabetes mellitus as a contributory factor in oral candidosis. Diabet Med. 2006;23(5):455–9.

Stoves J, Connolly J, Cheung CK, et al. Electronic consultation as an alternative to hospital referral for patients with chronic kidney disease: a novel application for networked electronic health records to improve the accessibility and efficiency of healthcare. Qual Saf Health Care. 2010;19(5):e54.

Taylor GW. The effects of periodontal treatment on diabetes. J Am Dent Assoc. 2003;134:41S–8. Review.

Taylor GW, Borgnakke WS. Periodontal disease: associations with diabetes, glycemic control and complications. Oral Dis. 2008;14(3):191–203. Review.

Ueta E, Osaki T, Yoneda K, et al. Prevalence of diabetes mellitus in odontogenic infections and oral candidiasis: an analysis of neutrophil suppression. J Oral Pathol Med. 1993;22(4):168–74.

van der Waal I, Schulten EA, Pindborg JJ. Oral manifestations of AIDS: an overview. Int Dent J. 1991;41(1):3–8.

Vissink A, Burlage FR, Spijkervet FK, et al. Prevention and treatment of the consequences of head and neck radiotherapy. Crit Rev Oral Biol Med. 2003;14(3):213–25.

Wann LS, Curtis AB, Ellenbogen KA, et al. ACCF/AHA/HRS focused update on the management of patients with atrial fibrillation (update on dabigatran): a report of the American College of Cardiology Foundation/American Heart Association task force on practice guidelines. J Am Coll Cardiol. 2011;57(11):1330–7. Epub 2011 Feb 14.

WHO Towards universal access: scaling up priority HIV/AIDS interventions in the health sector progress report. 2010. http://www.who.int/hiv/pub/2010progressreport/en/index.html.

Wilson W, Taubert KA, Gewitz M, et al. Prevention of infective endocarditis: guidelines from the American Heart Association. Circulation. 2007;116(15):1736–54.

Zintzaras E, Voulgarelis M, Moutsopoulos HM, et al. The risk of lymphoma development in autoimmune diseases: a meta-analysis. Arch Intern Med. 2005;165(20):2337–44.

Matching Patients to Achieve Unique Patient Identification

Blakely T, Salmond C. Probabilistic record linkage and a method to calculate the positive predictive value. Int J Epidemiol. 2002;31(6):1246–52.

Gill L, Goldacre M, Simmons H, Bettley G, Griffith M. Computerised linking of medical records: methodological guidelines. J Epidemiol Community Health. 1993;47(4):316–9.

Liu S. Development of record linkage of hospital discharge data for the study of neonatal readmission. Chronic Dis Can. 1999;20(2):77–81.

Roos LL, Wajda A. Record linkage strategies. Part I: estimating information and evaluating approaches. Methods Inf Med. 1991;30(2):117–23.

Theis MK, et al. Case study of linking dental and medical healthcare records. Am J Manag Care. 2010;16(2):e51–6.

Improved Electronic Healthcare Technologies (EHT) Through the Harmonization of Application Design and Clinician Needs

Allen M, Currie LM, Graham M, Bakken S, Patel VL, Cimino JJ. The classification of clinicians' information needs while using a clinical information system. AMIA Annu Symp Proc. 2003;2003:26–30.

Armijo D, McDonnell C, Werner K. Electronic health record usability: interface design considerations. AHRQ Publication No. 09(10)-0091-2-EF. Rockville: Agency for Healthcare Research and Quality; 2009.

Covell DG, Uman GC, Manning PR. Information needs in office practice: are they being met? Ann Intern Med. 1985;103(4):596–9.

Horsky J, Kuperman GJ, Patel VL. Comprehensive analysis of a medication dosing error related to CPOE. J Am Med Inform Assoc. 2005;12(4):377–82.

Koppel R, Metlay JP, Cohen A, Abaluck B, Localio AR, Kimmel SE, Strom BL. Role of computerized physician order entry systems in facilitating medication errors. JAMA. 2005;293(10): 1197–203.

Electronic Decision Support in Medicine and Dentistry

Bader JD, Shugars DA. What do we know about how dentists make caries-related treatment decisions? Community Dent Oral Epidemiol. 1997a;25(1):97–103.

Bader JD, Shugars DA. A case for diagnoses. J Am Coll Dent. 1997b;64(3):44–6.

Bankowitz RA, et al. A computer-assisted medical diagnostic consultation service. Implementation and prospective evaluation of a prototype. Ann Intern Med. 1989;110(10):824–32.

Crespo KE, Torres JE, Recio ME. Reasoning process characteristics in the diagnostic skills of beginner, competent, and expert dentists. J Dent Educ. 2004;68(12):1235–44.

Ledley RS, Lusted LB. Reasoning foundations of medical diagnosis; symbolic logic, probability, and value theory aid our understanding of how physicians reason. Science. 1959; 130 (3366):9–21.

Melkos AB. Advances in digital technology and orthodontics: a reference to the invisalign method. Med Sci Monit. 2005;11(5):PI39–42.

Mendonca EA. Clinical decision support systems: perspectives in dentistry. J Dent Educ. 2004;68(6):589–97.

Okuda T, Yoshida T, Hotta M. A dental condition prediction system with artificial neural networks and fuzzy inference systems. Orlando: IEEE; 1997.

Rudin JL. DART (diagnostic Aid and resource tool): a computerized clinical decision support system for oral pathology. Compendium. 1994;15(11):1316, 1318, 1320 passim.

Sciubba JJ. Improving detection of precancerous and cancerous oral lesions. Computer assisted analysis of the oral brush biopsy. U.S. Collaborative OralCDx Study Group. J Am Dent Assoc. 1999;130(10):1445–57.

Shortliffe EH. Medical informatics: computer applications in health care and biomedicine. 2nd ed. New York: Springer; 2001. p. xxvii, 854 p.

Sox HC. Medical decision making. Boston: Butterworths; 1988, 406 p.

Walker GF. Cephalometrics and the computer. J Dent Res. 1967;46(6):1211.

Warner HR, Toronto AF, Veasy LG. Experience with Baye's theorem for computer diagnosis of congenital heart disease. Ann N Y Acad Sci. 1964;115:558–67.

Weed LL. Knowledge coupling: new premises and new tools for medical care and education. New York: Springer; 1991. p. xxv, 362 p.

White SC. Computer-aided differential diagnosis of oral radiographic lesions. Dentomaxillofac Radiol. 1989;18(2):53–9.

White SC. Decision-support systems in dentistry. J Dent Educ. 1996;60(1):47–63.

Chapter 3
Metrics and Measurements

Valerie J.H. Powell, Amit Acharya, Andrea Mahnke, Franklin M. Din, and Thankam P. Thyvalikakath

3.1 Performance and Quality Measures

Valerie J. Harvey Powell

In this era of care accountability, patient-centered care, prevention-focused care initiatives, performance measures are widely applied.

A typical performance measure consists of, in the format used by the National Quality Measures Clearinghouse (NQMC 2011) of the U.S. Agency for Healthcare Research and Quality (AHRQ), these components:

- Title,
- Description,
- Rationale (which may refer to the applicable standards of care of a healthcare professional organization)
- Primary clinical component,
- Sampling frame (such as patient associated with provider),
- Denominator description,
- Numerator description, and

V.J.H. Powell (✉)
Department of Computer and Information Systems Department and Clinical Data Integration Project, Robert Morris University, Moon Township, PA, USA
e-mail: powell@rmu.edu

A. Acharya • A. Mahnke
Biomedical Informatics Research Center, Marshfield Clinic Research Foundation, Marshfield, WI, USA

F.M. Din
HP Enterprise Services, Global Healthcare, Camp Hill, PA, USA

T.P. Thyvalikakath
Center for Dental Informatics, School of Dental Medicine, University of Pittsburgh, Pittsburgh, PA, USA

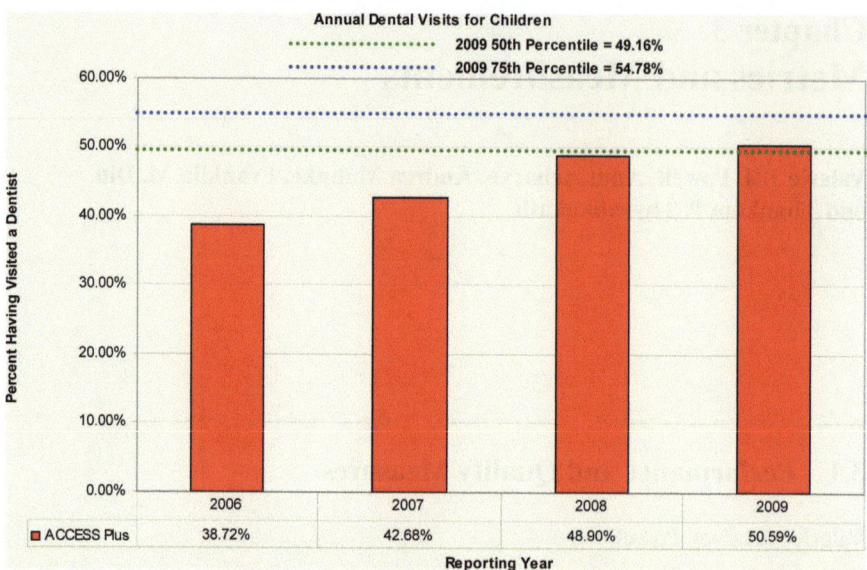

Fig. 3.1 Annual dental visits for children (Source: Pennsylvania DPW, 2010)

- Other categories of documentation relating to evidence, use, data collection, and computation (including interpretation to identify better quality of care and also stratification, as, for example, by age, gender, or language).

The denominator identifies the population, such as patients or members of a given health or dental plan within a specified age range, and specifies the applicable time period within which data can be gathered for the measure.

The numerator identifies a healthcare service received (or benefit, in health plan terms), such as a healthcare visit, an immunization, a medical test, a treatment, a new diagnosis, or a screening. The numerator may be constrained, for example, to those members of the population with a certain set of behaviors, a certain kind of lesion or wound, or a certain diagnosis.

The result is a percent of the designated population who received the service or benefit (which was a treatment, screening, visit, immunization) or demonstrate the outcome (meeting a certain goal). In quality improvement initiatives charts based on service and outcome measures are used to assess success or failure at improving the quality of care. An example is chart for Annual Dental Visits for Children, graciously provided by the Pennsylvania Department of Public Welfare (DPW). This chart shows that the number of dental visits increased each year from 2006 through 2009, finally meeting the first goal of the 50th percentile in 2009 (Fig. 3.1).

This chart used Health Effectiveness Data and Information Set (HEDIS®) dental data for children under 21 in the Pennsylvania Access Plus program from 2006 to 2009. The HEDIS® measure used by Pennsylvania as a basis for collecting dental visit data and interpreting them can be viewed online at the web site of the National Quality Measures Clearinghouse (NQMC 2011) of the Agency for Healthcare Research and Quality (AHRQ), and computes the percentage of members the Pennsylvania DPW 2010 Access Plus Plan aged 2 through 21 years who had at least one dental visit during the particular measurement year. Consulting the National Quality Measures Clearinghouse (NQMC) of the Agency for Healthcare Research and Quality (AHRQ) reveals a number of measures related to dental care quality of the quality of dental education. Most of these originated with the U.S. Agency for Healthcare Research and Quality, regarding dental plans members' experiences, or with the Australian Council on Healthcare Standards (ACHS).

The (HEDIS®) measures provided by the National Committee on Quality Assurance (NCQA) are among the best known performance measures in the U.S. today. The purpose of HEDIS® codes is to furnish a consistent definition for collecting data to evaluate the effectiveness of health plans. NCQA then publishes annual reports of the "State of Health Care Quality" based on HEDIS® data. Through this process, NCQA endeavors to help the U.S. (1) provide necessary care, (2) avoid delivering wrong care, and (3) to avoid delivering care that is not needed. NCQA has existed since 1990. By its very structure, NCQA has no mission to include oral health care in the definition of health care, since the NCQA was established by health plans, which, with a few exceptions, do not reimburse routine preventive dental care. Certain oral health provider procedures for Oral and Maxillofacial Surgery, Oral and Maxillofacial Radiology, and Oral and Maxillofacial Pathology are likely billed through medical insurance. Benefits for routine preventive and restorative dental care would ordinarily be provided by dental plans, which are not related organizationally to NCQA. The NCQA's establishment appears to be based on an assumption that the totality of health care is supported by medical insurance payers. All benefits relevant to health care quality are provided by a carrier (medical) who works with NCQA. Dental benefits and care are implicitly irrelevant to HEDIS® performance measures unless associated with a member health plan's benefit schedule (Fig. 3.2).

While NCQA supports a pediatric "access" performance measure for an annual dental visit, it has not so far chosen to include referral for a dental visit among the measures for comprehensive diabetes care. The NCQA has had an opportunity to add dental referral to the HEDIS® measures for comprehensive diabetes care as formal requests was submitted to NCQA for including a HEDIS® measure for dental referral including periodontal screening (NCQA, 2009, NCQA Tracking Numbers 28565 (for submissions regarding dental referral in Amer Diabetes Assn 2009 standards of care. Integration of medical and dental care lacking in diabetes measures), 29629, 29728, and 34203, personal communication, January 20, 2009, February 18, 2009).

One cannot say that NCQA is unaware of dental care, since there is a HEDIS® dental care measure assessing "the percentage of members 2 through 21 years of age who had at least one dental visit during the measurement year" (NQMC 2009). This measure makes it possible to assess the level of access to pediatric dental visits for health plans which offer such dental benefits. The age range for the NCQA measure cited here reveals that it relates to Medicaid pediatric benefits (NCQA (2011a, b, c)). Examples of health plans that offers dental benefits related to chronic illness care are Aetna (Albert et al. 2006); CIGNA (2006), "CIGNA Dental today announced the expansion of its Oral Health Integration Program to include new initiatives promoting the treatment of gum disease for members with diabetes and cardiovascular disease." A CIGNA study was recently announced at the 2011 International Association for Dental Research meeting in which "medical costs for patients with type II diabetes and periodontal disease were compared for those patients who had

Fig. 3.2 Assumption that medical health comprises the totality of healthcare

M = Medical Care
D = Dental Care
H = Health Care

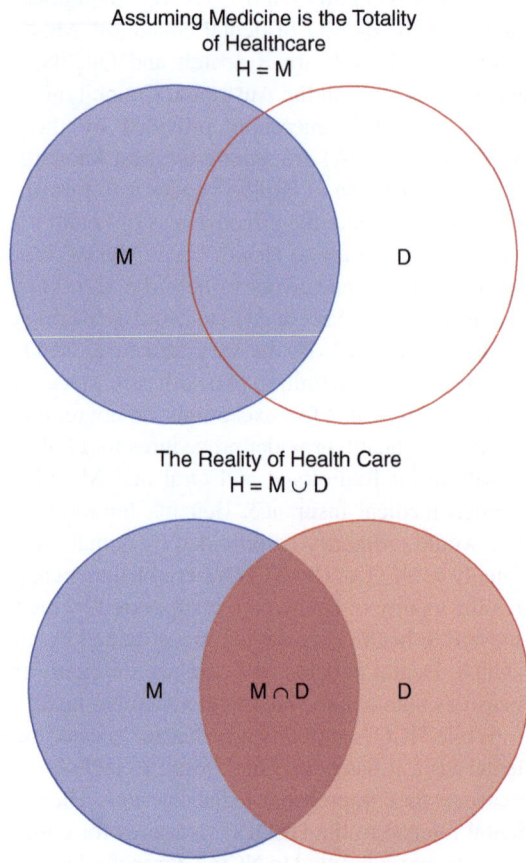

their periodontal disease treated and received maintenance therapy with controls who did not have complete therapy." According to Jeffcoat (2011, personal communication, June 20, 2011), a "savings of $2,483.51 per patient per year was realized in the group who received the periodontal treatment."

It is possible that the impact of the NCQA HEDIS® diabetes measure set configuration on quality improvement efforts can be gauged by examining the diabetes quality measures used by health collaborative, such as the Wisconsin Collaborative for Health Quality (WCHQ). The WCHQ Diabetes Recognition Program includes two categories of measure, one for medical groups and one for health plans. Health plan measures are all HEDIS® measures. Medical Group measures were all developed by WCHQ. Both sets include HbA1c, LDL-C, and blood pressure. The WCHQ health plan group also includes medical attention for nephropathy and a retinal eye exam (both HEDIS® measures). The medical group includes a measure for kidney function and an "all-in-one" composite measure (Nolan and Berwick 2006).

What would be the reasoning behind expecting WCHQ or any other health collaborative to include an oral health measure in their diabetes quality effort? First of all, the "Standards of Medical Care in Diabetes – 2011" list "dental disease" under the "History of diabetes-related conditions," and "Dental Examination" is included in Table 8, the "components of the comprehensive diabetes examination" (American Diabetes Association 2011). "Dental Examination" has been included in the ADA standards of medical care at least since 2008. Beyond the ADA standards and within the same state, the Wisconsin Diabetes Mellitus Essential Care Guidelines of the Wisconsin Diabetes Advisory Group (WDAG) include "simple inspection of gums and teeth for signs of periodontal disease" by the primary care provider on diagnosis and then a "dental exam by general dentist or periodontal specialist." (WDAG 2011) The Wisconsin essential diabetes guidelines have been in place since at least 2004, and have been updated twice since then.

There is in general a tendency not to go beyond the HEDIS® diabetes measures in designing chronic illness care initiatives. In the case of Wisconsin, it is solely speculation to suppose that performance measure choices were constrained by the set available as NCQA HEDIS® measures. In the case of establishing the Pennsylvania collaborative, performance measures were restricted to HEDIS® diabetes measures (Siminerio et al. 2009), even though a "dental referral" diabetes measure was proposed on more than one occasion. Siminerio et al. explicitly state under "Decision Support" that the Performance Measure Subcommittee "required [sic] the following NCQA measures." Thus, unintentionally the very structure of U.S. health care reimbursement by which medical and dental care are not reimbursed within the same plans effectively subverts diabetes quality initiatives and contributes to inhibiting optimal, evidence-based diabetes performance measures from being adopted.

Outside the HEDIS® framework, the U.S. Health Resources Services Administration (HRSA) has a diabetes measure that assesses the percent of diabetic patients in the clinical information system who obtained a dental exam in the last 12 months. The HRSA measure is suitable for the U.S. federally sponsored network of community health centers (CHCs), which, by statute, have co-located medical and dental care delivery.

Performance measures that check whether a goal has been achieved or not obviously have a dichotomous (two-valued), rather than scaled, response pattern. A scaled response pattern reveals more about the content of care. So far the oral health performance measures discussed are dichotomous. Here is an example of a performance measure from the ACHS, using a scaled (percent) measure: "children: percentage of teeth requiring repeat fissure sealant treatment within 24 months of the initial fissure sealant treatment." ACHS has numerous measures using percents regarding such topics as education, treatment, screening examinations, and health plan member experiences. Also, even measures with dichotomous patterns use scaled values such as medical test result values (blood tests for HbA1c, creatinine level) to indicate the extent to which outcome goals were met. With regard to outcomes, the IOM publication (IOM 2006) favors composite (all-or-none) measures as evidence of optimal chronic illness management, citing examples from HealthPartners, Inc., in Minnesota, and specifying in which circumstances composite measures are to be preferred (identifying poor performance) or avoided (making comparisons).

A question that has been raised is whether there are any scaled measures than could be utilized in oral health quality efforts. Well-known metrics in oral health include *decayed, missing*, and *filled teeth* (DMFT), *decayed, missing*, and *filled surfaces* (DMFS), and the Significant Caries Index (SIC) for caries and probing depth (PD) and clinical attachment level (CAL) for periodontal disease. Ditmyer et al. (2011) compare the DMFT and SIC, showing the difference between DMFT and SIC scores for the state of Nevada for an 8-year period. Page and Eke (2007) compare PD and CAL for purposes of surveillance and ultimately find value in both, since although "CAL is considered a more accurate measure than PD, and CAL is accepted as the gold standard for disease severity and progression," a "patient or tooth with periodontitis can be treated successfully or the disease can resolve spontaneously without a return of CAL to normal." Please note that Page and Eke's survey follow the NHANES protocols for interviews and clinical examination and include a "full-mouth clinical examination." Bassani et al. (2006) compare results of using full and partial Community Periodontal Index of Treatment Needs (CPITN) examinations for population periodontitis screening. Page and Eke emphasize that full-mouth exams are resource intensive and costly. An outcome measure based on the dental record can include information on the prevalence of periodontal disease in a population (Mattila et al. 2002). Keller et al. (2009) describe using a survey of insured patients to support "comparison of plan performance, as evaluated by dental patients."

There has been criticism of claims-based measures, since they only account for that part of a population of people treated in a healthcare system, namely those who have a commercial or public (Medicaid) payer. According the Wisconsin Collaborative for Healthcare Quality (WCHQ), physicians, "data analysts and quality specialists from the WCHQ membership have developed ambulatory care specifications that capture all patients and all payers. By uniting claims, clinical and patient data, WCHQ tracks each provider's entire practice. This comprehensive approach enables WCHQ to create a sophisticated measure set that evaluates both clinical processes and intermediate outcomes, like A1c, blood pressure and LDL control." WCHQ characterizes its approach as "All Patients, All Payers." The technical problem in trying to integrate medical and dental claims data in processing performance measures is that health plans and dental plans in the U.S. have separate claim streams with separate patient identifiers, posing a serious barrier to any effort to combine data from the two domains of care delivery, except for patients of CIGNA, Aetna, the Veterans Health Administration, the Indian Health Service, and the U.S. military. Should WCHQ choose to include "dental checkup" among its diabetes performance measures, it would have to address the technical challenge of reconciling claims (with respect to patient identification) from the systems of two different plans, medical and dental.

Given, for example, the practice alert of the American Association of Critical Care Nurses (AACN 2010) regarding "Oral Care for Patients at Risk for Ventilator-Associated Pheumonia," one would expect ICU performance measures, especially composite measures, to include a specific oral health measure.

3.2 The Meaningful Use of Certified Electronic Health Records in Dentistry

Amit Acharya, Andrea Mahnke, and Franklin M. Din

3.2.1 Introduction

On February 17th, 2009, the American Recovery and Reinvest Act (ARRA) of 2009 was signed into on law by the United States' federal government. The ARRA allocated an amount of $787 Billon, included under this is a portion of $19.2 Billion with an intention to incentivize the physicians and hospitals for the adoption of the Electronic Health Record (EHR). Incentive payments range from a maximum of $ 44,000 under the Medicare incentive option or $ 64,000 under the Medicaid option for each qualifying physician. This portion of the bills was called, the Health Information Technology for Economic and Clinical Health Act or the HITECH Act. As a result of the HITECT Act and the incentive involved for the eligible providers and hospitals for adopting the EHR, the healthcare arena in Unites States is witnessing a lot of activities. The majority of the providers and organizations are currently in a transitional phase in an effort to automate the entire process of clinical documentation and management of patient data. Although the HITECH act does include Dentist as an Eligible Professionals (EPs), the reimbursement is only for those who accept Medicare and Medicaid patients. For dental providers, only the Medicaid incentives apply since only Medicaid covers typical dental treatment.

The Office of National Coordinator (ONC) for Health Information Technology located within the Department of Health and Human Services (HHS) was legislatively mandated in the ARRA. As part of the HITECH Act, the ONC came up with an initial set of Health Information Technology (HIT) standards and the definition of "Meaningful Use" of certified EHR technology. The Center for Medicare and Medicaid Services (CMS) was charged with providing reimbursements for EPs and hospital providers.

3.2.2 Priorities for Health Outcomes Policy

Released in a staged approach, the Meaningful Use criteria will be presented in three stages to focus on healthcare that is patient-centered, evidence-based, prevention-oriented, efficient and equitable. Meaningful Use calls for Certified EHR technology to be used in a meaningful way. The proposed regulations outline five priorities for health outcomes policy:

- Improve quality, safety, efficiency, and reducing health disparities;
- Engage patients and families in their health care;
- Improve care coordination;
- Improve population and public health; and
- Ensure adequate privacy and security protections for personal health information.

3.2.3 Stage I Meaningful Use Objectives

Each priority comes with several specific care goals and, in turn, objectives and measures are aligned with each of those goals. Meaningful Use Final Ruling was published July 13th, 2010 for Stage I. Important to those wishing to ensure they meet the goals of this first set of regulations are the objectives of Stage I, which CMS clarifies as:

- Electronically capturing health information in a coded format;
- Using that information to track key clinical conditions and communicating that information for care coordination purposes;
- Implementing clinical decision support tools to facilitate disease and medication management;
- Reporting clinical quality measures and public health information.

3.2.4 Meaningful Use Stage I Core and Menu Objectives

CMS presents 15 objectives, representing actions that meaningful users must take in order to demonstrate meaningful use. In addition to these "core" objectives, providers must also choose five objectives from a menu of ten offered by CMS. For the menu-based measures, one of the two public health criteria must be chosen (Table 3.1 and 3.2).

3.2.5 Meaningful Use Clinical Quality Measures

As part of the core objective *'Report clinical quality measures to CMS or States'*, EPs must report on three required 'Core' Clinical Quality Measure (CQM), and if the denominator of one or more of the required core measures is 0, then EPs are required to report results for up to three 'Alternate Core' CQM. In addition, EPs also must select three additional CQM from a set of 38 CQM (other than the core/alternate core measures). In sum, EPs must report on six total measures: three required core measures (substituting alternate core measures where necessary) and three additional measures (Table 3.3–3.9).

Table 3.1 Summary of meaningful use core objectives

Core objective	Measure
1. Record patient demographics (gender, race, ethnicity, date of birth, preferred language) (patient reminder preference collection note)	More than 50% of patients' demographic data recorded as structured data
2. Record vital signs and chart changes (height, weight, blood pressure, body-mass index growth charts for children)	More than 50% of patients 2 years of age or older have height, weight, and blood pressure recorded as structured data
3. Generate and transmit permissible prescriptions electronically (eRx)	More than 40% of all permissible prescriptions written by the EP are transmitted electronically using certified EHR Technology
4. Implement drug-drug and drug-alergy interaction checks	The EP has enabled this functionality for the entire EHR reporting period
5. Maintain active medication allergy list	More than 80% of patients have at least one entry recorded as structured data
6. Maintain active medication list	More than 80% of patients have at least one entry recorded as structured data
7. Implement one clinical decision support rule relevant to specialty or high clinical priority along with the ability to track compliance with that rule	Implement one clinical decision support rule
8. Maintain up-to-date problem list of current and active diagnoses	More than 80% of patients have at least one entry recorded as structured data
9. On request, provide patients with an electronic copy of their health information (including diagnostic test results, problem list, medication lists, medication allergies, and discharge summary and procedures)	More than 50% of requesting patients receive electronic copy within three business days
10. Implement capability to electronically exchange key clinical information among providers and patient-authorized entities	Perform at least *one test* of EHR's capacity to electronically exchange information
11. Protect electronic health information created or maintained by the certified EHR technology through the implementation of appropriate technical capabilities	Conduct or review a security risk analysis per 45 CFR 164.308(a)(1) of the certified EHR technology, and implement security updates and correct identified security deficiencies as part of its risk management process
12. Provide clinical summaries for patients for each office visit	Clinical summaries provided to patients for more than 50% of all office visits within three business days
13. Record smoking status for patients 13 years of age or older	More than 50% of patients 13 years of age or older have smoking status recorded as structured data
14. Report clinical quality measures to CMS or States	For 2011, provide aggregate numerator and denominator through attestation; for 2012, electronically submit measures

(continued)

Table 3.1 (continued)

Core objective	Measure
15. Use CPOE for medication orders directly entered by any licensed healthcare professional who can enter orders into the medical record per state, local, and professional guidelines	More than 30% of all unique patients with at least one medication in their medication list seen by the EP during the EHR reporting period have at least one medication entered using CPOE

Table 3.2 Summary of meaningful use menu objectives

Menu objective	Measure
1. Implement drug formulary checks	Drug formulary check system is implemented and has access to at least one internal or external drug formulary for the entire reporting period
2. Generate lists of patients by specific conditions to use for quality improvement, reduction of disparities, research, or outreach	Generate at least one listing of patients with a specific condition
3. Submit electronic immunization data to immunization registries or immunization information systems	Perform at least one test of data submission and follow-up submission (where registries can accept electronic submissions).
4. Submit electronic syndromic surveillance data to public health agencies	Perform at least one test of data submission and follow-up submission (where public health agencies can accept electronic data).
5. Incorporate clinical laboratory test results into EHRs as structured data	More than 40% of clinical laboratory test results whose results are in positive/negative or numerical format are incorporated into EHRs as structured data.
6. Provide patients with timely electronic access to their health information (including lab results, problem list, medication lists, medication allergies) within four business days of the information being available to the EP.	More than 10% of all unique patients seen by the EP are provided timely (available to the patient within four business days of being updated in the certified EHR technology) electronic access to their health information subject to the EP's discretion to withhold certain information.
7. Perform medication reconciliation between care settings	Medication reconciliation is performed for more than 50% of transitions of care
8. Send reminders to patients per patient preference for preventive/follow up care	More than 20% of all unique patients 65 years or older, or 5 years old or younger, were sent an appropriate reminder during the EHR reporting period

Table 3.2 (continued)

Menu objective	Measure
9. Use EHR technology to identify patient-specific education resources and provide those to the patient as appropriate	More than 10% of patients are provided patient-specific education resources
10. The EP who transitions their patient to another setting of care or provider of care or refers their patient to another provider of care should provide summary care record for each transition of care or referral	Summary of care record is provided for more than 50% of patient transitions of care and referrals

Table 3.3 Core clinical quality measure

NQF measure number & PQRI implementation number	Clinical quality measure title
NQF 0013	Hypertension: Blood Pressure Measurement
NQF 0028	Preventive Care and Screening Measure Pair: (a) Tobacco Use Assessment (b) Tobacco Cessation Intervention
NQF 0421 PQRI 128	Adult Weight Screening and Follow-up

Table 3.4 Alternate Core clinical quality measure clinical quality measure

NQF measure number & PQRI implementation number	Clinical quality measure title
NQF 0024	Weight Assessment and Counseling for Children and Adolescents
NQF 0041 PQRI 110	Preventive Care and Screening: Influenza Immunization for Patients 50 Years Old or Older
NQF 0038	Childhood Immunization Status

Table 3.5 Additional clinical quality measure: diabetes

	Clinical quality measure title
Diabetes	Hemoglobin A1c Poor Control
	Low Density Lipoprotein (LDL) Management and Control
	Blood Pressure Management
	Diabetic Retinopathy: Documentation of Presence or Absence of Macular Edema and Level of Severity of Retinopathy
	Diabetic Retinopathy: Communication with the Physician Managing Ongoing Diabetes Care
	Eye Exam
	Urine Screening
	Foot Exam
	Hemoglobin A1c Control (<8.0%)

Table 3.6 Additional clinical quality measure: heart disease

	Clinical quality measure title
Heart Disease	Heart Failure: Angiotensin-Converting Enzyme (ACE) Inhibitor or Angiotensin Receptor Blocker (ARB) Therapy for Left Ventricular Systolic Dysfunction (LVSD)
	Heart Failure: Warfarin Therapy Patients with Atrial Fibrillation
	Heart Failure: Beta-Blocker Therapy for Left Ventricular Systolic Dysfunction (LVSD)
	Coronary Artery Disease: Beta-Blocker Therapy for CAD Patients with Prior Myocardial Infarction (MI)
	Coronary Artery Disease: Drug Therapy for Lowering LDL-Cholesterol
	Coronary Artery Disease: Oral Antiplatelet Therapy Prescribed for Patients with CAD
	Ischemic Vascular Disease: Blood Pressure Management
	Ischemic Vascular Disease: Use of Aspirin or Another Antithrombotic
	Ischemic Vascular Disease: Complete Lipid Panel and LDL Control

Table 3.7 Additional clinical quality measure: asthma

	Clinical quality measure title
Asthma	Asthma Pharmacologic Therapy
	Asthma Assessment
	Use of Appropriate Medications for Asthma

Table 3.8 Additional Clinical Quality Measure: cancer

	Clinical quality measure title
Cancer	Oncology Breast Cancer: Hormonal Therapy for Stage IC-IIIC Estrogen Receptor/Progesterone Receptor (ER/PR) Positive Breast Cancer
	Oncology Colon Cancer: Chemotherapy for Stage III Colon Cancer Patients
	Prostate Cancer Patients
	Breast Cancer Screening
	Colorectal Cancer Screening
	Cervical Cancer Screening

3.2.6 How Does the Meaningful Use Requirement Affect Dentistry?

3.2.6.1 Certified EHR

One of the basic prerequisites to participating in the Meaningful Use Incentive payments is the need to use a "certified" EHR. Unfortunately, there are no "certified" EDRs. Hence all discussions about MU are theoretical at this time. In anticipation of a certified EDR, the following MU discussion is relevant.

3 Metrics and Measurements

Table 3.9 Additional clinical quality measure: others

	Clinical quality measure title
Others	Pneumonia Vaccination Status for Older Adults
	Anti-depressant medication management: (a) Effective Acute Phase Treatment,(b) Effective Continuation Phase Treatment
	Primary Open Angle Glaucoma (POAG): Optic Nerve Evaluation
	Appropriate Testing for Children with Pharyngitis
	Smoking and Tobacco Use Cessation, Medical assistance: (a) Advising Smokers and Tobacco Users to Quit, (b) Discussing Smoking and Tobacco Use Cessation Medications, (c) Discussing Smoking and Tobacco Use Cessation Strategies
	Initiation and Engagement of Alcohol and Other Drug Dependence Treatment: (a) Initiation, (b) Engagement
	Prenatal Care: Screening for Human Immunodeficiency Virus (HIV)
	Prenatal Care: Anti-D Immune Globulin
	Controlling High Blood Pressure
	Chlamydia Screening for Women
	Low Back Pain: Use of Imaging Studies

3.2.6.2 The Challenges of Meeting Meaningful Use Core Measures with EDR (Table 3.10 and 3.11)

While there may be an EDR that differs from the table above, in general, EDRs will require significant improvements to meet these metrics.

3.2.6.3 Specific Concerns on Existing Meaningful Use Objective in Dentistry

Clinical Decision Support

Applying clinical decision support (CDS) at the point of care is highly unlikely for dentistry since EDR is still primitive at this time. Further, there is no adequate determination of what constitutes appropriate CDS. Using CDS to advice on treatment based on diagnostic criteria is essentially useless since:

- EDR lack robust collection of diagnostic information (usually no labs, no ICD codes, clinical indicators are not standardized)
- Treatment options are limited and a single treatment, like a filling, is the treatment of choice for a wide range of diagnostic conditions.
- No clear best practices to determine the use of alternative treatments, for example, when do you use a three-fourths crown versus a full crown.

A better method of implementing CDS is to provide a decision function that takes medical conditions into account and how the medical condition may affect dental disease and treatment. This approach allows the EDR to provide functionality and knowledge that the provider may lack or prevent the provider from overlooking a critical systemic condition. This later use of CDS also helps with justifying the effort to integrate medical and dental data to benefit the patient.

Table 3.10 Summary of MU core measures and EDR compliance

Core objective	Likelihood of EDR compliance
1. Record patient demographics (gender, race, ethnicity, date of birth, preferred language) (patient reminder preference collection note)	Likely. EDRs must review the demographic data elements and make the necessary changes to comply. In most cases, compliance should be a straight forward replacement of Free text fields with a structured field.
2. Record vital signs and chart changes (height, weight, blood pressure, body-mass index growth charts for children)	Unlikely. Dentistry will need to be allowed to omit or replace some irrelevant data. For instance, replace "body-mass index growth charts for children" with a "dentition growth chart for children".
3. Generate and transmit permissible prescriptions electronically (eRx)	Unlikely. eRx capability will need to be added to EDR functionality
4. Implement drug-drug and drug-alergy interaction checks	Unlikely. EDR developers will need to add this capability to EDR. Dentists tend to prescribe a small subset of medications and it may be difficult to extract a subset of interactions from existing drug-drug and drug-allergy knowledgebase.
5. Maintain active medication allergy list	Unlikely. Will require the EDR to capture this information as structured data.
6. Maintain active medication list	Unlikely. Will require the EDR to capture this information as structured data.
7. Implement one clinical decision support rule relevant to specialty or high clinical priority along with the ability to track compliance with that rule	Unlikely. A detailed discussion on CDS follows.
8. Maintain up-to-date problem list of current and active diagnoses	Unlikely. EDR don't capture diagnosis as structured data. A detailed discussion on Problem Lists follows.
9. On request, provide patients with an electronic copy of their health information (including diagnostic test results, problem list, medication lists, medication allergies, and discharge summary and procedures)	Unlikely. EDR must add capability to issue a complete CDD. Many of the components of the CCD are not available in the EDR.
10. Implement capability to electronically exchange key clinical information among providers and patient-authorized entities	Unlikely. EDR must add capability to participate in a standardized data exchange, like participation in a health information exchange. A detailed discussion on clinical data sharing follows.
11. Protect electronic health information created or maintained by the certified EHR technology through the implementation of appropriate technical capabilities	Unlikely. EDR are unsophisticated relative to EMR.
12. Provide clinical summaries for patients for each office visit	Likely. Even if this needs to be developed, the task is straightforward.
13. Record smoking status for patients 13 years of age or older	Likely. Even if this needs to be developed, the task is straightforward.

Table 3.10 (continued)

Core objective	Likelihood of EDR compliance
14. Report clinical quality measures to CMS or States	Unlikely. The clinical quality measures are medical specific. A detailed discussion on clinical quality follows.
15. Use CPOE for medication orders directly entered by any licensed healthcare professional who can enter orders into the medical record per state, local, and professional guidelines	Unlikely. EDR must add CPOE capability. The rationale for this functionality for dentists is questionable.

Table 3.11 Summary of meaningful use menu objectives and EDR compliance

Menu objective	Likelihood of EDR compliance
1. Implement drug formulary checks	Unlikely. EDR are not connected to drug formularies.
2. Generate lists of patients by specific conditions to use for quality improvement, reduction of disparities, research, or outreach	Likely. Even if this needs to be developed, the task is straightforward.
3. Submit electronic immunization data to immunization registries or immunization information systems	Unlikely. Dentistry is not involved with immunizations.
4. Submit electronic syndromic surveillance data to public health agencies	Unlikely. Dentists cannot legally diagnose systemic conditions that are applicable to syndromic surveillance.
5. Incorporate clinical laboratory test results into EHRs as structured data	Unlikely. Dentist rarely need to order lab tests.
6. Provide patients with timely electronic access to their health information (including lab results, problem list, medication lists, medication allergies) within four business days of the information being available to the EP.	Unlikely. EDR must add the capability to generate a CCD and then provide a secure electronic access to this information.
7. Perform medication reconciliation between care settings	Unlikely. EDR must develop the capability to exchange standardized medication data.
8. Send reminders to patients per patient preference for preventive/follow up care	Likely. EDR must develop the capability to send reminders electronically. A detailed discussion on patient reminders follows.
9. Use EHR technology to identify patient-specific education resources and provide those to the patient as appropriate	Likely.
10. The EP who transitions their patient to another setting of care or provider of care or refers their patient to another provider of care should provide summary care record for each transition of care or referral	Unlikely. EDR must add the capability to generate a CCD and then provide a secure electronic access to this information.

Quality Improvement and Public Reporting

The uniqueness of dentistry requires that the metrics developed to improve quality must be specific to dentistry. For instance, there is no systemic equivalent to a dental crown. So to track and analyze the quality of crowns must track specific data, like the presence of recurrent caries, loss of cementation and recementation, cracked facings, localized periodontal disease, radiographic evidence of fit, number of occlusal adjustments, etc. None of these are typical of medical quality analysis.

For public reporting, there are no mandated oral health reportable conditions. There will need to be an effort to identify reportable conditions, like STD signs. This may require policy or legal changes.

Up-to-Date Problem List

One of the objectives of the stage 1 meaningful use are to maintain an up-to-date problem list of current and active diagnoses based on ICD-9-CM or SNOMED CT®. "Problem list" is described as a list of current and active diagnoses as well as past diagnoses relevant to the current care of the patient.

Generally, ICD 9 is not suitable for dental diagnosis. ICD-10 has just a few more dental diagnoses when compared to ICD9 and the utility and completeness of ICD-10 has not been proven. So ICD-10 may also be inadequate to developing a robust problem list. SNOMED CT, while larger may also be inadequate to use to populate a problem list. If it is used, great effort must be made to create a Dental subset to avoid concept overload. The ADA created SNODENT many years ago but this terminology has many flaws and gaps, and has not been maintained/updated in years. Hence it is inadequate to the task. ADA was supposed to undertake an update of SNODENT in 2008 but there is no public announcement on progress.

If the problem list is to be created, to meet meaningful use requirements, it must be with the understanding that the problem list may have gaps that will take time to correct (requires a submission to IHTSDO to add/modify a concept).

Last complicating factor is that Dentistry has generally never used coded terminologies outside of CDT for dental procedures. This is a huge cultural change.

Patient Reminders

One of meaningful use objective calls for sending reminders to patients per patient preference for preventive/follow-up care. Patient preference refers to the patient's choice of delivery method between internet based delivery or delivery not requiring internet access.

While dentistry has always valued the need to send reminders for ongoing dental check-ups, it is usually limited to setting up an appointment well into the future or a periodic scheduled phone or mail reminder. The addition of an electronic maintenance communication is spotty at best among existing EDRs.

Implement five clinical decision support rules relevant to specialty or high clinical priority, including for diagnostic test ordering, along with the ability to track compliance with those rules.

We believe greater clarification is required around the concept of "clinical decision support". We propose to describe clinical decision support as health information technology functionality that builds upon the foundation of an EHR to provide persons involved in care processes with general and person-specific information, intelligently filtered and organized, at appropriate times, to enhance health and health care.

If the CDS is built to advise provider on systemic health effects on dental care, then five CDS can be constructed. For instance a medical history of severe liver problems should trigger a CDS warning about increased bleeding.

Exchange Key Clinical Information

This objective focuses on the capability to exchange key clinical information (for example, problem list, medication list, allergies, and diagnostic test results), among providers of care and patient authorized entities electronically. Dental EDR are currently not designed to generate an interoperable record. Work is needed to help EDR vendors develop a CCD or an HL7 2.x message.

3.2.6.4 Potential Measures That Could Be Considered for Assessing Meaningful Use in Dentistry (Thyvalikakath and Schleyer 2009)

- % of pediatric patients who receive caries-preventive interventions, such as fluoride varnish or sealants
- % of patients who are seen at patient-specific recall intervals
- % of high-risk patients screened for oral pre-malignant lesions or oral cancer
- % of patients with improving/stable/deteriorating periodontal disease trends for decayed/missing/filled teeth by individuals and population cohorts
- % of medications prescribed that are checked against authoritative medication/allergy list for interactions/contraindications
- % of patient referrals made as a consequence of potential oral-systemic health interactions, such as periodontal disease leading to low pre-term birth weight or periodontal disease leading to cardiovascular disease
- % of systemic conditions, such as diabetes, cardiovascular disease and hematologic disorders, discovered in the course of dental diagnosis/treatment

Table 3.12 Summary of focus group participants

Center	Dentists	Hygienists	Dental assist.	Other	
Center 1	3	3	3	3	
Center 2	1	2	3	2	
Center 3	1	2	2	2	
Center 4	2	2	3	1	
Center 5	1	2	2	3	
Center 6	3	3	0	2	
Center 7	4	2	3	2	**Total**
	15	16	16	15	62

3.2.7 Marshfield Clinic Dental Centers' Perspective on Meaningful Use (MU) Stage 1 Objectives: Focus Group Sessions

Marshfield Clinic conducted a series of focus groups to investigate the operational changes that would be required by all dentists and their staff at all its dental centers to meet the meaningful use objectives. Focus groups were conducted at all seven Marshfield Dental Centers both to educate staff about meaningful use requirements and to collect feedback about their perceptions of having to comply with the sets of requirements. In particular, another goal of the focus groups was to find out if they felt that adopting the meaningful use requirements would impact their daily workflow and if so, how.

Focus groups were conducted from January 10 to February 7, 2011. They were conducted over the lunch hour and lunch was provided. All focus groups were audio and video recorded. Groups consisted of a mix of dental staff including dentists (15), dental hygienists (16) and dental assistants (16), as well as appointments coordinators, patient financial staff and managers (15) (Table 3.12).

The focus groups were moderated by an usability analyst and a dental informatics scientist. The moderators started by giving a brief overview of meaningful use, providing background information to the participants. This was followed by an item by item review of the core, menu and clinical quality measures objectives. A number of themes that came out of focus groups are listed below.

3.2.7.1 Medications Requirements

The dental staffs were already comfortable with the medications requirements. This was due to the fact that the EHR medication component, medications manager, was already capturing the majority of these requirements. Overall the staffs were satisfied with how medications manager was working.

3.2.7.2 Environmental Challenges

It was apparent to the staff that some of the meaningful use requirements would require changes to their working environments and in some cases work flow as well.

In the case of recording the patient's weight and height, they stated that they would need not only scales, but scales that would accommodate people in wheel chairs. They bring back 20–30 patients an hour and traffic flows the same for all patients and they predicted that bottlenecks could form. They also questioned how they would record the weight because they do not work with tablet computers like medical staffs do. Comments were also made that patient privacy should be respected and questioned taking their weight in a public area.

> We would have to have a place to put the scale when we are walking the patient back. Right now it's sort of in the middle of the clinic. There are so many of us walking back at the same time. People want that to be private.

3.2.7.3 Time/Priorities

Dental staff felt strongly that they already are pressed for time to complete the existing tasks they need to complete. Adding any new task(s) was perceived as putting them behind schedule. Hygienists in particular, have just 1 h and often run short on time completing everything they currently need to do. Regarding the patient education resources, staff felt it was their priority to educate patients on oral health topics. Hygienists in particular already felt challenged with educating patients on brushing once a day. Staff felt that if they were spending more time meeting MU requirements that production would drop – they would not to be able to see as many patients in a day.

> I look at what we are going to be asked to do in a shorter amount of time. Do I want them to talk about brushing, their area of expertise, or a foot exam? We are already doing so much. Biggest problem is time. They decrease the time hygienists have with patients.

3.2.7.4 Patient Resistance

Dental staff felt that patients would be resistant to some of actions that would be necessary to meet meaningful use requirements. This was especially true for recording the patient's weight and providing weight related educational information and counseling to both children and adults. Because these dental clinics serve under insured and uninsured populations, they have a 10–12% no show rate. Staff felt that it is already a challenge to get patients to come in for their appointments. Taking their weight and discussing weight related health issues with patients were seen as deterrents for patients to keep future appointments. Staff also felt that their patients were not going to make the connection between dental health and weight issues. They also felt that in the case of children/adolescents, parents of these patients would be offended if a dentist attempted to counsel them about their child's weight issues. Also, some patients are seen up to six times a month – should weight be recorded at every appointment? The Marshfield Clinic dental centers already record blood pressure and several staff indicated that many patients were resistant to having their blood pressure taken. They expected even more resistance from patients when asked to have their weight recorded.

> I'm worried about the comfort level of a lot of adults getting weighed at a dental office. It would be really nontraditional. Patients are just getting used to having blood pressure taken.

3.2.7.5 Role

Dental staff did not feel comfortable crossing the line from dentistry and counsel in other areas. For example, since they did not feel they qualified as dieticians. In the case of decision support, staff did not feel that they should take blood pressure at an appointment to then compare to BMI and make a diabetes diagnosis. They felt it was a fine line where they cross from educating, which is acceptable, to diagnosing, which is unacceptable.

> When we take blood pressure at the beginning of the appointment, it's not to diagnose. If we are looking at BMI and blood pressure. In dentistry we run the risk; it's a fine line, we are not supposed to be diagnosing.

3.2.7.6 Changes to Electronic Medical Record

Since the current electronic medical record didn't have the capability to capture some of the meaningful use requirements; it was a bit hard for the staff to conceptualize how it would fit into their workflow. In the case of recording smoking status and problem list, they were recording at some level. They felt it would be important to record in a more structured manor. Changes to the EHR would need to be made to allow recording of more structured data. Staff felt that it would be great to provide patients with a summary of their visit, but they did not have the capability to easily provide that information.

3.2.7.7 Information Overload

Staff was worried that patients would suffer from information overload in the case of tailored educational materials. They wanted to maintain focus on dental education. They felt that their patients were already inundated with so much information and more information, especially regarding numerous medical issues would be a deterrent for patients returning for future appointments. Educating patients about why things were being done and giving them options was seen as important.

> I would worry about information overload. If we're getting flagged to provide them with five different brochures and four of those are medical related, are we the best place to provide that? Maybe, maybe not. It's not getting down to the focus of the care we are here to give"

3.2.7.8 Additional Staff or New Role

It was frequently mentioned that in order to meet the meaningful use criteria, there may need to be additional staff in order to do this. Perhaps a new role would be created, like a patient liaison or care facilitator. This role could do things like record weight and blood pressure, provide tailored educational material and possibly

3 Metrics and Measurements

coordinate any medical appointments. These comments dovetail with the time/priority, role, and information overload themes.

> May require another role, like a care facilitator that could do education and possibly appointments.

3.2.7.9 Non-representation of Dental Practice in MU Requirements

The staff felt that the MU use requirements in general did not necessarily represent dental practices. In particular, regarding the CQM requirements, they noticed holes. For example, cancer screenings, diabetic oral exams and 6 month cleanings are routinely done, but were not present on the list.

3.2.7.10 Data Availability to Staff and Patients

Dental staff thought it would be very helpful to be able to identify patients by condition, especially in the case of diabetes and heart disease. They felt this would be very helpful for outreach and scheduling follow up appointments. They also thought it would be helpful to identify children that fall out of the schedule and don't come back for years when they have lots of problems. Another example stated was having the ability to identify periodontal patients in order to send reminders. Staff thought is would be helpful to electronically provide patients with their dental information, or at least a subset of it. They did not feel that patients would need to see clinical notes. Managers indicated that many patients were already requesting to see their information online, especially in order to request and view appointments. Marshfield Clinic patients already have the ability to see their medical information online via a patient portal, so an expectation already exists. Appointment summaries were seen to be helpful for example in the event of a child with divorced parents.

> Yes, I can think of a lot. Diabetics, pregnant patients, every age really. We looked at patients under 18 who hadn't been seen in 18 months. We had a huge list that hadn't been seen in 18 months and they should be seen every six months. Periodontal patients, to do reminders.

3.2.8 Summary

At the beginning of the millennium, about 85% of all United States (US) general dentists used computers in their office (American Dental Association Survey Center 2001). However, only 25% of those dentists used the computer in a clinical environment. A land mark study in 2006 which focused on clinical computing in dentistry (Schleyer et al. 2006) reported that only 1.8% of all US general dentists maintain patient information in a complete electronic format. A more recent survey from the state of California focused on the Health Information Technology (HIT) in dental practices (Loeb et al. 2010). About 23% of the California dentists reported that they have fully implemented Electronic Dental Records (EDRs) in their practice and about 15% were in the process. There has been a gradual rise in the adoption of the Electronic Health Records in Dentistry; however, there are some unique barriers for adoption of EDR which has to be resolved.

As the majority of the dentists in the United States do not accept Medicare and/or Medicaid patients for various reasons, the HITECT Act does not provide the necessary push for adopting the Electronic Dental record (EDR) among dentists. Dentistry as a clinical practice has its own needs and hence "Meaningful Use" criteria defined for the EHR would not be completely relevant for the EDR. It would be wrong to apply a 'one size fits all' approach.

Even to begin realizing the "Meaningful Use" of EDR, a standardized content of the EDR has to be in place. The design of the dental record should represent and adequately document the patient care process in dentistry. EDR has the potential to become an integral part of clinical practice as dental healthcare transforms to the new era of managing the patients' health data through an electronic medium.

3.3 Significance of Using Risk Assessment Tools for Periodontal Disease in Practice

Thankam P. Thyvalikakath

3.3.1 Introduction

Recent research has significantly expanded our understanding of the etiology and pathogenesis of periodontal disease. Studies have identified many risk factors for periodontal disease (Elter et al. 1999; Genco 1996; Papapanou 1996; Pihlstrom 1994), including smoking; stress; poor diet; inadequate oral hygiene; medical conditions such as diabetes mellitus, osteoporosis and AIDS; certain medications; female hormone levels; and genetic factors. Diagnosing and treating periodontal disease successfully requires clinicians to perform a thorough patient examination and to integrate the findings into an accurate and valid assessment of the current disease state and future disease risk (Pihlstrom 2001). This assessment is a precondition for the selection of appropriate preventive and therapeutic interventions.

However, many dental diseases, including periodontal disease, are being managed using a reparative model, under which dentists and hygienists concentrate on the clinically obvious that requires immediate intervention and focusing less attention on preventing future disease (Page et al. 2005). Using this model, the treatment is essentially the same for all patients with identical clinical presentation.

This approach to care ignores individual variation in the susceptibility and risk for disease, with the consequence that not all patients receive optimal treatment. The new, risk-based approach requires clinicians to assess the patient's current disease status and risk of developing disease in the future and predominantly to manage it by preventive methods. Thus, individual patients are much more likely to receive the most appropriate treatment. The polarized distribution of diseases such as periodontal disease compels us to develop a well-defined strategy that targets preventive management for high-risk patients (Vanobbergen et al. 2001; Stamm et al. 1991). The personalization of treatment can result in appropriate use of dental resources and lower dental costs for individuals with low disease risk (Page et al. 2005; Axelsson et al. 1991, 2000, 2004; Axelsson and Lindhe 1981; Axelsson 2002; Patel et al. 2001; Stamm et al. 1991). Through long-term studies, Axelsson has found that oral health status can be improved with a net savings of 50% in treatment costs by targeting the needs of individual patients (Axelsson et al. 1991, 2000, 2004; Axelsson and Lindhe 1981; Axelsson 2002; Page et al. 2005; Midwest Business Group on Health, Juran Institute, I., and The Severyn Group, I 2003).

Recognizing this significant challenge faced by general dentists in diagnosing and treating periodontal diseases, the American Academy of Periodontology (AAP) recently developed guidelines for the management of patients with periodontal disease. The guidelines are intended to help clinicians identify patients with periodontal disease in a timely manner and consider factors that may influence future disease progression (Krebs and Clem 2006). Various multi-factorial risk assessment models have been proposed in an attempt to identify individuals at high risk for periodontal disease (Beck 1994; Tonetti 1998; Page et al. 2002; Persson et al. 2003b; Renvert and Persson 2004). The Previser Risk Calculator developed by Page et al. is based on AAP guidelines (oral communication with Dr. John Martin, Chief Scientific Officer, PreViser Corp.). Despite emerging evidence of the validity and clinical utility of risk-based diagnosis and treatment in dentistry and, specifically, periodontology, little evidence suggests that these approaches are adopted broadly in general practice (Helminen et al. 1999).

3.3.2 Description of Previser Risk Calculator

Based on the scientific evidence of the importance of risk factors in periodontal disease, Page et al. (2002) developed a computer-based risk assessment tool, the Previser Risk Calculator (PRC) (PreViser Corp., Mount Vernon, WA). The tool calculates the patient's disease score and risk score based on a mathematical algorithm that assigns relative weights to nine factors: patient age; smoking history; diagnosis of diabetes; history of periodontal surgery; pocket depth; furcation involvement; restorations or calculus below the gingival margin; and radiographic bone lesions (see Fig. 3.3).

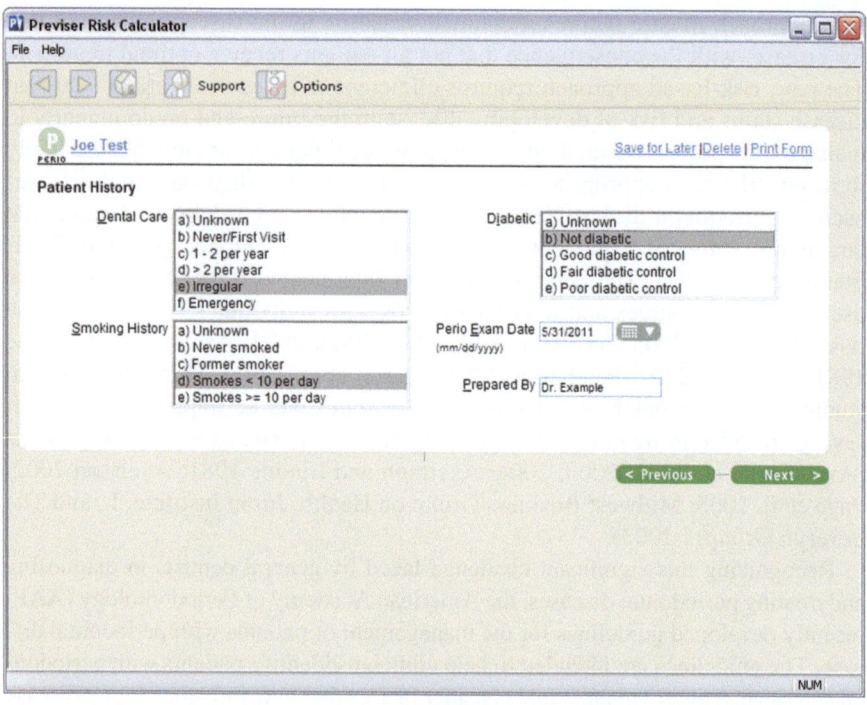

Fig. 3.3 Screenshot of Previser Risk Calculator (PRC) that shows the health history questions PRC asks about to assess patient's risk of periodontal disease

The disease score ranges from 0 (no disease) to 100 (severe periodontitis), and the risk score from 1 (lowest) to 5 (highest) (see Fig. 3.4).

The PRC was validated in a retrospective study involving 523 male participants over a period of 15 years (Page et al. 2003). Information from baseline examinations was entered into the risk calculator, and risk scores for periodontal deterioration were calculated for each subject. Actual periodontal status in terms of alveolar bone loss, determined using digitized radiographs, and tooth loss, determined from clinical records, was assessed at years 3, 9 and 15. The risk scores at baseline were found to be strong predictors of future periodontal status as measured by increasing severity and extent of alveolar bone loss and loss of periodontally affected teeth. The study concluded that risk scores that the PRC calculated from information gathered during a standard periodontal examination predicted future periodontal status with a high level of accuracy and validity. In a subsequent study, clinician subjective assessment was compared with the PRC (Persson et al. 2003a). The risk scores assigned by the expert clinicians were heterogeneous and were lower than the scores generated by the PRC. Expert clinicians assigned more subjects to the PRC low-risk group and fewer to the PRC high-risk group than did the PRC. Thus, expert clinicians varied greatly in evaluating risk, and, relative to the PRC, they appeared to underestimate the risk for periodontal disease, especially in high-risk patients.

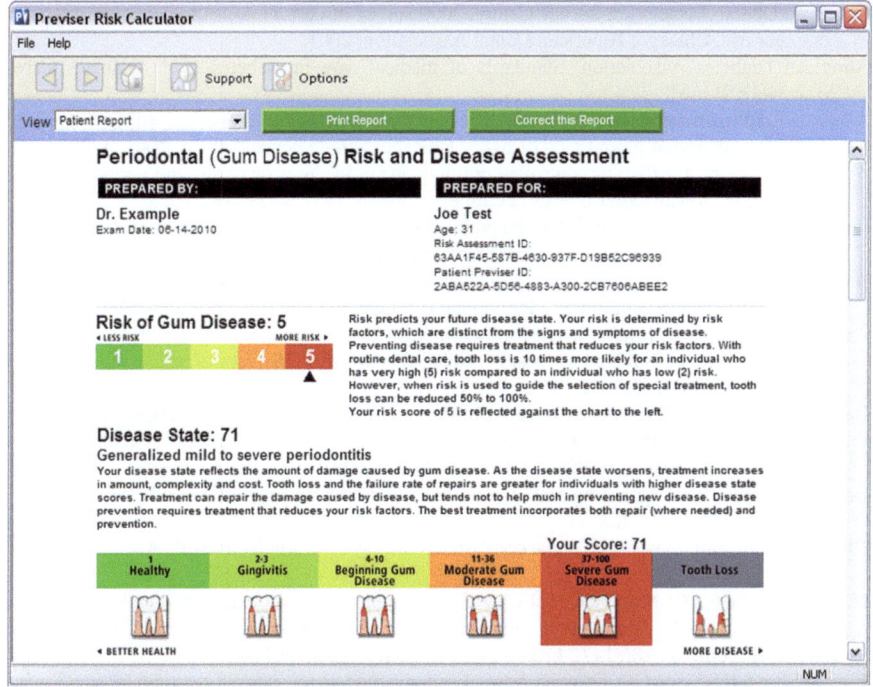

Fig. 3.4 Screenshot of Previser Risk Calculator (PRC) that shows the disease score ranging from 0 (no disease) to 100 (severe periodontitis) and the risk score ranging from 1 (lowest) to 5 (highest)

3.3.3 Summary

However, multiple barriers exist to the adoption and use of a risk-based approach for managing periodontal disease in general dental practice. Barriers to the adoption and use of a risk-based approach for managing periodontal disease include the following: (1) lack of awareness of risk-based diagnostic and treatment approaches; (2) difficulty in calculating risk without a computer algorithm; (3) progressive complexity of risk assessment algorithms; and (4) lack of integration of existing risk-based tools with computer-based patient records and practice operations.

References

AACN. Oral care for patients at risk for ventilator associated pneumonia. 2010. http://www.aacn.org/WD/Practice/Docs/PracticeAlerts/oral%20care%2004-2010%20final.pdf. Accessed 28 Jun 2011.

Albert DAA, Sadowsky D, Papapanou P, Conicella ML, Ward A. An examination of periodontal treatment and per member per month (PMPM) medical costs in an insured population. BMC Health Serv Res. 2006;6:103. Continued analysis of retrospective study proves sustained results, Aetna Health Analytics.

American Dental Association Survey Center. 2000 survey of current issues in dentistry: dentists' computer use. Chicago: American Dental Association; 2001.

American Diabetes Association. Standards of medical care in diabetes-2011. Diabetes Care. 2011;34(1):S11–61.

Axelsson P. Diagnosis and risk prediction of periodontal diseases. In: Axelsson P, editor. Diagnosis and risk prediction of periodontal diseases. Chicago: Quintessence Pub Co; 2002. p. 287.

Axelsson P, Lindhe J. Effect of controlled oral hygiene procedures on caries and periodontal disease in adults. Results after 6 years. J Clin Periodontol. 1981;8:239–48.

Axelsson P, Lindhe J, Nystrom B. On the prevention of caries and periodontal disease. Results of a 15-year longitudinal study in adults. J Clin Periodontol. 1991;18:182–9.

Axelsson P, Paulander J, Svärdström G, Kaijser H. Effects of population based preventive programs on oral health conditions. J Parodontal d'Implantol Orale. 2000;19:255–69.

Axelsson P, Nystrom B, Lindhe J. The long-term effect of a plaque control program on tooth mortality, caries and periodontal disease in adults. Results after 30 years of maintenance. J Clin Periodontol. 2004;31:749–57.

Bassani DG, da Silva CM, Oppermann RV (2006) Validity of the Community Periodontal Index of Treatment Needs (CPITN) for population periodontitis screening Cadernos de Saúde Pública 22(2):277–283. doi: 10.1590/S0102-311X2006000200005.

Beck JD. Methods of assessing risk for periodontitis and developing multifactorial models. J Periodontol. 1994;65:468–78.

CIGNA. 2006. http://newsroom.cigna.com/article_display.cfm?article_id=629. Accessed 19 Jun 2011.

Ditmyer M, Dounis G, Mobley C, Schwarz E. Inequalities of caries experience in Nevada youth expressed by DMFT index vs. Significant Caries Index (SiC) over time. BMC Oral Health. 2011;11:12. doi:10.1186/1472-6831-11-12. Accessed 18,Jun 2011.

Elter JR, Beck JD, Slade GD, Offenbacher S. Etiologic models for incident periodontal attachment loss in older adults. J Clin Periodontol. 1999;26:113–23.

Genco RJ. Current view of risk factors for periodontal diseases. J Periodontol. 1996;67:1041–9.

Helminen SE, Vehkalahti M, Ketomaki TM, Murtomaa H. Dentists' Selection of measures for assessment of oral health risk factors for Finnish young adults. Acta Odontol Scand. 1999;57:225–30.

IOM. Performance measurement: accelerating improvement. Washington DC: National Academies Press; 2006.

Keller S, Martin GC, Evenson CT, Mitton RH. The development and testing of a survey instrument for benchmarking dental plan performance: using insured patients' experiences as a gauge of dental care. J Am Dent Assoc. 2009;140:229–37.

Krebs KA, Clem DS. Guidelines for the management of patients with periodontal diseases. J Periodontol. 2006;77:1607–11.

Loeb P, McGibony R, Yeung P. Health information technology in California dental practices: survey findings. California Healthcare Foundation. 2010. http://www.chcf.org/~/media/Files/PDF/H/PDF%20HealthITInCADentalPracticesSnapshot.pdf. Accessed 18 May 2011.

Mattila ML, Rautava P, Paunio P, Ojanlatva A, Hyssälä L, Helenius H, et al. Children's dental healthcare quality using several outcome measures. Acta Odontol Scand. 2002;60(2):113–6.

Midwest Business Group on Health, Juran Institute, I., and The Severyn Group, I. Reducing the costs of poor quality health care through responsible purchasing leadership. Chicago: Midwest Business Group on Health; 2003.

NCQA. HEDIS® Criteria. 2011a. http://www.lacare.org/files/English/file/HEDIS/HEDIS%20CDC%20Tool_2011.pdf. Accessed 18 June 2011.

NCQA. National committee for quality assurance comments on the initial core set of children's healthcare quality measures for voluntary use by medicaid and CHIP Programs: CMS proposed rule CMS-2474–NC. 2011b. http://www.ncqa.org/Portals/0/Public%20Policy/NCQA%20public%20comment%20on%20CHIPRA%20core%20set.pdf. Accessed 18 June 18, 2011.

NCQA. NCQA diabetes recognition program. 2011c. http://www.ncqa.org/tabid/139/Default.aspx. Accessed 17 June 17, 2011.

Nolan T, Berwick DM. All-or-none measurement raises the bar on performance. J Am Med Assoc. 2006;295(10):1168–70. Accessed 18 June 2011.

NQMC. 2009. http://www.qualitymeasures.ahrq.gov/content.aspx?id=14998&search=dental. Accessed 17 Jun 2011.

NQMC. 2011. http://www.qualitymeasures.ahrq.gov/search/search.aspx?term=dental. Accessed 17 June 2011.

Page RC, Eke PI. Case definitions for use in population-based surveillance of periodontitis. J Periodontol. 2007;78:1387–99. doi: 10.1902/jop.2007.060264. Accessed 18 June 2011.

Page RC, Krall EA, Martin J, Mancl L, Garcia RI. Validity and accuracy of a risk calculator in predicting periodontal disease. J Am Dent Assoc. 2002;133:569–76.

Page RC, Martin J, Krall EA, Mancl L, Garcia R. Longitudinal validation of a risk calculator for periodontal disease. J Clin Periodontol. 2003;30:819–27.

Page RC, Martin JA, Loeb CF. The Oral Health Information Suite (OHIS): its use in the management of periodontal disease. J Dent Educ. 2005;69:509–20.

Papapanou PN. Periodontal diseases: epidemiology. Ann Periodontol. 1996;1:1–36.

Patel VL, Arocha JF, Diermeier M, How J, Mottur-Pilson C. Cognitive psychological studies of representation and use of clinical practice guidelines. Int J Med Inform. 2001;63:147–67.

Pennsylvania DPW 2010. Access Plus Clinical Quality Measures Based on HEDIS® 2010 Specifications. http://www.accessplus.org/Files/AccessPlusClinicalQualityMeasures2010.pdf. Accessed 4 June 2011.

Persson GR, Mancl LA, Martin J, Page RC. Assessing periodontal disease risk: a comparison of clinicians' assessment versus a computerized tool. J Am Dent Assoc. 2003a;134:575–82.

Persson GR, Matuliene G, Ramseier CA, Persson RE, Tonetti MS, Lang NP. Influence of interleukin-1 gene polymorphism on the outcome of supportive periodontal therapy explored by a multi-factorial periodontal risk assessment model (PRA). Oral Health Prev Dent. 2003b;1:17–27.

Pihlstrom BL. People at risk for periodontitis. J Periodontol. 1994;65:464–563.

Pihlstrom BL. Periodontal risk assessment, diagnosis and treatment planning. Periodontol 2000. 2001;25:37–58.

Renvert S, Persson GR. Supportive periodontal therapy. Periodontol 2000. 2004;36:179–95.

Schleyer TK, Thyvalikakath TP, Spallek H, Torres-Urquidy MH, Hernandez P, Yuhaniak J. Clinical computing in general dentistry. J Am Med Inform Assoc. 2006;13(3):344–52.

Siminerio L, Wagner EH, Gabbay R, Zgibor J. Implementing the chronic care model: a statewide focus on improving diabetes care for Pennsylvania. Clin Diab. 2009;27(4):153–9.

Stamm JW, Stewart PW, Bohannan HM, Disney JA, Graves RC, Abernathy JR. Risk assessment for oral diseases. Adv Dent Res. 1991;5:4–17.

Thyvalikakath T, Schleyer T. Underserved and medicaid providers panel – dentists. 2009. http://healthit.hhs.gov/portal/server.pt/community/healthit_hhs_gov__policy_past_meetings/1814. Accessed 18 May 2011.

Tonetti MS. Cigarette smoking and periodontal diseases: etiology and management of disease. Ann Periodontol. 1998;3:88–101.

Vanobbergen J, Martens L, Lesaffre E, Bogaerts K, Declerck D. The value of a baseline caries risk assessment model in the primary dentition for the prediction of caries incidence in the permanent dentition. Caries Res. 2001;35:442–50.

WCHQ. Diabetes, all regions. http://www.wchq.org/reporting/measures.php?topic_id=11. Accessed 18 Jun 2011.

WDAG. 2011. http://www.dhs.wisconsin.gov/health/diabetes/guidelines.htm. Accessed 18 June 2011.

Chapter 4
Broader Considerations of Medical and Dental Data Integration

Stephen Foreman, Joseph Kilsdonk, Kelly Boggs, Wendy E. Mouradian,
Suzanne Boulter, Paul Casamassimo, Valerie J.H. Powell, Beth Piraino,
Wells Shoemaker, Jessica Kovarik, Evan(Jake) Waxman, Biju Cheriyan,
Henry Hood, Allan G. Farman, Matthew Holder,
Miguel Humberto Torres-Urquidy, Muhammad F. Walji, Amit Acharya,
Andrea Mahnke, Po-Huang Chyou, Franklin M. Din, and Steven J. Schrodi

S. Foreman
Health Economics, Robert Morris University, Pittsburgh, PA, USA

J. Kilsdonk • K. Boggs
Division of Education, Marshfield Clinic, Marshfield, WI, USA

P. Casamassimo
Division of Pediatric Dentistry, The Ohio State University College of Dentistry,
Columbus, OH, USA

Center for Clinical and Translational Research, Nationwide Children's Hospital,
Columbus, OH, USA

B. Piraino
Renal Division, Department of Medicine, University of Pittsburgh Medical School,
Pittsburgh, Pennsylvania, USA

W. Shoemaker
California Association of Physician Groups, Sacramento, California, USA

E. Waxman
Department of Ophthalmology, University of Pittsburgh, Pittsburgh, PA, USA

J. Kovarik
School of Medicine, University of Pittsburgh, Pittsburgh, Pennsylvania, USA

B. Cheriyan
Holy Cross Hospital, Kottiyam and Caritas Hospital, Kottiyam, Kerala, India

H. Hood
Department of Orthodontic, Pediatric and Geriatric Dentistry,
University of Louisville School of Dentistry, Louisville, KY, USA

Underwood and Lee Clinic, Louisville, KY, USA

A.G. Farman
Department of Surgical and Hospital Dentistry,
University of Louisville School of Dentistry, Louisville, KY, USA

M. Holder
Underwood and Lee Clinic, Louisville, KY, USA

American Academy of Developmental Medicine and Dentistry, Louisville, KY, USA

M.H. Torres-Urquidy (✉)
Department of Biomedical Informatics,
University of Pittsburgh, Pittsburgh, PA, USA

M.F. Walji
Dental Branch, University of Texas,
Houston, Texas, USA

A. Acharya • A. Mahnke • P.-H. Chyou
Biomedical Informatics Research Center,
Marshfield Clinic Research Foundation, Marshfield, WI, USA

F.M. Din
HP Enterprise Services, Global Healthcare, Camp Hill, PA, USA

S.J. Schrodi
Center for Human Genetics, Marshfield Clinic Research Foundation, Marshfield, WI, USA

W.E. Mouradian
Department of Pediatric Dentistry, Schools of Dentistry, Medicine and Public Health,
University of Washington, Seattle, WA, USA

S. Boulter
Department of Pediatrics, Dartmouth Medical School, Hanover, NH, USA

V.J.H. Powell
Department of Computer and Information Systems, Clinical Data Integration Project,
Robert Morris University, Moon Township, PA, USA

4.1 Economics of Clinical Data Integration

4.1.1 A Cost Benefit Analysis of Expanding Dental Insurance Coverage

Stephen Foreman

4.1.1.1 Introduction

Dental health insurance coverage in the United States is either nonexistent (Medicare and the uninsured), spotty (Medicaid) and limited (most employer-based private benefit plans). Perhaps as a result, dental health in the United States is not good. What public policy makers may not appreciate is that this may well be impacting medical care costs in a way that improved dental benefits would produce a substantial return to investment in expanded dental insurance coverage.

On the surface, it would appear to be politically and economically difficult or impossible to expand dental insurance coverage at this time. Health insurance costs have been rising at double digit rates. Most employers have been dropping health care coverage rather than expanding it (Kaiser Family Foundation 2010). Medicare trust funds are bankrupt (Social Security and Medicare Boards of Trustees 2011). Adding coverage would exacerbate an already alarming problem. Medicaid funding is a major source of state government deficits. Many states are slashing Medicaid coverage during this time of crisis (Wolf 2010). Improving Medicaid dental coverage during times of budget crisis would meet substantial political resistance.

Strikingly, strong and increasing evidence suggests relationships between oral health and a range of chronic illnesses. For example, recent findings show relationships between periodontal inflammatory conditions and diabetes, myocardial infarction, coronary artery disease, stroke, preeclampsia and rheumatoid arthritis. This suggests that improved oral health may well have the potential to reduce the incidence of chronic diseases as well as their complications. If chronic disease incidence is reduced it may be possible to avoid medical care costs related to treating them. It would be important to know more about the extent to which improved oral health could reduce health care costs and improve lives.

There are few, if any, studies of the costs of providing Medicare dental benefits, the costs of improving the Medicaid dental benefit or the cost of providing dental insurance to the uninsured. There are a few studies that indicate that periodontitis increases medical care costs, perhaps by as much as 20% (Ide et al. 2007; Albert et al. 2006).[1] Ideally there should be a controlled study to assess the benefit of providing dental coverage through a government payer system. For a preliminary inquiry we can consider work already done and using some cost and benefit estimates, determine whether it is possible that benefits of extending dental coverage may outweigh costs.

4.1.1.2 Dental Insurance and Coverage in the United States

The failure of Medicare to cover dental care has engendered some (albeit not much) public debate. In 2003, Congress enacted the Medicare Prescription Drug, Improvement, and Modernization Act (Medicare Part D). By 2009 Medicare provided $56.6 billion in benefit payments for outpatient prescription drugs and Medicaid paid 15.7 billion for outpatient prescription drugs (Center for Medicare and Medicaid Services 2010). Beneficiaries provided billions more in the form of monthly Part D premiums. The expense of the Medicare prescription drug program and the controversy surrounding its enactment may well have eroded public support for increased Medicare coverage. So while there has been no shortage of effort paid to improving Medicare, the one common theme in all of the recent initiatives is that dental care has been conspicuously

---

[1] A new study by Hedlund, Jeffcoat, Genco and Tanna funded by CIGNA of patients with Type II diabetes and periodontal disease found that medical costs of patients who received maintenance therapy were $2483.51 per year lower than patients who did not. CIGNA, Research from CIGNA Supports Potential Association between Treated Gum Disease and Reduced Medical Costs for People with Diabetes, http://newsroom.cigna.com/NewsReleases/research-from-cigna-supports-potential-association-between-treated-gum-disease-and-reduced-medical-costs-for-people-with-diabetes.htm, March 29, 2011, accessed June 23, 2011; Jeffcoat M (2011). Personal communication, 20 June 2011.

omitted. As a result, 43 million Medicare recipients in 2009 (US Census Bureau 2011) continue to have no dental insurance coverage through Medicare.[2]

Medicaid dental coverage is an optional benefit that states may or may not elect to provide. In Medicaid, both the State and the Federal government provide funds to cover healthcare services to eligible patients. The bulk of the money comes from the Federal government. Because the Medicaid dollars are limited and coverage for systemic diseases has precedence, Medicaid coverage of dental care has been spotty. Even where it has been provided, payments to dental providers have been so low as to make it difficult or impossible for Medicaid beneficiaries to obtain adequate dental care (Broadwater 2009). The 2008 recession increased the number of Medicaid eligible individuals nationwide. Further, the federal budget deficits of the past few years have reduced the federal contribution to state Medicaid programs. The combination of increases in the number of beneficiaries and diminished revenues has caused a number of states to eliminate or curtail Medicaid dental coverage (eHow 2011; Mullins et al. 2004). The result, 49 million Medicaid beneficiaries in the US (US Census Bureau 2011) in 2009 either had no dental insurance coverage or inadequate coverage.

Approximately 52 million people in the United States do not have health insurance (Kaiser Family Foundation 2010). Presumably, they have no dental insurance either. Further, not every employer provides dental insurance. A 1995 CDC survey found that 44.3% of adults do not have dental insurance coverage (Centers for Disease Control 1997). A 2006 Montana survey found that 53% of employers who offer health insurance do not offer dental insurance coverage (Montana Business Journal 2006). In 2009 there were approximately 202 million people enrolled in health insurance plans (US Census Bureau 2011). If half (a rough combination of the CDC and Montana percentages) of them do not have dental insurance it is likely that an additional 101 million (nonelderly, non-poor) people in the US do not have dental insurance coverage.

Finally, the term "dental insurance" is actually a misnomer.[3] Dental policies cover routine treatments, offer discounts for more complex treatment and impose a low yearly on total payments. In fact, it has been called "part insurance, part prepayment and part large volume discount" (Manski 2001). Effectively, many (if not most) people who have dental insurance find it coverage to be quite restrictive. For example, many impose a small yearly cap ($1,500 is common) or large coinsurance amounts (50% for orthodontia, for example) (Rubenstein 2005). Even with discounts it is easy for many people to exceed the annual limit.

Given the lack of dental insurance coverage it is not surprising that the status of oral health in the US is not particularly good. In 2002 approximately 26.5% of adults between the ages of 35 and 44 had untreated caries, 42% had decayed, missing and filled tooth surfaces and more than one-half of adults had gingival bleeding (Dental, Oral and Craniofacial Data Resource Center of the National Institute of Dental and Craniofacial Research 2002). Three fourths of adults in the US have gingivitis and 35% have periodontitis (Mealey and Rose 2008). If these levels of untreated disease were applied to most systemic diseases, there would be public outcry.

---

[2]Some of them may have dental insurance coverage through their retirement health insurance.
[3]Perhaps it might more accurately be called a dental plan.

4.1.1.3 The Relationship Between Dental Problems and Chronic Illness

Over the past decade evidence has been building that there is a relationship between dental disease, particularly periodontal disease, and chronic illnesses. Mealey and Rose note that there is strong evidence that "diabetes is a risk factor for gingivitis and periodontitis and that the level of glycemic control appears to be an important determinant in this relationship" (Mealey and Rose 2008). Moreover, diabetics have a six times greater risk for worsening of glycemic control over time compared to those without periodontitis and, periodontitis is associated with an increased risk for diabetic complications. For example, in one study more than 80% of diabetics with periodontitis experienced one or more major cardiovascular, cerebrovascular or peripheral vascular events compared to 21% of the diabetic subjects without periodontitis (Thorstensson et al. 1996). Also, a longitudinal study of 600 type 2 diabetics found that the death rate from ischemic heart disease was 2.3 times higher in subjects with severe periodontitis and the death rate from diabetic nephropathy was 8.5 times higher (Saremi et al. 2005). Clinical trials have demonstrated that treatment of periodontal disease improved glycemic control in diabetics (Miller et al. 1992). Moreover, investigations have found an association between periodontal disease and the development of glucose intolerance in non-diabetics (Saito et al. 2004). While it is difficult to establish causality and it is possible that other factors influence periodontal disease and medical complications, these studies suggest that treatment of periodontitis substantially improves health and greatly reduces medical complications related to diabetes.

Similarly, periodontitis is associated with cardiovascular disease and its complications including ischemia, atherosclerosis, myocardial infarction and stroke. A study by Slade and colleagues found both a relationship between periodontitis and elevated serum C- reactive protein levels (systemic marker of inflammation and documented risk factor for cardiovascular disease) as well as a relationship among body mass index, periodontitis and CRP concentrations (Slade et al. 2003). Hung and colleagues evaluated the association between baseline number of teeth and incident tooth loss and peripheral arterial disease. They determined that incident tooth loss was significantly associated with PAD, particularly among men with periodontal disease potentially implying an oral infection-inflammation pathway (Hund et al. 2003). The same group of researchers used the population enrolled in the Health Professionals' Follow-Up Study (41,000 men free of cardiovascular disease and diabetes at baseline) to assess the relationship between tooth loss and periodontal disease and ischemic stroke. Controlling for a wide range of factors including smoking, obesity, and dietary factors, the researchers found a "modest" Association between baseline periodontal disease history and ischemic stroke (Joshipura et al. 2003). As early as 1993 DeStefano and colleagues found that among 9760 subjects, those with periodontitis had a 25% increased risk of coronary heart disease relative to those without. The association was particularly high among young men. The authors questioned whether the association was causal or not, suggesting that it might be a more general indicator of personal hygiene and possibly health care practices (DeStefano et al. 1993). In 2000 Wu and colleagues used data from the First National Health and Nutrition Examination Survey and its Epidemiologic Follow-Up Study to examine the association between periodontal disease and cerebrovascular accidents. The study found that periodontitis was a significant risk factor for total CVA, in particular, for non-hemorrhagic stroke (Wu et al. 2000).

In addition to diabetes and coronary artery disease, associations have been found between periodontal disease and rheumatoid arthritis and respiratory disease. This is not surprising given the role of periodontal disease in the production of inflammation related proteins. Dissick and colleagues conducted a pilot study of the associate ion between periodontitis and rheumatoid arthritis using multivariate regression and chi square tests. They found that periodontitis was more prevalent in patients with rheumatoid arthritis than in the control group and that patients who were seropositive for rheumatoid factor were more likely to have moderate to severe periodontitis than patients who were RF negative and also that patients who were positive for anti-cyclic citrullinated peptide antibodies were more likely to have moderate to severe periodontitis (Redman et al. 2010). Paju and Scannapeico investigated the association among oral biofilms, periodontitis and pulmonary infections. They noted that periodontitis seems to influence the incidence of pulmonary infections, particularly nosocomial pneumonia in high-risk subjects and that improved oral hygiene has been shown to reduce the occurrence of nosocomial pneumonia. They found that oral colonization by potential respiratory pathogens, for possibly fostered by periodontitis and possibly by bacteria specific to the oral cavity contribute to pulmonary infections (Paju and Scannapeico 2007).

4.1.1.4 Implications for Health Policy

The implications for these findings are profound. Professionally, they suggest that managing patients with chronic illness and periodontal disease will require teamwork and a deeper knowledge base for dentists and for physicians (Mealey and Rose 2008). Dentists will need to be alert for early signs of chronic illness among their patients and physicians will need to be alert for signs of dental disease. Both will need to consider wider treatment options than their specialty indicates. Dentistry and medicine have operated as professional silos in the past. The relationship between dental disease and chronic medical conditions suggests that continued separation is detrimental to patient centered care.

Beyond treatment implications, there are extremely important health policy concerns. If treatment of periodontitis and other dental problems leads to reduced incidence of chronic illness, fewer complications from chronic diseases and reduced morbidity among chronically ill patients, increased access to dental services could significantly reduce health care costs.

The diseases associated with periodontitis are among the most common illnesses, the fastest growing and the most expensive diseases that we treat. A recent Robert Wood Johnson report notes that approximately 141 million Americans have one or more chronic conditions, that the number of people with chronic conditions is expected to increase by 1% per year for the foreseeable future and that the most common chronic conditions include hypertension, disorders of lipid metabolism, upper respiratory disease, joint disorders, heart disease, diabetes, cardiovascular disorders, asthma and chronic respiratory infections (Anderson 2010) (see Fig. 4.1).

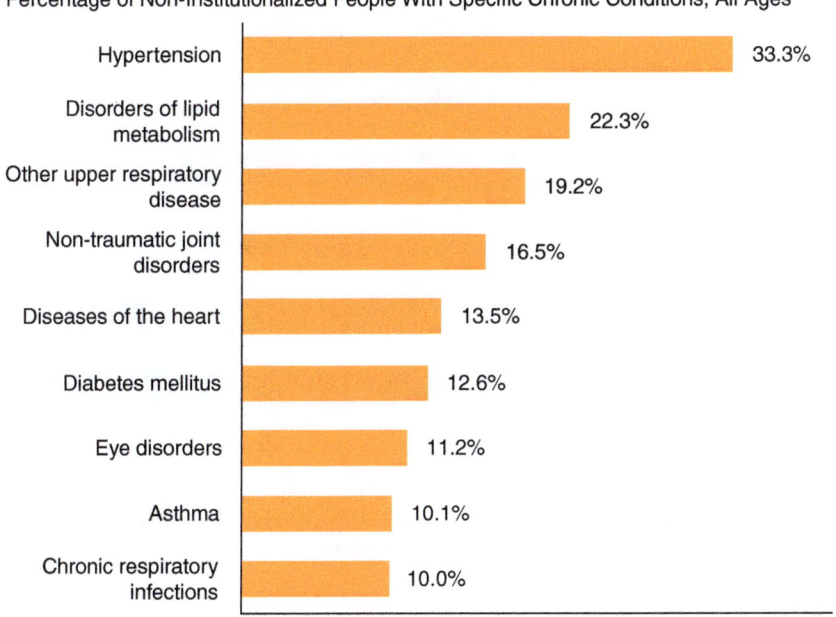

Fig. 4.1 Most common chronic US illnesses. Anderson (2010) (Copyright 2010. Robert Wood Johnson Foundation. Used with permission from the Robert Wood Johnson Foundation)

One in four Americans has multiple chronic conditions. Ninety-one percent of adults aged 65 and older have at least one chronic condition and 73% have two or more of them (Anderson 2010). People with chronic conditions account for 84% of all healthcare spending. Seventy eight percent of private health insurance spending is attributable to the 48% of privately insured persons with chronic conditions. Seventy three percent of healthcare spending for the uninsured is for care received by the one third of uninsured people who have chronic conditions. Seventy nine percent of Medicaid spending goes to care for the 40% of non-institutionalized beneficiaries who have chronic conditions (Anderson 2010) (see Fig. 4.2).

Further, health care spending increases with the number of chronic conditions (Anderson 2010) (see Fig. 4.3). More than three fifths of healthcare spending (two thirds of Medicare spending) goes to care for people with multiple chronic conditions. Those with multiple chronic conditions are more likely to be hospitalized, fill more prescriptions, and have more physician visits (Anderson 2010).

In 2002 the American Diabetes Association estimated direct medical expenditures for diabetes at $91.8 billion: $23.2 billion for diabetes care, $24.6 billion for chronic complications and $44.1 billion for excess prevalence of general medical conditions. Approximately 52% of direct medical expenditures were incurred by people over 65. Indirect expenditures included lost workdays, restricted productivity mortality and permanent disability – a total of $39.8 billion. All told, diabetes was found to be responsible for $160 billion of $865 billion in total

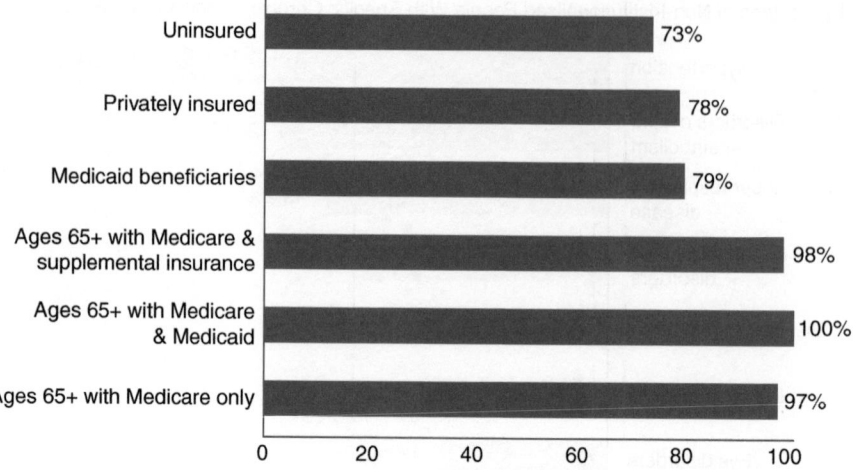

Fig. 4.2 Percentage of healthcare spending for individuals with chronic conditions by type of insurance – 2006. Anderson (2010) (Copyright 2010. Robert Wood Johnson Foundation. Used with permission from the Robert Wood Johnson Foundation)

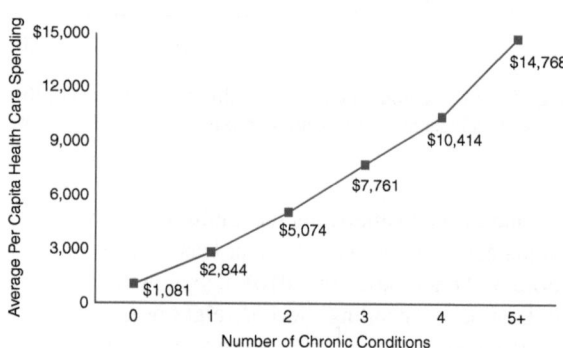

Fig. 4.3 Per capita healthcare spending and number of chronic conditions – 2006. Anderson (2010) (Copyright 2010. Robert Wood Johnson Foundation. Used with permission from the Robert Wood Johnson Foundation)

expenditures. Per capita medical expenditures totaled $13,000 annually for people with diabetes and $2600 for people without diabetes (Hogan et al. 2002). More recently, Dall and colleagues estimated that the US national economic burden of prediabetes and diabetes had reached $218 billion in 2007, $153 million in higher medical costs and $65 billion in reduced productivity. Annual cost per case was estimated at $2,900 for undiagnosed diabetes and 10,000 for type 2 diabetes (Dall et al. 2010).

The costs of caring for people with diabetes have risen both because the numbers of diabetics has been increasing and because the per capita costs of care have increased. The number of diabetics increased from 5.8 million on 1980 to 14.7 million in 2004 (Ashkenazy and Abrahamson 2006). A recent report by the UnitedHealth Group Center for Health Reform & Modernization provides a dire estimation – that more than 50% of adult Americans could have diabetes (15%) or prediabetes (37%) by 2020 at a cost of $3.35 trillion over the decade. This compares with current estimates of 12% of the population with diabetes and 28% with prediabetes, or 40%. These estimates conclude that diabetes and prediabetes will account for 10% of total healthcare spending in 2020 at an annual cost of $500 billion, up from an estimated $194 billion in 2010 (UnitedHealth Center for Health Reform and Modernization 2010). Average annual spending over the next decade by payer type is $103 billion for private health insurance, $204 billion for Medicare, $11 billion for Medicaid and $16.6 billion for the uninsured.

What about cardiovascular disease and rheumatoid arthritis? Among the top ten health conditions requiring treatment for Medicare beneficiaries in 2006 approximately 50% of beneficiaries suffered from hypertension, 25% from heart conditions, 33% had hyperlipidemia 24% had COPD, 23% had osteoarthritis and 22% had diabetes (Thorpe et al. 2010). The American Heart Association estimates the 2010 cost of cardiovascular disease and stroke to be $324 billion in direct expenditures and $41.7 billion for productivity losses due to morbidity and $137.4 billion in lost productivity due to mortality (present value of lost wages at 3%) (Lloyd-Jones et al. 2010). The Centers for Disease Control estimates that during 2007–2009 50 million Americans had self-reported doctor diagnosed arthritis, 21 million of them with activity limitations (Cheng et al. 2010). Cisternas and colleagues estimated that total expenditures by US adults with arthritis increased from $252 billion in 1997 to $353 billion in 2005. Most of the increase was attributable to people who had co-occurring chronic conditions (Cisternas et al. 2009). The Cisternas study appears to aggregate all medical care expenditures by people with arthritis (which would include expenditures to treat diabetes and cardiovascular disease). An earlier CDC study focused on the direct and indirect costs in 2003 attributable to arthritis that estimated $80.8 billion in direct costs (medical expenditures) and $47 billion in indirect costs (lost earnings) (Yelin et al. 2007).

In short, current cost estimates for direct health care expenditures (excluding productivity losses) related to diabetes are approximately $190 billion, for cardiovascular treatment, $324 billion, and for rheumatoid arthritis, approximately $111 billion (estimating that the $80.8 billion in 2003 costs have grown approximately 6% per year), a total of $625 billion of the $2.6 trillion that will be spent in the US in 2010. Moreover, given current growth in the prevalence of diabetes, the UnitedHealth estimate of $500 million in 2020 spending for diabetes alone is not unreasonable. If health care costs attributable to diabetes, cardiovascular disease and rheumatoid arthritis only increase by 100% over the next decade (even given added demand produced by the aging baby boomer population), annual costs of these chronic diseases will exceed $1.2 trillion in 2020.

If we use the UnitedHealth estimates for the proportions of diabetes costs paid by private insurance (48%), Medicare (38%), Medicaid (6%) and the uninsured (8%) and estimate total costs based on the 2010 studies projecting a 50% increase in 5 years and a 100% increase in 10 years we can obtain an estimate of future costs for treating diabetes, cardiovascular disease and arthritis. Table 4.1 set forth below, summarizes these cost estimates. By 2020 Medicare costs for these chronic illnesses

Table 4.1 US Medical care cost estimates for diabetes, cardiovascular disease and arthritis (millions of dollars)

			2010	2015	2020
	Diabetes		190	285	380
	Cardiovascular		324	486	648
	Arthritis		111	167	222
	Total		**$625**	**$938**	**$1,250**
Private		0.48	300	450	600
Medicare		0.38	238	356	475
Medicaid		0.06	38	56	75
Uninsured		0.08	50	75	100

would be approximately $475 billion. The estimated costs to Medicaid will be approximately $75 billion. The costs for the uninsured will be approximately $100 billion. Any intervention that has the potential to substantially reduce these costs will produce meaningful results.

Unfortunately, even though there had been a substantial numbers of studies that show relationships between dental disease and chronic illness that are have been very few studies that actually test whether improved dental treatment reduces the incidence of chronic illness and complications due to chronic illness. The potential for large health care cost savings through an active and aggressive program of dental care is so large that such studies are clearly indicated.

4.1.1.5 Potential Benefits of an Aggressive Dental Treatment Plan

Suppose, for example, that 10% of all medical care costs required to treat diabetes, cardiovascular disease and arthritis could be avoided through an active aggressive program of dental care.[4] What this would mean is that in 2020 private health insurers could see a $60 billion reduction in healthcare costs, Medicare would see a $47.5 billion reduction and Medicaid pay $7.5 billion reduction. Recent health reform has provided for the issuance of health insurance to the uninsured by state exchanges. Aggressive dental care that saved 10% of costs attributable to diabetes, cardiovascular disease and arthritis could save the exchanges $10 billion per year. And, if greater proportions of costs can be saved or if the 2020 estimates of costs are low, potential benefits will be even larger. Once again, it would be important to know whether aggressive dental care could produce such savings and how much.

---

[4]Ide and colleagues found that people who were treated for periodontitis incurred 21% higher health care costs than those who were free of periodontal disease (Ide et al. 2007). Similarly, Albert, et al., found medical costs associated with diabetes, cardiovascular disease and cerebrovascular disease were significantly higher for enrollees who were treated for periodontitis than for other dental conditions (Albert et al. 2006). Additional studies of this nature would be important to support a measured approach to expanding dental coverage.

4.1.1.6 Costs of an Aggressive Dental Treatment Plan

So what do we mean by an aggressive dental treatment plan? Suppose we were to provide dental insurance to all Medicare beneficiaries at the level of current private dental insurance coverage and strongly encourage beneficiaries to receive dental treatment. Suppose we were to provide for Medicaid payment for all beneficiaries at the level of current private dental insurance coverage. Suppose health care insurers provided dental coverage in order to reduce their costs and that such coverage was consistent with current private dental insurance coverage. Suppose health insurance companies, understanding the benefits from dental care, were to require their private employer customers to cover the costs of dental care. How much would all of this cost? How would it compare to the benefits that may be available?

In order to estimate the potential costs of providing enhanced coverage for dental care we start use the CMS estimates of national health care spending for dental services and Statistical Abstract of the US estimates for Medicare enrollment, Medicaid enrollment, private health insurance enrollment and uninsured persons. Based on the estimate that half of private employers with health insurance provided dental insurance coverage we estimate that of the private health insurance enrollment one half would have dental insurance coverage and one half would not. Table 4.2 sets forth the national health care expenditures for dental services in millions and enrollment in private dental plans, Medicare, Medicaid, the uninsured without health insurance and dental insurance, the uninsured with health insurance and dual eligibles.

From this we derive a cost per enrollee for private dental insurance, Medicare dental benefits and Medicaid dental benefits. Table 4.2 also sets forth the calculations for 2000–2009. For example, per beneficiary costs in 2009 for private health dental insurance was $494.66. As expected given the lack of Medicare coverage and the low level of Medicaid coverage, per beneficiary expenditures in 2009 were $6.73 for Medicare beneficiaries and $146.75 for Medicaid beneficiaries.

In order to estimate the annual cost of providing full dental coverage to Medicare beneficiaries we subtracted dual eligibles (who receive some dental insurance) from total Medicare enrollees to determine the number of persons who would need coverage. In our 2009 example there were 43 million Medicare beneficiaries including 9 million dual eligibles. Accordingly, the estimates would cover the 34 million Medicare beneficiaries that are not dual eligible at a cost equal to the per capita cost of private dental insurance ($494.66) less amounts that Medicare is already paying for dental services ($6.73 per person). The result provides an estimate of the cost of covering all Medicare beneficiaries for dental services at a level equivalent to private health insurance. Using the 2009 example the cost of providing full dental insurance coverage to Medicare beneficiaries would have been $16.6 billion.

In addition, we used the CMS national health expenditure figures to determine administrative costs for private health insurance, Medicare and Medicaid as a percentage of program expenditures for medical care. We found that the administrative costs of the Medicare program were 6.2% on average for 1966–2009. In order to fully estimate the cost of Medicare dental coverage we added 6.2% to the cost

Table 4.2 Estimated cost to provide full dental coverage

Spending/millions	2000	2001	2002	2003	2004	2005	2006	2007	2008	2009
Private	31,175	34,158	36,464	37,359	40,472	42,871	45,137	47,836	49,142	49,960
Medicare	81	86	79	70	71	86	103	164	222	290
Medicaid	2,312	3,124	3,467	3,745	4,005	4,229	4,378	4,758	5,818	7,147
Enrollment in millions										
Private dental coverage	101	100	100	99	100	101	101	101	101	101
Medicare	38	38	38	40	40	40	40	41	43	43
Medicaid	30	32	33	36	38	38	38	40	43	49
Uninsured	40	41	44	45	44	45	47	46	46	50
Uninsured w/health cov	101	100	100	99	100	101	101	101	101	101
Dual eligible	12	11	11	11	8	9	9	9	9	9
Per enrollee cost										
Private	310	342	366	378	403	426	448	476	487	495
Medicare	2	2	2	2	2	2	3	4	5	7
Medicaid	78	99	104	105	105	111	114	120	137	147
Pct cost increase										
Private		10.2%	7.2%	3.0%	6.7%	5.8%	5.0%	6.3%	2.2%	1.7%
Medicaid		26.2%	5.6%	0.7%	0.2%	5.3%	3.0%	5.1%	13.7%	7.5%

Cost to cover/millions										
Medicare	7,913	9,268	9,839	10,559	12,635	13,314	13,929	15,340	16,368	16,589
Medicaid	6,835	7,675	8,700	9,696	11,305	12,007	12,764	14,091	14,909	16,943
Uninsured	12,340	14,080	15,978	16,990	17,526	19,091	21,036	21,752	22,527	24,881
Uninsured w/health cov	31,175	34,158	36,464	37,359	40,472	42,871	45,137	47,836	49,142	49,960
Cost incl admin										
Medicare 6.2%	8,404	9,843	10,450	11,214	13,419	14,139	14,792	16,291	17,382	17,618
Medicaid 7.6%	7,354	8,258	9,361	10,433	12,164	12,919	13,734	15,162	16,042	18,231
Uninsured-exchanges 7.6%	13,278	15,150	17,193	18,281	18,858	20,542	22,634	23,405	24,240	26,772
Uninsured w/health cov	33,545	36,754	39,235	40,199	43,548	46,129	48,567	51,471	52,877	53,757

estimates. In 2009, for example the added cost of providing full dental insurance coverage to 34 million Medicaid beneficiaries would have been $17.6 billion.

Similarly, we calculated the per person cost of bringing Medicaid payment for dental services up to the level of private dental insurance. To do this we deducted the per capita amounts provided to Medicaid beneficiaries for dental services from the amounts paid on behalf of private health insurance beneficiaries and multiplied the difference by the number of Medicaid beneficiaries in the US. For example, in 2009 there were 48.7 million Medicaid beneficiaries. The cost of upgrading their dental insurance benefits which have been 48.7 million times $494.66 less $146.75 or $16.9 billion. After adding administrative costs of 7.6% the cost of upgrading Medicaid to private insurance levels in 2009 would have been $18.2 billion.

Health insurers will be in the same position as Medicare and Medicaid regarding dental coverage. If quality dental coverage saves health care costs attributable to diabetes, cardiovascular disease and rheumatoid arthritis then the exchanges will have an incentive to provide quality dental coverage to reduce costs. Accordingly, we estimated the cost of providing dental coverage equivalent to private dental insurance coverage through the exchanges. Again we assume that the costs of such coverage will be equivalent to the number of uninsured persons multiplied by the annual per capita cost of coverage.[5] For the 2009 example, this would reflect coverage for 52 million people at $494.66 per person, a total of $24.9 billion. With administrative costs, the cost of providing dental insurance coverage to the uninsured at a level equivalent to private dental coverage would be $26.8 billion.

Finally, given the evidence that improved dental care has the potential to reduce health care costs private health insurers may wish to expand health insurance to cover dental care.[6] Here, we estimate the cost of providing dental insurance to the 50% of the workforce whose employers currently do not provide dental insurance benefits. Once again, we multiply the number of covered lives by the estimated annual per capita cost. For the 2009 example we estimate 101 million adults will receive dental coverage at $495 per person: $50 billion for dental services and $3.8 billion for administrative costs or a total of $53.8 billion.

Of course, as noted a number of times above, these estimates are based on providing full "universal" dental insurance coverage at levels equivalent to current benefit levels for private dental insurance. It may be that an appropriate package of dental services that deals specifically with periodontitis can be provided for less than the full cost of private dental insurance. Once again, further research should provide better information.[7]

---

[5]The health reform law does not attempt to provide coverage to all 52 million people without health insurance. Estimates are that only 31 million people will be covered by the bill. Even though this is the case we prepare our estimates using all 52 million uninsured Americans.

[6]Indeed, the failure of 50% of employers to cover dental services may well constitute a classic externality in the market for health insurance. Internalizing this externality may well provide better efficiency.

[7]It is also possible that dental care for persons with greater incidence of chronic illness as is the case with Medicare beneficiaries may require even higher levels of spending per beneficiary. Again, it would be good to know scientifically if this is the case.

Table 4.3 Estimated medical care costs, expanded dental coverage costs and percent of medical costs that would need to be saved to justify coverage

	Medical care costs	Insurance costs	Percent medical
Private	300	53.8	17.9%
Medicare	238	17.6	7.4%
Medicaid	38	18.2	48.5%
Uninsured	50	26.8	53.6%

4.1.1.7 Comparing Costs and Benefits

As noted in Sect. 6 above, 2010 costs for diabetes, cardiovascular disease and arthritis will be $300 billion for private health insurance, $238 billion for Medicare, $38 billion for Medicaid and $50 billion for the uninsured. Costs of providing "full" dental coverage will be $17.6 billion for Medicare, $18.2 billion for Medicaid, $26.8 billion for the uninsured and $53.8 billion for private health insurance. Given this, if 7.4% or more of the Medicare costs can be "saved" through improved dental care, Medicaid dental insurance will pay for itself and will provide a positive return on investment. See Table 4.3. Similarly, private health insurers could justify providing dental insurance coverage to employees who do not have it so long as they spend 17.9% or more of their chronic care costs for diabetes, cardiovascular disease and arthritis. On the other hand, it would appear that Medicaid expansion would require cost savings of approximately 48% and that health care insurance coverage of the uninsured would require savings of approximately 54% in order to justify coverage. While it is possible, it may not be likely that full dental coverage would be justified for these programs.

Of course, these estimates do not consider indirect costs in the form of lost wages or premature death. These costs are externalities to the health insurance programs. To the extent that they represent a social benefit that a national dental insurance program might internalize, it would be appropriate to consider their impact in the cost-benefit analysis.

In any event, better understanding of the potential for deriving savings in health insurance costs related to chronic diseases like diabetes, cardiovascular disease and arthritis would be crucial to any determination whether to expand insurance coverage for dental care.

4.1.1.8 Expanded Dental Insurance Coverage

Heretofore the case for expanding Medicare coverage to include dental care has taken the form of "benefit" to patients rather than benefit to health insurance programs and society and has been cast in emotional and political terms. For example, Oral Health America grades "America's commitment to providing oral health access to the elderly" (Oral Health America 2003). In truth, there is no American commitment to providing oral health access to any age group, much less the elderly. Rubenstein notes that "at least one commentator has suggested that the dental profession should join with senior citizen groups when the time is right to ask Congress to expand Medicare to cover oral health" (Rubenstein 2005). Rubenstein emphasizes that "calls for action" are "mere words" unless they are accompanied by political actions that health policy professionals and the dental profession must help promote (Rubenstein 2005). Another commentator has suggested that "as soon as the debate over Medicare prescription drug coverage and, the debate to provide dental care coverage for the elderly may soon begin" (Manski 2001). Rubenstein, again suggests that "the dental community must convince Americans, and particularly aging boomers, that oral health is integral to all health, and for that reason, retiree dental benefits are an important issue".

In truth, a decade of deficit spending and public distaste for out of control program costs in the Medicare and Medicaid programs as well as the unpopularity of the process that was used to provide Medicare prescription drug coverage (with perceived abuses by the health insurance and drug lobbies) and national health reform makes it unlikely that the public would be willing to approve expansions in insurance coverage for dental care "for its own sake" or "as the right thing" or to "benefit seniors." What this political climate has produced is an arena in which a good idea that could provide appropriate return on investment for society might well be rejected out of hand based on political history of health insurance coverage. As a result, it is incumbent on policymakers, medical and dental research scientists and health economists to investigate and confirm the potential savings that expansion of dental insurance coverage has the potential to produce and to develop hard evidence regarding potential costs of the expansion prior to, not as a part of, political efforts aimed at dental coverage expansion. A responsible, well informed effort to expand dental coverage may well go far to restore public confidence in the health policy process.

4.1.2 Economics of Clinical Data Integration

Joseph Kilsdonk and Kelly Boggs

4.1.2.1 Introduction

The adage of "putting your money where your mouth is" is often referenced when being challenged about public statements or claims. In this instance, we use it literally. In 2008 health care costs in US were $2.2 Trillion. There have been numerous reports on health disparities, the burden of chronic diseases, increasing healthcare costs and the need for change. Long-term economic benefits associated with the cost of care are dependent upon integrating oral health with medicine. This is particularly true as it relates to the management of those conditions which impact the economics of healthcare the most. As examples, 96% of Medicare costs and 83% of Medicaid costs are in managing chronic health conditions (Partnership for Solutions National Program Office 2004). More than 40% of the U.S. population has one or more chronic condition (Cartwright-Smith 2011) and in 2006, 76% of Medicare spending was on patients with five or more chronic diseases (Swartz 2011). Effective management of health care resources and information are critical to the economic well-being of our healthcare system. We can no longer afford to manage care in isolation. Integration of care between medicine and dentistry holds much promise in terms of reducing the cost of care and an integrated Medical-Dental Electronic Healthcare Record (iEHR) is the vehicle that will lead to downstream cost savings.

4.1.2.2 The Economics of Integrated Decision Making

In the United States the Center for Medicare & Medicaid Services (CMS) has conducted demonstration projects around chronic disease management. Section 121 of the Benefits Improvement and Protection Act of 2000 mandated CMS to conduct a disease management demonstration project. April 1, 2005, as an effort to reduce the cost of care and improve quality associated with chronic diseases, CMS partnered with ten premier health systems to effectively manage chronic diseases in a Medicare Physician Group Practice Demonstration (PGP). It was the first pay-for-performance initiative for physicians under the Medicare program (Center for Medicare and Medicaid Services 2010). It involved giving additional payments to providers based on practice efficiency and improved management of chronically ill patients. Participants included ten multispecialty group practices nationwide, with a total of more than 5,000 physicians, who care for more than 200,000 Medicare beneficiaries (Frieden 2006). The chronic diseases that were targeted were based on occurrence in the population and included diabetes, heart failure, coronary artery disease, and hypertension (Frieden 2006). The partners CMS selected were; Billings Clinic, Billings, Montana Dartmouth-Hitchcock Clinic, Bedford, New Hampshire; The Everett Clinic, Everett, Washington; Forsyth Medical Group, Winston-Salem, North Carolina; Geisinger Health System, Danville, Pennsylvania; Marshfield Clinic, Marshfield, Wisconsin; Middlesex Health System, Middletown, Connecticut; Park Nicollet Health Services, St. Louis Park, Minnesota; St. John's Health System, Springfield, Missouri; University of Michigan Faculty Group Practice, Ann Arbor, Michigan. Under the PGP, physician groups continued to be paid under regular Medicare fee schedules and had the opportunity to share in savings from enhancements in patient care management. Physician groups could earn performance payments which were divided between cost efficiency for generating savings and performance on 32 quality measures phased in during the demonstration as follows: year 1, 10 measures, year 2, 27 measures and years 3 and 4 having 32 quality measures. For each of the 4 years only the University of Michigan Faculty Group Practice and Marshfield Clinic, earned performance payments for improving the quality and cost efficiency of care. A large part of the success of this project was attributed to being able to extract, evaluate, and monitor key clinical data associated with the specific disease and to manage that data through an electronic health record (Table 4.4).

During the third year of the demonstration project Marshfield Clinic, using a robust electronic health record succeeded in saving CMS $23 million dollars; that's one clinic system in 1 year. As a result of such demonstration projects and as of this

Table 4.4 A table of the quality measures from the PGP initiative

Diabetes mellitus	Congestive heart failure	Coronary artery disease	Preventive care
HbA1c management	Left ventricular function assessment	Antiplatelet therapy	Blood pressure screening
HbA1c control	Left ventricular ejection fraction testing	Drug therapy for lowering LDL cholesterol	Blood pressure control
Blood pressure management	Weight management	Beta-Clocker therapy – prior MI	Blood pressure control plan of care
Lipid measurement	Blood pressure screening	Blood pressure	Breast cancer screening
LDL cholesterol level	Patient education	Lipid profile	Colorectal cancer screening
Urine protein testing	Beta-blocker therapy	LDL cholesterol level	
Eye exam	Ace inhibitor therapy	Ace inhibitor therapy	
Foot exam	Warfarin therapy for patients HF		
Influenza vaccination	Influenza vaccination		
Pneumonia vaccination	Pneumonia vaccination		

writing, CMS is looking to establish Accountable Care Organization's as the medical front runners to new care delivery methods for quality and cost control. Accountable Care Organization (ACO) is a term used to describe partnerships between healthcare providers to establish accountability and improved outcomes for the patients. In a CMS workshop on October 5, 2010, Don Berwick, the administrator of CMS, stated "An ACO will put the patient and family at the center of all its activities..." An emerging model of an ACO is the patient-centered medical home (PCMH). PCMH is at the center of many demonstration projects. ACOs were derived from studies piloted by CMS. Since funds provided by CMS, do not cover routine dental care as part of the patient management or quality and cost objectives CMS ACO studies are limited if they become models for the PCMH, due to the exclusion of dental.

More recently, organizations representing the major primary care specialties – the American Academy of Family Practice, the American Academy of Pediatrics, the American Osteopathic Association, and the American College of Physicians – have worked together to develop and endorse the concept of the "patient-centered medical home," a practice model that would more effectively support the core functions of primary care and the management of chronic disease (Fisher 2008). In 2011 Geisinger Health System, Kaiser Permanente, Mayo Clinic, Intermountain Healthcare and Group Health Cooperative announced they will be creating a project called the Care Connectivity Consortium. This project is intended to exchange patient information. Although progressive in their approach their project does not include dental.

These benefits however, are yet to be adapted in the arena of oral health. As of this writing, dentistry remains largely separate from medical reimbursement mechanisms such as shared billing, integrated consults, diagnosis, shared problem lists, and government coverage. For example, CMS does not cover routine dental care. Dentistry is also working to establish its own "dental home" with patients. However to reap the economic benefits of integrated care, a primary care "medical-dental" home is what needs to be created.

According to an Institute of Oral Health Report (2010) it is widely accepted across the dental profession that oral health has a direct impact on systemic health, and increasingly, medical and dental care providers are building to bridge relationships that create treatment solutions. The case for medical and dental professionals' co-managing patients has been suggested for almost the past century, in 1926 William Gies reported that "The frequency of periodic examination gives dentists exceptional opportunity to note early signs of many types of illnesses outside the domain of dentistry" (Gies 1926). As described by Dr. Richard Nagelberg, DDS "The convergence of dental and medical care is underway. Our patients will be the beneficiaries of this trend. For too long, we have provided dental care in a bubble, practicing – to a large degree – apart from other health-care providers. Even when we consulted with our medical colleagues, it was to find out if premedication was necessary, get clearance for treatment of a medically compromised patient, or find out the HbA1c level of a diabetic individual, rather than providing true patient co-management. We have made diagnoses and provided treatments without the benefit of tests, reports, metrics, and other information that predict the likelihood of disease development and progression, as well as favorable treatment outcomes. We have practiced in this manner not due to negligence, but because of the limitations of tools that were available to us" (Nagelberg 2011). Integrated medical/dental records need to be a tool in a providers' toolbox. In the case of Marshfield Clinic, dental was not included in their past CMS demonstration project as dental is not a CMS covered benefit, and thus not part of the demonstration. However, as a leader in healthcare, the Marshfield Clinic recognizes the importance of data integration for both increased quality and cost savings. "Marshfield Clinic believes the best health care comes from an integrated dental/medical approach," said Michael Murphy, director, Business Development for Cattails Software. Integration enhances communication between providers and can ultimately lead to better management of complex diseases with oral-systemic connection, avoidance of medical errors, and improved public health.

While the CMS PGP and other demonstration projects along with independent studies have shown to improve quality and reduce costs through integration, greater results may be afforded if studies are not done in isolation from dental data. In fact, if healthcare does not find a way to manage the systemic nature of the 120 pathogens known to the oral cavity the economic impact and cost savings around chronic disease management will hit a ceiling. The economic opportunity of having clinical data for integrated decision making is readily identified by the insurance industry. The effective management of clinical data around chronic and systemic oral and medical disease as part of an iEHR is the greatest healthcare cost savings opportunity associated with such a tool.

4.1.2.3 Insurance Industry Studies Show the Way

The insurance industry sustains itself through risk management [obtaining best outcomes] using actuarial analysis [data] and controlling costs [reduction of costs] in order to ensure coverage [profitability]. As such they have pursued the economic and outcome benefits of integrated medical – dental clinical decision making. As an example, in 2009 there was a study conducted by the University of Michigan, commissioned by the Blue Cross Blue Shield of Michigan Foundation (2009), the study included 21,000 Blue Cross Blue Shield of Michigan members diagnosed with diabetes who had access to dental care, and had continuous coverage for at least 1 year. With regular periodontal care, it was observed diabetes related medical costs were reduced by 10%. When compounding chronic health complications were also examined, the study showed a 20% reduction in cost related to the treatment of cardiovascular disease in patients with diabetes and heart disease. A 30% reduction in cost related to treatment of kidney disease for patients with diabetes and kidney disease. And a 40% reduction in costs related to treating congestive heart failure for patients with diabetes and congestive heart failure. According to a joint statement by lead researchers, and Blue Cross Blue Shield of Michigan executives, "Our results are consistent with an emerging body of evidence that periodontal disease…it addresses quality of care and health care costs for all Michigan residents."

Also, at the Institute for Oral Health conference in November 2007 Joseph Errante, D.D.S., Vice President, Blue Cross Blue Shield of MA reported that 2003 Blue Cross Blue Shield of Massachusetts claims data showed medical costs for diabetics who accessed dental care for prevention and periodontal services averaged $558/month, while medical costs for diabetics who didn't get dental care were about $702/month (Errante 2007). Similarly insured individuals with cardiovascular diseases who accessed dental care had lower medical costs, $238/month lower than people who did not seek dental treatment (Errante 2007). The cost is $144 less per visit for those diabetics who accessed prevention and periodontal services. Those savings could be translated into access to care or additional benefits for more individuals.

In the case of neonatal health there is similar research. Over 12% of all births in the U.S. are delivered preterm, with many infants at risk of birth defects (Martin et al. 2009). According to a January 2006 statement issued by Cigna, announcing their CIGNA Oral Health Maternity Program, "the program was launched in response to mounting research indicating an increased probability of preterm birth for those with gum disease. These research-based, value-added programs are designed to help improve outcomes and reduce expense" (CIGNA 2006). The program was initially designed to offer extended dental benefits free of charge to members who were expecting mothers, citing "research supporting the negative and costly impact periodontal disease has on both mother and baby." According to research cited by CIGNA, expecting mothers with chronic periodontal disease during the second trimester are seven times more likely to deliver preterm (before 37th week), and the costs associated with treating premature newborns is an average of 15 times more during their first year, and premature newborns have dramatically more healthcare challenges throughout their life. CIGNA also cited the correlation between periodontal disease and low birth weight, pre-eclampsia, gestational diabetes as additional rationale to support extended dental benefits to expecting mothers. Six months later CIGNA initiated Well Aware for Better Health, an extended benefits free of charge program for diabetic and cardiovascular disease patients aimed at "turning evidence into action by enhancing dental benefits for participants in disease management" programs. It is interesting to note, not only does CIGNA offer extended dental benefit to targeted groups, they also reimburse members for any out-of-pocket expenses associated to their dental care (co-pays, etc.)

In 2006, Columbia University researchers conducted a 2-year retrospective study of 116,306 Aetna PPO members with continuous medical and dental insurance, exhibiting one of three chronic conditions (diabetes mellitus, coronary artery disease, and cerebrovascular disease) (Aetna 2008). Researchers found members who received periodontal treatments incurred higher initial per member per month medical costs, but ultimately achieved significantly lower health screening (Episode Risk Group/ERG) risk scores than peers receiving little or no dental care. Convinced by the data and understanding lower risk scores ultimately leads to healthier people and cost savings, Aetna initiated the Dental/Medical Integration (DMI) Program in 2006. Aetna's DMI program offers enhanced benefits in the form of free-of-charge extended benefit dental care to Aetna's 37.2 million Indemnity, PPO and Managed Choice medical plan members, specifically targeting members deemed at-risk, including those who are pregnant, diabetic, and/or have cardiovascular disease and have not been to a dentist in 1 year As a result of various outreach methods during the pilot, 63% of at-risk members who had not been to a dentist in the previous 12 months, sought dental care (Aetna 2008). "The findings from this latest study we conducted continue to show that members with certain conditions who are engaged in seeking preventive care, such as regular dental visits, can improve their overall health and quality of life," said Alan Hirschberg, head of Aetna Dental (Aetna 2008).

Delta Dental of Wisconsin understands the connection between oral and systemic health and has created a program that is designed to offer members with certain chronic health conditions the opportunity to gain additional benefits. More than 2,000 groups now offer Delta Dental of Wisconsin's Evidence-Based Integrated Care Plan (EBICP) option (Delta Dental of Wisconsin 2011). EBICP provides expanded benefits for persons with diseases and medical conditions that have oral health implications. These benefits include increased frequency of cleanings and/or applications of topical fluoride. They address the unique oral health challenges faced by persons with these conditions, and can also play an important role in the management of an individual's medical condition. EBICP offers additional cleanings and topical fluoride application for persons who are undergoing cancer treatment involving radiation and/or chemotherapy, persons with prior surgical or nonsurgical treatment of periodontal disease and persons with suppressed immune systems. The EBIC offers additional cleanings for persons with diabetes and those with risk factors for IE, persons with kidney failure or who are on dialysis and for women who are pregnant.

The iEHR provides the insurance industry in partnership with the healthcare industry an integrated tool to facilitate these health and subsequently economic outcomes across medicine and dentistry.

4.1.2.4 Economic Benefits of Increased Efficiency and Patient Safety Through iEHR

In addition to the anticipated savings through better outcomes using integrated clinical data, an example of a positive economic outcome associated with an integrated record as related to increased efficiency and patient safety is found in the United States Veterans Administration (VA) hospitals and clinics. The VA is one of the few institutions that have implemented the shared electronic medical–dental record successfully. The VA has the ability to be the "one stop shop" for their patients. An April 2010 press release published on the Department of Veterans Affairs website highlighted the success of VA's health information technology in terms of cost reductions and "improvements in quality, safety, and patient satisfaction" (Department of Veterans Affairs 2010). The press release spotlighted a recent study conducted by the public health journal, Health Affairs, which focused on VA's health IT investment from 1997 to 2007. The study confirmed that while VA has spent $4 billion on their technology initiative, a conservative estimate of cost savings was more than $7 billion. After subtracting the expense of the IT investment, there was a net savings of $3 billion for the VA during the 10 years covered by the study (McBride 2011). Furthermore, the study estimated that "more than 86 percent of the savings were due to eliminating duplicated tests and reducing medical errors. The rest of the savings came from lower operating expenses and reduced workload." Independent studies show that the VA system does better on many measures, especially preventive services and chronic care, than the private sector and Medicare. VA officials say "its [integrated] technology has helped cut down hospitalizations and helped patients live longer" (Zhang 2009).

Recently, the Journal of Obstetrics and Gynecology reported on a tragic loss of life due to the systemic nature of oral health. A study found oral bacteria called Fusobacterium nucleatum was the likely culprit in infecting a 35-year-old woman's fetus through her bloodstream (Carroll 2010). The doctors determined that the same strain of oral bacteria found in the woman's mouth was in the deceased baby's stomach and lungs. Integrated records would provide critical data to the Obstetrician including oral health issues and when the patient had her last dental exam. How does one measure the economic impact of a life not lived and another derailed by such tragedy?

In a randomized controlled study, Lopez et al. (2005) determined that periodontal therapy provided during pregnancy to women with periodontitis or gingivitis reduced the incidence of preterm and of low birth weight. The institute of Medicine and National Academies estimate that preterm births cost society at least $23billion annually (Albert et al. 2011). Data integration of the iEHR enables the effective management between the dentist and obstetrician to ensure proper periodontal therapy has been provided during pregnancy. Such management based on the Lopez et al. study, will have direct impact in reducing the prevalence per preterm births leading to reduced health care costs.

There have also been studies indicating a correlation between poorer oral hygiene or deficient denture hygiene and pneumonia or respiratory tract infection among elderly people in nursing homes or hospitals (Rosenblum 2010; Ghezzi and Ship 2000; Scannapieco 2006). One such study of 141 elderly persons in two nursing homes in Japan (Adachi et al. 2002) concluded that "the number of bacteria silently aspirating into the lower respiratory tract was lower in the group who received professional oral care, which resulted in less fatal aspiration pneumonia in that group." Over the 24 month period of the study, of the 77 patients receiving professional oral care, 5% died of pneumonia versus 16.7% of the 64 patients that died of the same cause who maintained their own oral hygiene. Lack of access is certainly a key factor to consider. However, lack of available data respective to the interrelationship between oral health and systemic health also contributed to the apathy in these cases.

As identified above, complications are correlated to cost. As conditions compound, costs go up. Marshfield Clinic, as part of their iEHR is creating a shared problem list that identifies both oral and medical conditions and history to recent visits and medication lists for monitoring at point of care [be it a medical or dental visit], such cross access to clinical data and care management milestones serves as a tool to prevent conditions from compounding and escalating costs such as those described above.

4.1.2.5 Other Areas of Economic Impact Relative to iEHR Clinical Data

Several other areas of economic impact will be seen as iEHR's become broadly deployed. Some of these are listed as follows:

- Medication management. A great deal of provider and allied support time is spent obtaining medication information between dentistry and medicine [and vice versa] including current medications, contraindications, tolerances, etc. Marshfield Clinic Cattails software has created a dashboard that readily identifies this for both the medical and dental providers. Not is time saved but chances for complications or escalation of conditions is reduced [both of which impact cost]. For example an integrated record allows medical providers treating respiratory infections to include or exclude oral flora as the possible source of the infection which would lead to more knowledgeable prescribing decision on the antibiotic used.
- Coordination of care has a direct impact on cost for the system and the patient. For example, in 2008 55.6% of the US population aged 2 years and older that was diagnosed diabetes had been to the dentist in the past year (Healthy People 2020 (2010)). The US government's program Healthy People 2020 includes an initiative to increase the proportion of people with diagnosed diabetes who have at least an annual dental examination. The American Diabetes Association recommends that diabetic patients be seen semi-annually and more if bleeding gums or other oral issues are present. The American Diabetes Association also recommends the consultation between the dentist and doctor to decide about possible adjustments to diabetes medicines, or to decide if an antibiotic is needed before surgery to prevent infection. The target from the Healthy People 2020 is a 10% improvement at 61.2%. Integrated medical/dental records could allow for the coordination of efforts between providers to include communication of treatment plan and services leading to quicker resolution, increased patient compliance, and less patient time away from work or home and potentially less travel.

- Similarly, integrated records also create a platform to integrate clinical appointing between medicine and dentistry. As such, combative patients or severely disabled patients needing anesthesia in order for care to be delivered can be treated with one hospital sedation vs. multiple sedations. Family Health Center of Marshfield, Inc. (FHC) Dental Clinics shares an iEHR with Marshfield Clinic and uses it integrated scheduling feature to complete dental care, lab work, ENT care, woman's health, preventive studies, all in one visit.
- Follow up care management can be more focused and coordinated. For example, without the knowledge or dental conditions, medical providers could spend months attempting to control diabetes with periodontal disease. However, with access to an iEHR, the practitioner or allied care manager can determine patient's oral health status immediately to determine possible influence of periodontal disease.
- Similarly an iEHR with a shared patient data dashboard brings to light history and physical examination data without having to have patients be the historian to their physician on their last dental visit or for the dentist to have to rely on the patient's recall of medications or medical diagnosis. For example, if an integrated record saved providers 5 min per hour of patient care, that would be 40 min per day. Imagine giving a physician or dentist 40 min more a day. In a capitated system, this allows for more patients to be seen in a day for roughly the same amount of expenditure. In a production based clinic this allows more patients to be seen and more charges per day. In either case, the investment into informatics is covered. In an underserved area, more patients get care quicker, which creates the opportunity for quicker resolution, which can lead to a healthier society, which in turn may lead them back to a productive livelihood sooner.
- An iEHR results in one system for acquisition, orientation, training and support. PC based owners who also own a Mac and Mac owners who also have to operate a PC can relate. Need we say more? Imagine if your PC function just like a Mac [or your Mac function just a PC]. No cross learning of software quirks. Not having to purchase two separate units to begin with. Reduced costs, increased space. Not having to jump from one computer to the other computer to get data from one data from another to create a report. Not having to call two separate computer companies for service or updates.
- Third Party Coordination. Having an iEHR creates a platform for interfacing with third party payers. A common system and language for timely reimbursement. In part, the result of an iEHR is driving the diagnostic coding for dentistry. Such an integrated interface provides a tool to bridge with healthcare payors that historically kept payment as segregated as the oral and medical health professions. The iEHR overcomes that limitation. Timely payment, consolidation of payment, expansion of covered patient and provider benefits based on clinical integration, and a viable system for interfacing are all potential economic benefits of iEHR clinical data.
- The iEHR creates new horizons for research that will lead to cost saving discoveries. As example, knowing the benefits of research, Marshfield Clinic Research Foundation (MCRF) has created an Oral and Systemic Health Research Project

(OSHRP). The creation of OSHRP, led by Dr. Murray Brilliant, will allow MCRF to capitalize on its existing and growing strengths in the areas of complex disease interactions and Personalized Health Care (PHC) to advance oral health and the health of the rest of the body. The OSHRP has three specific goals:

- Understand the connections between oral and systemic health (diabetes, heart disease, pre-term births)
- Understand the causes of oral diseases and determine the effect of genetics, diet, water source (well/city + fluoridation) and microbiome.
- Understand how improving oral health aids systemic health (comparative effectiveness) and bring Personalized Health Care (PHC) to the dental arena.

- The OSHRP research resource will be unique in the nation. As MCRF has done with other projects, it will share this resource with qualified investigators at other academic institutions both within and outside of Wisconsin. OSHRP will advance scientific knowledge, improve healthcare and prevention, reduce the cost of oral healthcare, and create new economic opportunities. Such knowledge will have a direct economic impact on the cost of care and care management.
- The iEHR creates an ability to have an integrated patient portal to comprehensively maintain their health. Portals are becoming more and more popular in the healthcare industry as a means to helping maintain compliance with care management recommendations and preventative procedures. Portals provide patents a tool to stay up to date on their care and recommendations. Portals can take iEHR clinical data, adapt it through programming, and provide creative visual reinforcement for patients as they monitor their health status. The more patients engage in owning their health status, the more preventative services are followed through with. The more medicine and dentistry can leverage the prevention potential [which insurance companies have come to realize] the more likely costly conditions can be avoided.

4.1.2.6 Conclusion

The link between oral health and systemic health is well documented. The separation of dental and medical is not a sustainable model in modern healthcare delivery. A new model of integrated care is necessary. Aristotle said, "The whole is greater than the sum of its parts." Increased access to combined medical and dental histories and diagnosis at the providers' fingertips makes vital information available. Shared diagnosis between physicians and dentists could aid in formulating interventions and to accelerate decision making abilities by allowing for prioritizing of medical/dental procedures. Clinical management and treatment of the patient would be expedited with immediate access to both records. Quality could be improved through a complete picture of the patient through the dashboard. All of which have a direct or indirect economic benefit.

The iEHR will be the tool that facilitates such delivery and the studies and scenarios described in these pages point to significant economic benefits to patients, payors, and providers. If increased access, multi-provider monitoring, shared problems lists with enhanced decision making abilities from iEHR could reduce healthcare costs. The greatest cost reduction will be with using the iEHR to manage chronic disease. A combined dental-medical electronic record with a shared data informatics platform is most likely to yield the best long-term economic solution while maintaining or enhancing positive patient outcomes.

4.2 Provider Viewpoints

This section reveals viewpoints from a variety of medical and dental providers. One section focuses on optimal use of ophthalmic imaging, which should show how that the challenges of clinical data integration go beyond those encountered in the effort to bring oral health and systemic health together.

4.2.1 Integration of Pediatric Medical and Pediatric Dental Care

Wendy E. Mouradian, Suzanne Boulter, Paul Casamassimo,
and Valerie J. Harvey Powell

Oral health is an important but often neglected part of overall health. Historically separate systems of education, financing and practice in medicine and dentistry fuel this neglect, contributing to poorer health outcomes for vulnerable populations such as children, while increasing costs and chances for medical error for all patients. Advances in understanding the impact of oral health on children's overall health, changing disease patterns and demographic trends strengthen the mandate for greater integration of oral and overall healthcare, as reviewed in two recent Institute of Medicine reports (IOM 2011a, b). The pediatric population could realize substantial benefit from oral disease prevention strategies under a coordinated system of care enhanced by integrated electronic health records (EHR). This approach would benefit all children but especially young children and those from low socioeconomic, minority and other disadvantaged groups who are at higher risk for oral disease and difficulties accessing dental care.

This section focuses on the pediatric population and the need for close collaboration of pediatric medical and dental providers. First we consider how a child's developmental position and their parents' level of understanding might affect oral health outcomes. Next we address the importance of children's oral health and the urgency of seizing missed opportunities to prevent disease. We then briefly outlines some steps to preventing early childhood oral disease utilizing some of the many health providers that interact with families. Finally we examine one pediatric hospital's approach to choosing an integrated EHR technology.

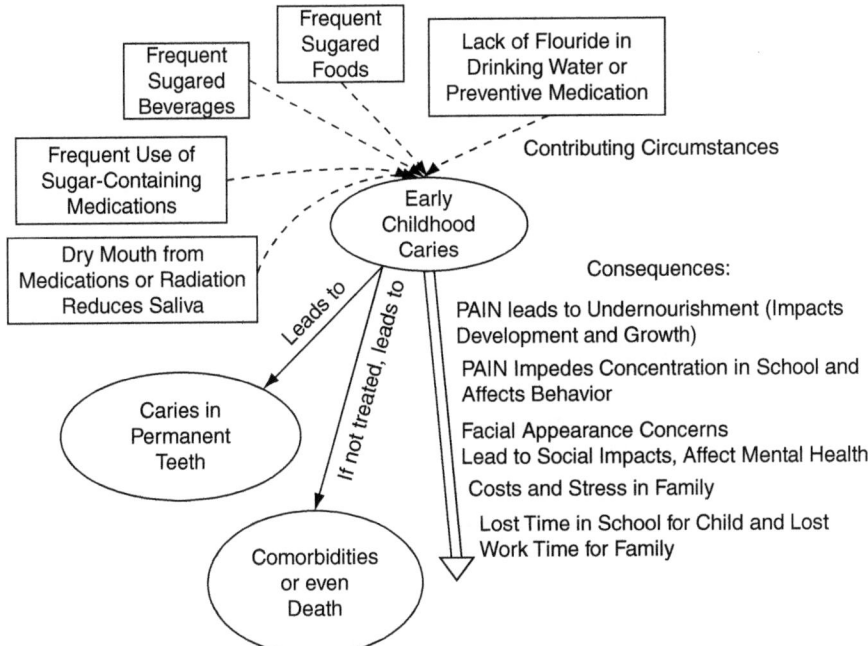

Fig. 4.4 Delivering oral healthcare to a child

4.2.1.1 A Childs-Eye View of Oral Health

Children have unique characteristics which distinguish their needs from those of adults. Children's developmental immaturities may increase their risks for poor oral health outcomes (Fig. 4.4). For example, a child…

- May not be able to communicate pain, discomfort and other symptoms,
- May not recognize a particular sensation or lesion as a symptom or sign of disease,
- May not grasp the consequences of poor oral health habits,
- May not realize the consequences of consuming quantities of sugared foods or beverages,
- Likely does not realize the consequences of chronic use of sugared medications,
- Does not understand the long-term consequences of early childhood caries,
- Does not know the potential for systemic spread of disease from a toothache, or for liver damage due to overuse of acetaminophen or other analgesics,
- Must learn good oral health habits from parents/caregivers
- Must trust parents/caregivers to judge the appropriateness of and necessity for health care, and
- Does not understand how the health care system works and cannot access care without an adult.

All children, but especially young children, are limited in their ability to care for their own health and must depend upon adults. A child's parent/caregiver may also lack basic oral health knowledge and an awareness of their child's oral health needs, and/or suffer from poor oral health themselves. Low oral health literacy is prevalent among patients and health professionals alike in America; individuals of low socioeconomic status or from ethnically diverse backgrounds may be at particular risk for low oral health literacy (IOM 2011a). Without appropriate education, a parent....

- May not correctly interpret a child's symptoms or signs of oral disease
- May not know that caries is an infectious disease that can be spread to a child by sharing spoons, for example,
- May not know the potential value of chewing gum with Xylitol,
- May not fully grasp the importance of good oral health hygiene habits,
- May not grasp the consequences of a child consuming quantities of sugared foods or beverages,
- May have difficulty controlling the child's consumption of sugared foods or beverages in or out of the home,
- May not realize the consequences of chronic use of sugared medications,
- May not know the potential for systemic spread of disease from a toothache, or for liver damage due to overuse of acetaminophen or other analgesics,
- May not grasp the long-term consequences of early childhood caries,
- May live in a community without fluoride in the tap water and not know about alternative sources of fluoride,
- May overlook oral health due to the stress of living in poverty,
- May be fearful of dentists or oral health care due to their own experiences,
- May have difficulty locating a dental provider accepting public insurance, or have other problems navigating the health care system.

Parents in turn depend on access to medical and dental providers with current understanding of the most effective ways to prevent caries and promote the child's oral and overall health. An important element in helping families is the provision of culturally-sensitive care to a diverse population. Children are the most diverse segment of the population with 44% from minority backgrounds compared with 34% of the overall population (US Census Bureau 2010).

The separation of medical and dental systems and the lack of shared information can create additional barriers for families, especially for those with low health literacy or facing linguistic or cultural barriers. All pediatric health professionals have increased ethical and legal responsibilities to promote children's health, including advocacy for them at the system level (Mouradian 1999).

4.2.1.2 Children's Oral Health: Impact of Missed Opportunities

Although many factors can influence children's oral health outcomes, caries is largely a preventable disease. Despite this, national trends and other data on children's oral health attest to this persistent national problem (Mouradian et al. 2009). Some important facts include the following....

- Caries is the most prevalent chronic disease of childhood,
- Caries is a preventable disease unlike many chronic diseases of childhood,
- Yet according to (NICDR 2011) 42% of children 2–11 have had dental caries in their primary teeth; 23% of children 2–11 have untreated dental caries. Further, "21% of children 6–11 have had dental caries in their permanent teeth; 8% of children 6–11 have untreated decay." Overall "[c]hildren 2–11 have an average of 1.6 decayed primary teeth and 3.6 decayed primary surfaces,"
- The latest epidemiologic evidence shows increasing rates of caries for youngest children, reverse from the Healthy People 2010 goal of decreasing caries. According to (NICDR 2011), overall "dental caries in the baby teeth of children 2–11 declined from the early 1970s until the mid 1990s. From the mid 1990s until the most recent (1999–2004) National Health and Nutrition Examination Survey, this trend has reversed: a small but significant increase in primary decay was found. This trend reversal was more severe in younger children."
- Disparities in children's oral health and access to care persist by age, income level, race and ethnicity, and parental education level (Edelstein and Chinn 2009). Of concern, the latest increase was actually in a traditionally low-risk group of young children (Dye and Thornton-Evans 2010).
- The human and economic costs of early childhood caries are substantial (Casamassimo et al. 2009). According to Catalanotto (2010), health consequences include...
  – extreme pain,
  – spread of infection/facial cellulitis, even death (Otto 2007)
  – difficulty chewing, poor weight gain
  – falling off the growth curve (Acs et al. 1999)
  – risk of dental decay in adult teeth (Broadbent et al. 2005; Li and Wang 2002)
  – crooked bite (malocclusion)
- Children with special health care needs (CSHCN) may be at higher risk for oral disease and difficulties accessing care. Analyzing data from the National Survey of Children with Special Health Care Needs, (Lewis 2009) found that "CSHCN are more likely to be insured and to receive preventive dental care at equal or higher rates than children without special health care needs. Nevertheless, CSHCN, particularly lower income and severely affected, are more likely to report unmet dental care need compared with unaffected children." Children who were both low-income and severely affected had 13.4 times the likelihood of unmet dental care needs,
- Dental care is the highest unmet health care need of children; 4.6 million children had unmet dental care needs because families could not afford care compared with 2.8 million with unmet medical needs for the same reasons (CDC 2008),
- According to the National Survey of Children's Health, children are 2.6 times as likely to lack dental as medical insurance (Lewis et al. 2007),

- There is evidence that children who get referred to a dentist early may have lower costs of care and disease. Savage et al. (2004) reported that children "who had their first preventive visit by age 1 were more likely to have subsequent preventive visits but were not more likely to have subsequent restorative or emergency visits" and concluded that preschool "children who used early preventive dental care incurred fewer dentally related costs,"
- Ramos-Gomez and Shepherd (1999), in their "Cost-effectiveness Model for Prevention of Early Childhood Caries," conclude that preventive ECC interventions could reduce ECC by 40–80% for a particularly vulnerable population of children, and that part of the costs of interventions will be offset by savings in treatment costs.

As these facts convey, and the deaths of more than one child from consequences of untreated caries make painfully clear, there is an urgent need for more attention to the oral health needs of children. A more coordinated system for oral health care including integrated EHR would be an important advance.

4.2.1.3 A Model for Intervention: Creating a System of Care

A glance at Table 4.5, an ideal model, reveals that intervention should begin before birth and that a range of medical and oral health professionals can contribute to the child's oral health. Early intervention is necessary because of the transmissibility of cariogenic bacteria from mother/caregiver to infant, and importance of oral health practice in preventing disease. The following professionals may be involved:

- *pediatric medical provider*family physician
    - pediatrician
    - pediatric nurse
    - nurse practitioner in pediatric/family practice
    - physician assistant in pediatric /family practice
- obstetrician
- obstetric nurse/nurse midwife
- general dentist
- pediatric dentist
- pediatric dental hygienist
- pharmacist
- other appropriate allied health professionals

The availability of some of these professionals can be affected socioeconomic status, health insurance, place of residence, or by a child's special health care need.

One obvious limitation on developing a "relay" as in Table 4.5, with a "hand-off" from family care to obstetric care to pediatric care is the education of the medical providers. As part of pre-conception and perinatal healthcare, providers should address oral health, but may lack the knowledge to do so. Additionally, as noted by Ressler-Maerlaender et al. (2005), "some women may believe that they or their

Table 4.5 Timeline of some oral health interventions to prevent early childhood caries (ECC) – birth to 3 years age (Marrs et al. 2011; Lannon et al. 2008; Han et al. 2010; Ezer et al. 2010; AAP 2008; Mouradian et al. 2000)

Child's age	Intervening professional(s)	Intervention, rationale, conditions and strategy
Planning conception, prenatal and perinatal	Family physician Obstetrician/nurse midwife Obstetric nurse General dentist	The physician and/or obstetric provider educates mother-to-be about good maternal oral hygiene and infant oral health issues, including transmissibility of caries. Mother's dentist assesses and treats caries, gingivitis or other oral health problems and educates the mother-to-be
Neonatal	Obstetric nurse	Obstetric nurse advises new mother to chew Xylitol gum, limit salivary contact between mother and infant, and help child avoid sugar intake (exposure) while asleep and from common sugar sources (medicines, sugared water, bottle feeding on demand at night with fluid other than water – following tooth eruption, certain foods), and to schedule dental exam at 1 year age
6 months	Pediatric medical provider	First dental examination recommended by AAPD *when the first tooth comes in, usually between 6 to 12 months*
	Pediatric/general dentist	Educate mother about optimal fluoride levels
	Dental hygienist or other allied dental professional	Anticipate window of infectivity: 17–36 months; period when deciduous teeth are erupting
		Caries- risk assessment tool[1]
		Presence of disabilities and other special health care needs may increase child's risk of disease
9 months	Pediatric medical provider refers to establish dental home for child	Assure child has dental home by 1 year
1 year	Pediatric medical	Pediatric or general dentist able to provide infant oral health care may not be available in rural areas or for families of lower socioeconomic status
	Professional provider delivers preventive oral healthcare if no pediatric /general dentist is available	Caries risk assessment tool[1]
		Anticipate that ECC can affect children as soon as teeth erupt

(continued)

Table 4.5 (continued)

Child's age	Intervening professional(s)	Intervention, rationale, conditions and strategy
2 years	Pediatric medical provider	Assure child has dental home
	Pediatric dentist	If no dental home, then administer oral health risk assessment
	Pediatric dental hygienist	Child may begin to use fluoride toothpaste with supervision
		Pediatric preventive care vital if pediatric dental care not available
		If primary water source is fluoride-deficient, consider fluoride supplementation or fluoride varnish
3 years	Pediatric medical provider	Assure child has dental home
	Pediatric/general dentist	Pediatric preventive care vital if pediatric dental care not available
	Pediatric dental hygienist	If primary water source is fluoride-deficient, consider fluoride supplementation or fluoride varnish

[1]Caries-Risk Assessment Tool (CAT) developed by the AAPD http://www.mchoralhealth.org/pocketguide/cat1.html

fetus could be harmed by treatment." During the prenatal visit, health care providers should:

1. assess the woman's oral health status, oral health practices, and access to a dental home;
2. discuss with the woman how oral health affects general health;
3. offer referrals to oral health professionals for treatment;
4. educate the woman about oral health during pregnancy, including expected physiological changes in the mouth and interventions to prevent and relieve discomfort; and
5. educate the woman about diet and oral hygiene for infants and children and encourage breastfeeding

New York and California have developed state guidelines for perinatal oral health to educate providers and patients (California Dental Association 2010; New York State Department of Health 2006).

A combination of anticipatory guidance, with continuity from prenatal and perinatal care to pediatric care, can help move infant oral health from "missed opportunities" to "seized opportunities." Others who may be of assistance to families in closing these gaps are professionals at the Women, Infants and Children's (WIC) supplemental nutrition program, Early Head Start/Head Start and Neurodevelopmental/Birth to Three programs. Together medical, dental and community professionals can help create a system of care to improve maternal and child oral health.

4.2.1.4 Capacity of the Workforce to Prevent Childhood Caries

For the envisioned model in Table 4.5 to be realized, the mother requires access to a general dentist with accurate information on her oral health during pregnancy and on her infant's oral health, including the need for an early dental visit. The mother and child then need access to a pediatric medical provider who will provide oral health screening/counseling, and who will guide the family to establishing the child's dental home by age 1. Success in dental referral requires access to a pediatric or general dentist willing and able to provide infant oral health. (dela Cruz et al. 2004), in a discussion of the referral process mentioned that among the factors in assessing the likelihood of a dental referral were the medical providers' "level of oral health knowledge, and their opinions about the importance of oral health and preventive dental care."

Since young children are much more likely to access medical than dental care, the medical provider plays an important role in promoting children's oral health. (Catalanotto 2010) recommends, as part of a pediatric well child checkup:

- an oral screening examination,
- a risk assessment, including assessment of the mother's/caregiver's oral health,
- application of fluoride varnish

- anticipatory guidance (parental education) including dietary and oral hygiene information,
- attempted referral to a dental home.

The AAP recommends that child healthcare providers be trained to perform an oral health risk assessment and triage all infants and children beginning by 6 months of age to identify known risk factors for early childhood caries (ECC). The oral health component of pediatric care is integrated into the AAP's "Recommendations for Preventive Pediatric Health Care (Periodicity Schedule)" (AAP 2008).

To what extent are medical and dental and providers aware of recommendations for a first dental visit for a child by age one, as recommended by the AAP, the American Academy of Pediatric Dentistry (AAPD), and the American Dental Association? (Wolfe et al. 2006) reported that 76% of licensed general dentists in Iowa were familiar with the AAPD age 1 dental visit recommendation and that most obtained the information through continuing education; 11% believed that the first dental visit should occur between 0 and 11 months of age. However, according to (Caspary et al. 2008), when pediatric medical residents were asked the age for the first dental visit, the average response was 2.4 years, while 35% reported received no oral health training during residency. In a national survey of pediatricians (Lewis et al. 2009) reported that less than 25% of had received oral health education in medical school, residency, or continuing education. Finally (Ferullo et al. 2010) surveyed allopathic and osteopathic schools of medicine and found that 69.3% reported offering less than 5 h of oral health curriculum, while 10.2% offered no curriculum at all.

Other workforce considerations relevant to preventing early childhood caries include the training of dentists in pediatric oral health (Seale et al. 2009), the number and diversity of the dental workforce, the number of pediatric dentists, and the use of alternative providers such as dental therapists, expanded function dental assistants and dental hygienists (Mertz and Mouradian 2009; Nash 2009).

Examples of integrated care models do exist, such as that presented by (Heuer 2007) involving school-linked and school-based clinics with an "innovative health infrastructure." According to Heuer, "Neighborhood Outreach Action for Health (NOAH)" is staffed by two nurse practitioners and a part-time physician to provide "primary medical services to more than 3,200 uninsured patients each year" in Scottsdale, Arizona. Heuer counts caries among the "top ten" diagnoses every year.

Mabry and Mosca (2006) described community public health training of dental hygiene students for children with neurodevelopmental/intellectual disabilities. They mentioned that the dental hygiene students had worked together with school nurses and "felt they had impacted the school nurses' knowledge of oral disease and care."

4.2.1.5 Paper Versus EHR: Planning Pediatric EHR Acquisition: the Decision to Acquire an integrated EHR

As pediatric clinicians (both medical and dental) work more closely together, they require appropriate EHR systems that integrate a patient's medical and dental records. Following is a set of local "best practices" from Nationwide Children's Hospital in Columbus, Ohio, which may help other children's hospitals in planning acquisition of an integrated pediatric EHR system. Integrated (medical-dental) EHR technologies are becoming more widely available outside the Federal government sector (see integrated models E1 and E2 in Fig. 1.3). Nationwide Children's 'drivers' for the acquisition process were, in 2011:

1. *Minimize registration and dual databases.* Patient registration takes time and requiring both a stand-alone dental *and* a medical patient registration inhibits cost-effective flow of services. Integration allows for the use of single demographics information for all clinics in the comprehensive care system serving the patient. Clinicians always have an updated health history on patients, if they have been a patient of record. If not, and for a dental clinic that sees walk-ins, a brief "critical" dental health history can be completed on paper by a parent and scanned into the eMR. In designing an integrated medical-dental record for patients of record, the system can sort essential health history elements into a brief focused dental history without the detail needed by other medical specialty clinics. Kiosk-driven electronic health histories for those children who are new to clinic similar to those used in airline travel could be considered if feasible in busy clinics.
2. *For charting, no more key/mouse strokes than with paper.* Some commercial dental record products try to accomplish too much. Moving from paper to electronics should be driven in part by efficiencies. The tooth chart, which is an essential part of any dental record, must be such that examination findings can be transferred quickly and accurately to either paper or electronic capture. A helpful exercise is visualization of the functionality of the charting process, including both the different types of entries (caries, existing restorations and pathology) and how these are entered in the paper world.

    If charting will be able to be used for research the system should be able to translate pictures to numerical values, often a complex programming function. Dental practitioners and faculty may want to use drawings of teeth or graphics of surfaces because that is their current comfort level. A true digital charting is possible with no images of teeth, but some habits are hard to change.
3. *Maximizing drop downs with drop down building possible.* Duplication of paper chart entries using drop downs which can be upgraded as more clinical entities are found is a staple of an EMR. The paper process usually relies on a clinician's wealth of medical-dental terms since inclusion of every possible, or even the most common findings, is prohibitive on a paper chart. The EMR drop down requires front-end loading of the most common clinical findings with opportunity for free-hand additions. Being able to add terms to any drop down is a needed capability.
4. *Don't design a system for uncommon contingencies, but for your bulk of work.* A pediatric dental record should be primarily designed around dental caries, with secondary emphases on oral-facial development (orthodontics) and a lesser capability to record traumatic injuries and periodontal findings. These second and third level characteristics can be hot-buttoned and should not drive the design of the basic system which is caries charting for 98% of our patients. Sadly in most

dental schools, the chart is slave to every teaching form, few of which ever exit with the DDS into practice! These forms may have little relationship to patient care and only create "signature black holes" that need to be addressed, usually *after* treatment is completed.

5. *Progress notes should be designed for the routine entries with free-hand modification possible.* Student learners tend to write too much and a carefully crafted progress note format with standard entries in required fields helps patient flow and record completion. In federally funded clinics and residencies, attending reconciliation of student/resident service delivery is a compliance requirement. A well-designed EMR system can "stack" required co-signing tasks on a computer screen, offer standard entries as well as free-hand options, and create a process far faster than paper records for an attending's validation (same as reconciliation?).

6. *Tie examination results to treatment planning and treatment planning into billing.* A good system allows easy transfer of clinical findings needing treatment into some problem "basket" and ideally in a tabulated format. An alternative is a split screen that allows a clinician to visualize clinical findings, radiographic findings while compiling a treatment plan. Again, in clinical settings where compliance to Medicaid/Medicare regulations is required, the design of the record should give attention to auditing principles and security. A good EMR system allows portals of entry for billing and compliance personnel.

7. *Plan for users of different skill levels and different periods of exposure.* The teaching hospital or dental school environment often involves learners and attendings with varying skill levels and computer experience who may be there for brief periods of time. This reality adds significant security and user-friendliness issues. Some medical record systems are far too complex for short-term or casual users. A well-integrated medical-dental EMR allows navigation of the depths of the medical side should a user want to explore, but should focus on the dental portion. Some suggestions in design:

- Initial opening or logging into the dental portion for dental users, rather than opening into the medical portion,
- Clearly indicated options for exploration of medical portions,
- Orientation of major dental component (examination, radiographs, treatment plan) in a logical dental treatment flow to replicate the way dentistry works rather than trying to reshape dentistry's normal flow to the record,
- Minimization of seldom-used functions on the main dental screen, such as specialty medical clinics, old laboratory tests and hyperfunctionalities like letter writing,
- Clear identification of existing non-caries dental portions like orthodontics or trauma, so a novice user need not randomly search to see if a patient has any of these records.

Unfortunately, many pediatric hospitals do not yet have an EHR system that supports convenient communication among a pediatric patient's medical and dental providers. Evidence of this state of affairs was provided unintentionally by

(Fiks et al. 2011). Some pediatric hospitals may have an awkward mix of systems serving physicians, dentists, and orthodontists and their shared patients.

4.2.1.6 Summary

This section demonstrates how closely medical and dental professionals must collaborate to deliver appropriate oral health care for infants and children. Such collaboration is especially important given the developmental vulnerabilities of children and the urgency of the oral health needs of many children, especially those from underserved populations. Collaboration is made more difficult by the long-standing separation of medical and dental systems and poor oral health literacy of parents and medical professionals alike.

Teamwork in the delivery of pediatric care requires appropriate electronic patient record technology to facilitate sharing of patient information, to avoid patient record discrepancies between systems, and to create efficiencies by maintaining only a single repository for patient demographics. Only comparatively recently have appropriate integrated systems become available to support a range of clinical sites from pediatric special needs clinics to the largest children's hospitals. Nationwide Children's has given practical examples of efficient decision-making in identifying an integrated system to acquire. Much more work will be needed to develop the means to move towards integrating office and community-based care for children through the sharing of electronic health records.

4.2.2 Periodontal Disease and Kidney Disease

Beth Piraino

Oral health is an oft neglected area in the care of patients who have chronic kidney disease. Furthermore, the provision of care by dentists and physicians to the same patient is fragmented as communication between the two health care providers is scant. Emerging data suggesting the periodontal disease is closely linked to chronic kidney disease highlights the importance of proper oral health and the importance of communication between dentists and physicians in the care of the patient.

Investigators used data from NHANES III, including information on 11, 211 adults who had an oral examination by a dentist who categorized each patient as having no periodontal disease, periodontal disease or edentulous to examine the relationship between numerous risk factors for moderate to severe chronic kidney disease, as determined by calculation of estimated GFR through use of the MDRD formula (Fisher et al. 2011). No chronic kidney disease was defined as an estimated GFR of 60 ml per min per 1.73 m^2. Three percent of the patients had CKD, 22.5% were hypertension and 4.4% had diabetes (2.4% with glycated hemoglobin of 7% or higher). Four models were constructed to examine the potential relationship between periodontal disease and CKD. In model one adults with either periodontal disease or edentulous had an adjusted odds ratio of 1.83 (with 95% confidence intervals of 1.31–2.55) of having CKD, independent of the other risk factors for CKD including of age above 60 years, ethnicity, hypertension, smoking status, female gender and C-reactive protein elevation. The fourth model contained 15 potential risk factors including the periodontal disease score and for every 1-unit increase in the score, the risk of having CKD increased by 1% controlling for the other risk factors. The authors hypothesized from their results that the relationship between periodontal disease and CKD was bidirectional in that CKD may increase the risk of periodontal disease which in turn increases the risk of CKD.

Grubbs et al. (2011) also used NHANES data to look more closely at the relationship between periodontal disease and CKD, using dental examinations obtained from 2001 to 2004 (n=6,199 adults, 21–75 years) (Grubbs V, et al. 2011). In this analysis edentulous subjects were excluded and those with albuminuria were included in the definition of CKD. In the entire population CKD was present in 10.6%, but in those with moderate to severe periodontal disease this increased to 21.6%. Other associations with moderate to severe periodontal disease were being older, male, nonwhite, less educated and poor. There was a strong relationship between periodontal disease and CKD (2.5 unadjusted odds ratio). When adjusted for age, gender, tobacco use, hypertension, diabetes, ethnicity, poverty and educational attainment, the odds ratio for the association of periodontal disease and CKD was still significant (1.55). In some groups (Mexican American, poor, and poorly educated) dental care was not received on an annual basis in the majority of this segment of the population.

Periodontal disease has been associated with an increased risk of death in hemodialysis patients (Kshirsagar et al. 2009). This relationship has been poorly studied in peritoneal dialysis patients. This requires further study but it appears possible that periodontal disease might hasten loss of residual kidney function and perhaps contribute to atherosclerosis in dialysis patients and therefore, contribute to the high mortality in this population.

Patients who desire a kidney transplant are required to undergo a thorough evaluation beforehand including an oral examination by a dentist. Some patients on dialysis have inadequate insurance which does not cover dental care, leading to a situation in which a kidney transplant is denied because the patient cannot afford the dental examination.

Communications between dentists and physicians in the care of the patient is scant. If oral surgery is required in a dialysis patient, the surgeon generally requires a brief summary from the nephrologist with recommendations. These might include suggestions for prophylactic antibiotics, avoidance of vasoconstrictor agents to an excess locally (which can elevate blood pressure) and the increased risk of bleeding of a dialysis patient. For more routine dental examinations no information is requested which could potentially lead to drug interactions or a dangerous situation.

Most nephrologists and health care providers in the dialysis unit do not inquire of the patient concerning dental health and examination of the mouth is quite uncommon. Although the dialysis patient is seen monthly at a minimum, there is little conversation or documentation of oral health.

Connecting the electronic health records of in-patient care, the out-patient dialysis unit and the dentists' office could potentially have a large impact in improving the care of those with end stage kidney disease.

4.2.3 What the Provider Needs to Know: Supporting Each Other's Efforts

Wells Shoemaker

Integrating medical and dental records in EHR's may or may not be the "golden ring." First, we need to integrate the clinical thinking...something we both realize is important, but not likely to be solved by an inert computer. I also think that integrated records will be very cumbersome, given the fact that the language used by the separate disciplines is so different, and the kind of detail required to support good decisions and good work is so different. It could be done...but for many professionals on either "side," they would never open the other module. To me, a more sensible solution may be to have a condensed "nugget" of information that could cross populate.

"Moderate periodontal disease" may be what the medical doctor needs to know, plus know what a treatment plan may include. She won't need to know the number of the teeth with the deepest pockets and erosions but will need to support the patient's determination to follow through. On the other hand, if the patient has shown remarkable initiative in gum care and has successfully migrated to a lower severity index, that would be important for congratulation and reinforcement...and also to encourage similar diligence in managing, let's say, the hypertension that is not optimally controlled.

In the other direction, the dentist should know that a patient has been erratic in clinical follow up, does not self-test blood glucose, uses hypoglycemic drugs only intermittently, and has failed several appointments for eye exams. This would lead to a rather different set of approaches from a highly motivated grandmother who is enrolled in a community cultural center's senior exercise club, and is learning to become a lay community teacher for diabetes.

Right now, I don't think even this superficial degree of information is exchanged. We need to support each other's efforts, but we probably do not need to share minute details.

4.2.4 Integrating Ophthalmic Imaging: Seeing the Big Picture in a Small Organ

Jessica Kovarik and Evan Waxman

The benefits of an electronic health record are well described. EHRs allow for legible standardized documentation and easier sharing of patient data between providers at multiple locations. They are less prone to loss and require much less space to store. They have the potential to result in a reduction in the cost of health care.

A distinct disadvantage of the EHR, in its current configuration, is the problem of information overload. Simply put, there is often too much information presented in a way that is difficult to review and digest. The EHR equivalent of thumbing through a chart quickly is not yet available. As a result we frequently see practitioners look only at the last note or two as they review a patient's history.

We require a way to communicate information directly relevant to patient diagnosis, treatment and prognosis among subspecialists and primary care providers. We require a way to identify subclinical cerebrovascular disease in a patient, independent of blood pressure and other traditional risk factors. We require a way to recognize which patients with cerebrovascular disease are two to four times more likely than average to develop a stroke in the next 3 years. We have a way – retinal imaging.

The eye is the one place in the body we can directly observe arteries, veins and a cranial nerve in a noninvasive manner. Routine imaging of the retina and optic nerve could allow primary care providers to assess retinal, and by proxy systemic, end organ damage from atherosclerosis in an efficient manner. The key to optimal use of the medical record and efficient yet effective communication among providers may lie with the familiar adage; a picture is worth a 1,000 words.

Traditionally, when ophthalmologists communicate with primary care providers they send brief letters regarding the findings seen during a yearly dilated examination and the presence, absence or progression of diabetic retinopathy. These letters end by exhorting the virtues of improved blood sugar, blood pressure and lipid control, a sentiment that the primary care provider likely shares. This system of communication does not provide particularly useful information for the primary care provider, except to serve as a notice that the standard of care screening guidelines have been met. The box has been checked.

If primary care providers, cardiologists, nephrologists had access to routine ophthalmic imaging, they would be able to directly visualize the effect that suboptimal blood sugar control is having on their diabetic patients. As importantly, they would be equipped with information directly predictive of congestive heart failure, stroke, and cardiovascular mortality for their patient with hypertension, hyperlipidemia and for those who smoke.

Large clinical studies have shown that assessment of retinal vascular changes such as retinal hemorrhages, microaneurysms and cotton wool spots provides important information for vasculopathy risk stratification. As an example, Wong et al. showed that the presence of retinopathy indicates susceptibility to and onset of preclinical systemic vascular disease, independent of and qualitatively different from measuring blood pressure or lipids (Wong and McIntosh 2005). In the Atherosclerosis Risk in Communities (ARIC) study, individuals with hypertensive retinopathy signs such as cotton wool spots, retinal hemorrhages and microaneurysms were two to four times more likely to develop a stroke within 3 years, even when controlling for the effects of blood pressure, hyperlipidemia, cigarette smoking and other risk factors (Wong et al. 2001). In a recent study by Werther et al., patients with retinal vein occlusions were found to have a two-fold increased risk of stroke compared to controls (Werther et al. 2011).

In addition, the ARIC study group reported that individuals with retinopathy were twice as likely to develop congestive heart failure as individuals without retinopathy, even after controlling for pre-existing risk factors (Wong et al. 2005a).

Interestingly, even among individuals without pre-existing coronary artery disease, diabetes or hypertension, the presence of hypertensive retinopathy was associated with a three-fold increased risk of congestive heart failure events (Wong et al. 2005a). In the Beaver Dam Eye Study, cardiovascular mortality was almost twice as high among individuals with retinal microaneurysms and retinal hemorrhages as those without these signs (Wong et al. 2003a, b). The ARIC and Beaver Dam Eye Studies have also shown that, independent of other risk factors, generalized retinal arteriolar narrowing predicts the incidence of type II diabetes among individuals initially free of the disease (Wong et al. 2002a, 2005b).

A primary care provider with access to patients' retinal photographs may therefore have the evidence needed to suggest which patient with either established systemic vascular disease or preclinical systemic vascular disease requires a more aggressive treatment and risk factor modification. They could do this without wading through the electronic equivalent of piles of records. One photograph could reflect both acute changes in blood pressure (retinal hemorrhages, microaneurysms and cotton wool spots) and chronic changes resulting from cumulative damage from hypertension (AV nicking and generalized arteriolar narrowing) (Sharrett et al. 1999; Wong et al. 2002a; Leung et al. 2004).

In Brown et al. 23 out of 24 patients, excluding those with known diabetes, that presented with a single cotton wool spot or a predominance of cotton wool spots on examination of the retina were found to have underlying systemic disease (Brown et al. 1985). Systemic work-up revealed diagnoses including previously undiagnosed diabetes, hypertension, cardiac valvular disease, severe carotid artery obstruction, leukemia, metastatic carcinoma, systemic lupus erythematosus, AIDS and giant cell arteritis (Brown et al. 1985). These findings illustrate the importance of retinal findings on a systemic level.

The utilization and integration of ophthalmic imaging may serve to achieve more effective communication among subspecialists and primary care providers and ultimately to provide improved diagnosis and treatment for delivery of optimal quality of patient care. Moreover, the improved integration and maximal use of resources may serve to reduce overall health care cost and perhaps decrease provider frustration with the electronic health record (Fig. 4.5).

There are cotton wool spots, exudates, intraretinal dot-blot hemorrhages and microaneurysms. AV nicking is also present especially along the superior arcade just as the vessel leaves the optic nerve (Fig. 4.6).

AV nicking, tortuosity of vessels, intraretinal hemorrhages and dry exudates are seen (Fig. 4.7).

There is edema of the optic nerve head, with cotton wool spots and flame shaped hemorrhage along the disc margin. There are several cotton wool spots along the vascular arcades and scattered dot hemorrhages throughout the posterior pole and periphery (Fig. 4.8).

Notice the cholesterol plaque in the vessel just as it exits the optic nerve head and the pallor in the superior macula corresponding to retinal ischemia and edema (Fig. 4.9).

Fig. 4.5 Nonproliferative diabetic retinopathy and hypertensive retinopathy

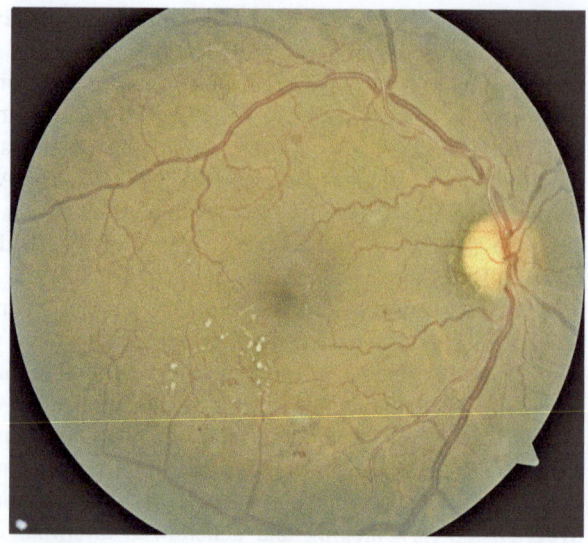

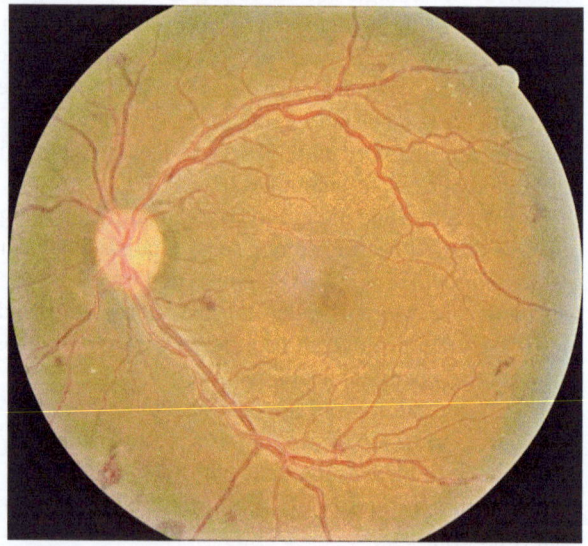

Fig. 4.6 Hypertensive retinopathy

The cholesterol embolus has resulted in lack of blood flow to the superior arcade (Fig. 4.10).

There is pooling of subretinal blood just superior to the optic disc with a central fibrin clot and associated vitreous hemorrhage (Fig. 4.11).

Optic disc edema, flame hemorrhages and venous congestion are seen in a patient with severe hypertension.

Fig. 4.7 Central retinal vein occlusion

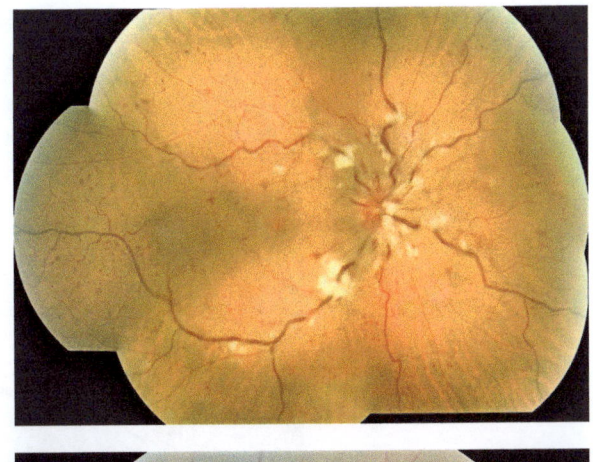

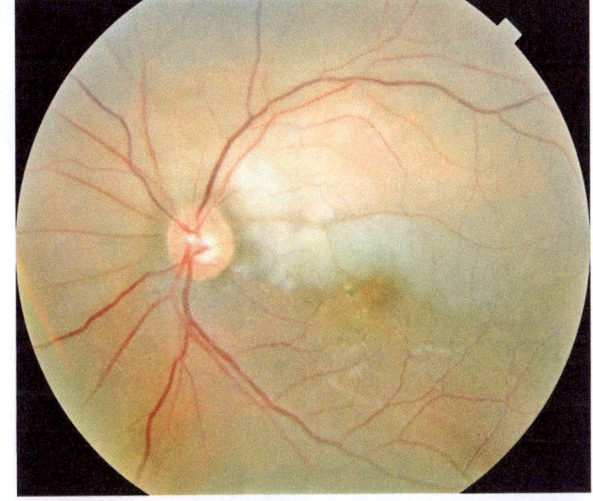

Fig. 4.8 Branch retinal artery occlusion

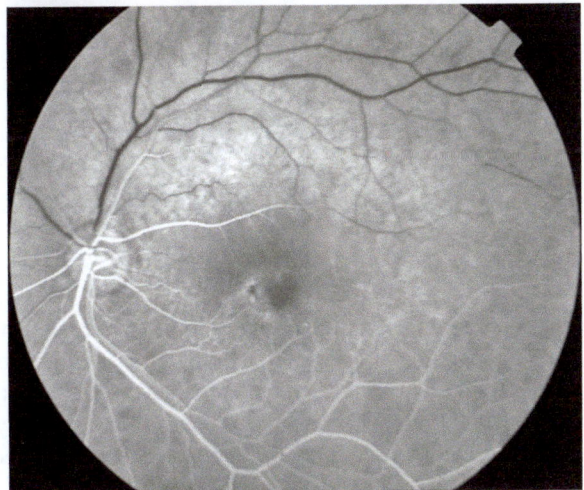

Fig. 4.9 Branch retinal artery occlusion, fluorescein angiogram

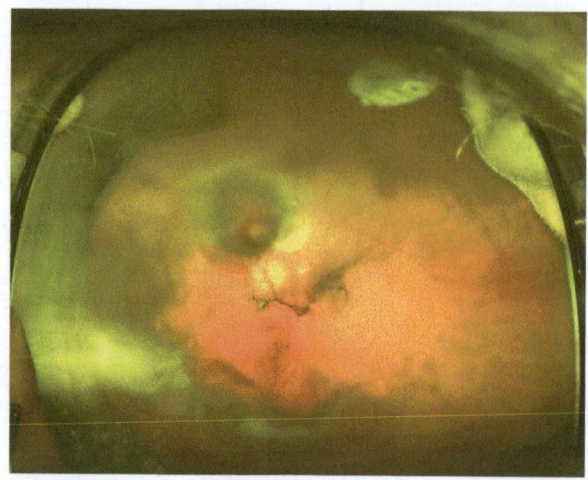

Fig. 4.10 Retinal macroaneurysm

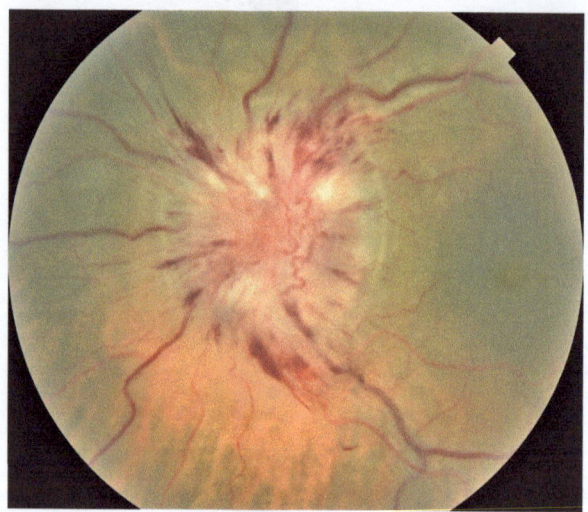

Fig. 4.11 Hypertensive optic neuropathy

4.2.5 Do Dentists and Otolaryngologists Need to Collaborate? If So Does Their Patient Record System Help Them Do It?

Biju Cheriyan

In clinical practice, an otolaryngologist often needs a dental consult not only because of the topographically adjacent nature of the structures but also because most structures are supplied by the same neurovascular bundle and therefore there is overlapping of symptoms. The converse scenario can also apply. Apart from this, there are many systemic medical conditions (for example: bleeding diatheses, diabetes) a dentist encounters throughout his or her practice which can determine the outcome of a successful treatment. Sometimes, providers may observe a cluster of diagnostic criteria which may have to a single source. In the sections below, I will explore a few of these scenarios and conditions, and indicate where and how an integrated electronic health record (EHR) could optimize delivery of health care by dentists and otolaryngologists.

4.2.5.1 Congenital Conditions

Cleft palate/Cleft lip: Cleft lip and cleft palate (CL/CP) are congenital conditions that require multidisciplinary management by dentists, oral and maxillofacial surgeons, orthodontists, otolaryngologists, speech pathologists and plastic surgeons A number of studies report that a multidisciplinary approach is essential for better treatment outcomes (Wangsrimongkol and Jansawang 2010) and for post operative rehabilitation (Furr et al. 2011). These multidisciplinary approaches may lead to new ways to manage and treat CL/CP patients (Salyer et al. 2009).

Hutchinson's teeth: Notching of the upper two incisors is typically seen in individuals inflicted with congenital syphilis.

Macroglossia refers to enlarged tongue in relation to oral cavity. Macroglossia is an important sign. It can indicate important systemic diseases like systemic amyloidosis, congenital hypothyroidism, acromegaly, or Down syndrome.

4.2.5.2 Headache

A common complaint that dentists and otolaryngologists encounter in their practice is the common headache. Because of the special nature of the neurovascular bundle of the head and neck this symptom can be presented to both dentists and otolaryngologists (Ram et al. 2009). Any sinus pathology can present as a headache to an otolaryngology practice. Since the maxillary sinus floor is in close proximity to the maxillary premolars and molars, it is imperative to obtain a dental evaluation in persistent cases of headache. There are a number of causes for headache from the dental and otolaryngology perspective. A mal-aligned denture patient with chronic headache, whom I saw in my practice was shuttled between departments and an array of investigations only to find at the end that an ill-fitting denture caused the intractable headache. In these cases, an integration of findings is extremely important in providing quality treatment to the patient and also saves money and time for the whole health care system. Hence it is important to have an integrated patient record for this particular symptom alone.

4.2.5.3 Trigeminal Neuralgia

Trigeminal neuralgia is facial pain of neurogenic origin experienced along the distribution of the trigeminal nerve(fifth cranial nerve). It can present as a dental pain and can also be triggered by brushing teeth among other trigger factors. As a result, patients with dental pain without obvious causes are required to have a physicians' consultation to rule out this obscure condition. Sometimes it is diagnosed by omission (Aggarwal et al. 2011; Rodriguez-Lozano et al. 2010; Spencer et al. 2008).

4.2.5.4 Tumors of Nasal Sinuses

Any tumor of the nasal sinuses (specifically maxillary and ethmoids) can erode the lower bony wall and present in the oral cavity (usually the maxillary arch) as dental pain, loose tooth, etc. Therefore, these are areas of interest to both dentists and otolaryngologists. Such tumors most commonly present first to a dentist or could also be an accidental finding. Cancers of the naso/oro/laryngo pharynx can also present as toothache to a dentist as these structures have a common nerve supply from cranial nerves 5,7 and 9. Therefore, an integration of the patient record may even help in early diagnosis of the tumor. The same principle applies to all oral tumors, tumors of the nasopharynx, the oropharynx etc. This is especially true of malignant lesions of the oral cavity as these may help in early detection and treatment of cancer. In these cases, an early biopsy and histopathology can save the life of the patient. Therefore, it is imperative to say that a collaborative patient record can save patients' lives.

4.2.5.5 Ulcers of the Oral Cavity

Ulcers of the oral cavity from aphthous ulcers to carcinomas can present both to a dentist and an otolaryngologist. Oral ulcers can be of dental origin. Contact ulcers from sharp edges of a mal-aligned tooth can result in intractable ulcers, where a simple smoothing of sharp edges may eradicate the ulcer and terminate it as a chronic condition and can even prevent the ulcer turning into a malignancy. If you have an integrated electronic health record (EHR) these problems are immediately addressed and managed. Otherwise, the condition will consume valuable time of both the patient and the physician concerned. In addition to this, there are a few conditions which require special attention: aphthous stomatitis (canker sore), which may indicate oral manifestation of deficiencies of iron, vitamin B12, folate deficiency and oral candidiasis, which can be a sign of diabetes mellitus or of an immunocompromised patient (e.g. AIDS).

4.2.5.6 Temporomandibular Joint Disorders

Temperomandibular joint (TMJ) disorders can present in a variety of symptoms to both dentists and otolaryngologists. They can present as a headache, earache, toothache, or as facial pain. There can be a number of causes for this including osteoarthritis of the TMJ, recurrent dislocation, bruxism, or even an ill fitting denture. There have been cases where patients have been subjected to removal of teeth for chronic toothache only to discover at the end that the symptom was a referred pain from TMJ! Therefore, an integrated EHR can prevent misdiagnoses and resulting impairment or disability to patients. Trismus (lock jaw) can indicate important diagnoses such as tetanus and rabies.It is due to a spasm of muscles of mastication, which is an important oral manifestation of widespread muscle spasm. Apart from these conditions, other causes of trismus are peritonsillar abscesses, and scleroderma.

Other problems dentists and otolaryngologists encounter in clinical practice are concurrent systemic diseases (patients with multiple problems): patients with bleeding diatheses, diabetes mellitus and a hidden primary malignancy. A non-healing ulcer in the oral cavity may hide a primary malignancy behind it. In these cases, you have to look for it specifically. Similarly, one has to be aware of oral manifestations of internal pathology. Some of them are Crohn's disease, ulcerative colitis and gastro-intestinal tract malignancies.

Often dentists see patients after a tooth extraction with intractable bleeding to find that they have a bleeding diathesis. So, this may be the first presentation of these patients' bleeding disorder. When this patient undergoes any elective procedure in future, it will be a great help to surgeons to be aware of this information to prevent any inadvertent complications. Therefore an integrated EHR can prevent unwanted complications where a patient's life may be in jeopardy.

4.2.5.7 Refered Otalgia (Earache)

The source of otalgia or earache can be from a number of sites other than ear itself. Technically ear lobe and ear canal are supplied by four different cranial nerve branches (5th, 7th, 9th, 10th). Therefore, an area with a common nerve supply can present as earache. Common dental problems which present as referred otalgia are (1) dental caries (2) oro-dental diseases or abscesses (3) an impacted molar tooth (which is a common cause) (4) malocclusion (5) benign and malignant lesions of oral cavity and tongue (Kim et al. 2007). Therefore, it is essential these two departments collaborate with each other in diagnosing and treating these diseases, and one way of facilitating it is through an integrated EHR system.

4.2.5.8 Halitosis (Bad Breath)

There is a lot of overlap between dentists and otolaryngologists in the diagnosis and treatment of patients with halitosis (Delanghe et al. 1999; Bollen et al. 1999). Poor oral hygiene is the most common cause for this common complaint. Oral causes include tooth caries, oral ulcers, periodontal diseases, unhealthy mucosa of the oral cavity. It is interesting to note that a simple oral ulcer can form an abcess eroding the floor of mouth and becoming a life-threatening oral cellulitis (Ludwig angina). Once the cellulitis has developed, it becomes a medical emergency. Therefore, it is essential to prevent it before it can progress into a life-threatening condition, which of course is possible. Causes pertaining to otolaryngologists include: chronic sinusitis or mucociliary disorder, chronic laryngitis or pharyngitis, pharyngeal pouches-related pathology, tumors or ulcers of naso/oro/laryngopharynx, diseases or conditions that impair normal flow of saliva such as salivary gland diseases or stones preventing flow of saliva, medications which cause dryness of mouth: antihistamines, antidepressants; local manifestation of systemic disorders: auto immune disorders, Sjögren syndrome, dehydration from any cause, diabetes mellitus and Gastro Esophageal Reflux Disorder (GERD).

GERD is caused by improper neuro-autonomy of the lower esophageal sphincter (LES). The LES does not close tightly after food intake which causes gastric content to enter the esophagus. Over time this can erode mucosa and cause various diseases even becoming cancerous (Friedenberg et al. 2010). This disorder is attributed to life style. Fast food consumption habits (oily fried foods) and eating habits (swallowing food without properly chewing) are partly responsible for this disorder (Lukic et al. 2010; Al-Humayed et al. 2010). Here again an early diagnosis can manage the disease process before it is fully developed.

At present there are no integrated EHR systems serving these specialties (dentistry and otolaryngology). An integrated EHR would facilitate efficient communication between a dentist and an otolaryngologist who are providing care to the same patient and addressing a problem with a shared focus between the two disciplines. Such integrated communication, may only require consulting the available medical or dental record of the patient, based on the particular circumstance. Even enabling this simple communication would avoid duplication of effort, clarify the context of certain symptoms and reduce stress endured by the patient. It also has the potential to reduce healthcare delivery costs, and in some cases, even contribute to saving the patient's life.

4.2.6 Providing Collaborative, Interdisciplinary Healthcare to Patients with Neurodevelopmental Disorders and Intellectual Disabilities

Henry Hood, Allan G. Farman, and Matthew Holder

In this chapter, the authors attempt to put forth a justification for precisely this kind of collaborative approach through a summary and discussion of a series of actual clinical cases. The protocols discussed in the management of each of these clinical cases illustrate the value in providing whole-person, interdisciplinary health care to this complex patient population.

4.2.6.1 Surveying the Landscape

There is arguably no single patient population for whom the provision of collaborative, interdisciplinary health care is more challenging than for patients with neurodevelopmental disorders and intellectual disabilities (ND/ID). In planning and delivering the generally-accepted standard of health care to this unique population, myriad biomedical, psychosocial and sociopolitical realities converge to create a landscape that is, at best, daunting for patients with these disorders, and for the clinicians who are charged with their care.

Anecdotal and scientific evidence suggest that this landscape has produced a paucity of physicians and dentists who are willing and able to provide care to patients with ND/ID, and that American medical and dental schools are providing little training focused on their care (Holder et al. 2009; Wolff et al. 2004).

In February of 2002, 16th Surgeon General David Satcher issued a report, which documented that Americans with ND/ID experience great difficulty accessing quality health care (Thompson 2002). In that same report, former Health and Human Services Secretary Tommy Thompson said, "Americans with mental retardation and their families face enormous obstacles in seeking the kind of basic health care that many of us take for granted." (Thompson 2002) The disparities identified by Dr. Satcher and Secretary Thompson require that physicians and dentists approach this population in a spirit of collaboration, compassion, and teamwork in order to produce positive health outcomes for them.

Perhaps, an even greater imperative driving the need for collaboration between medicine and dentistry in this arena is the fact that many patients with intellectual disabilities have developed this cognitive impairment as the result of an underlying neurodevelopmental disorder that is often undiagnosed. And it is this neurodevelopmental illness and the constellation of potentially devastating complications associated with that illness that create a biomedical fragility and a vulnerability that neither begins nor ends at the oral cavity, and that leaves these patients at risk in almost every aspect of their daily lives.

When, for example, patients with ND/ID are dependent upon publicly-funded programs for their health care, and when these systems fail to provide the health services that biomedically complex cases require because they fail to account for and accommodate the link between medical and dental pathologies, the risk of a negative outcome is greatly enhanced. Such was the case for an intellectually disabled woman in Michigan who, in October of 2010, was unable to access dental services through the state's public medical assistance program, and who fatally succumbed to a systemic bacteremia resulting from an untreated periodontal disease (Mich. Dent. Assoc. 2009).

4.2.6.2 Neurodevelopmental Disorders and Their Associated Primary Complications

The American Academy of Developmental Medicine and Dentistry (AADMD) defines a neurodevelopmental disorder as a disorder involving injury to the brain that occurs at some point between the time of conception and neurological maturation – approximately age 21 or 22 (Zelenski et al. 2008).

Examples of frequently-encountered neurodevelopmental disorders would include Fragile X syndrome, a genetically acquired neurodevelopmental disorder caused by a mutation at the distal end of the long arm of the X chromosome

Fig. 4.12 Fragile X syndrome

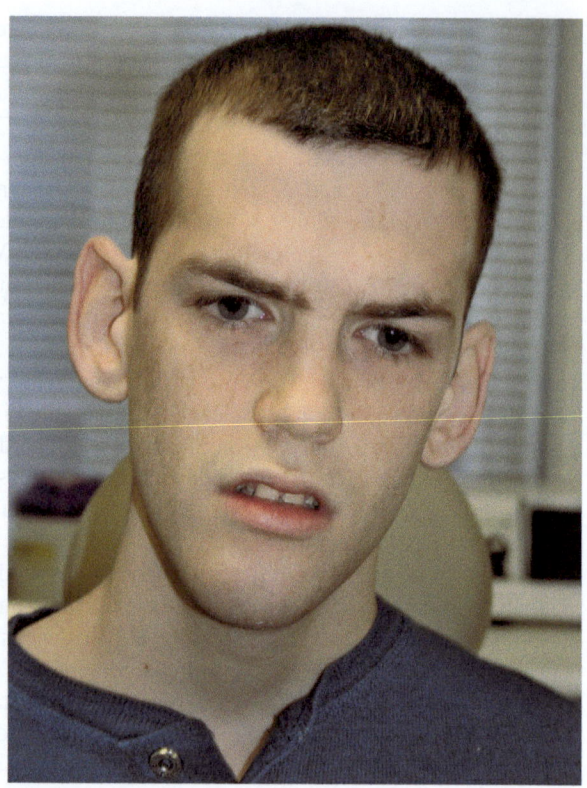

(see Fig. 4.12), Trisomy 21, another genetic disorder, which features extra genetic material at the chromosome 21 site (see Fig. 4.13), and Cerebral Palsy, a prenatal or perinatal, acquired neurodevelopmental disorder (see Fig. 4.14).

Patients with neurodevelopmental disorders tend to present clinically with one or more of five frequently-encountered, objective symptom complexes or primary complications. These five, classic primary complications include intellectual disability (aka: mental retardation), neuromotor impairment, seizure disorders, behavioral disturbances, and sensory impairment (AADMD).

Additionally, multiple secondary health consequences can derive from the five primary complications; and any one of these secondary health consequences, or a combination of them, can produce profound morbidity. An example of a common secondary health consequence seen in patients with ND/ID, which is derived from intellectual disability and / or neuromotor impairment, is the patient who is unable to care for his or her own mouth, and who develops ubiquitous caries and advanced periodontal disease as a result (See: Fig. 4.15). Another example would be the patient who suffers from the secondary health consequence of gastroesophageal reflux disease (GERD) as a result of the neuromotor impairment associated with multiple neurodevelopmental disorders; and whose tooth enamel and dentinal tissues become chemically eroded as a result of the chronic intraoral acidity produced by GERD (See: Fig. 4.16).

Fig. 4.13 Trisomy 21

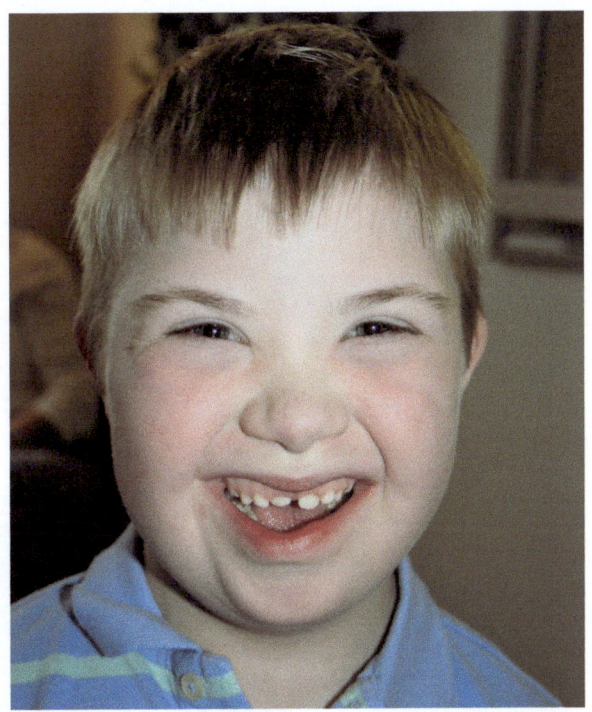

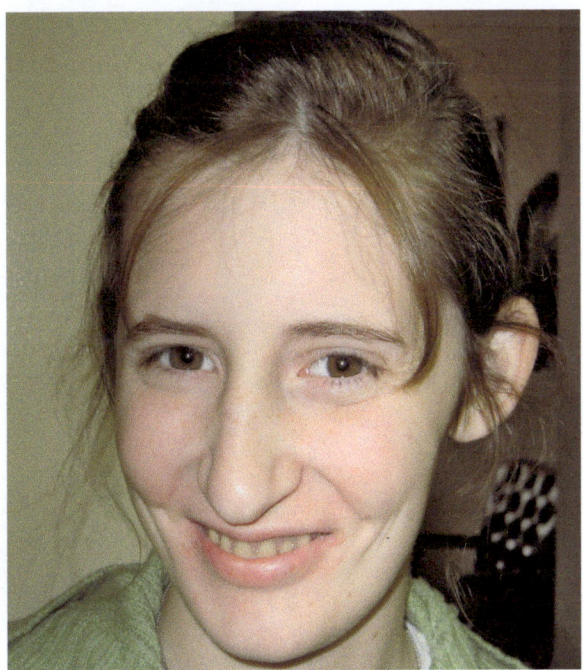

Fig. 4.14 Cerebral palsy

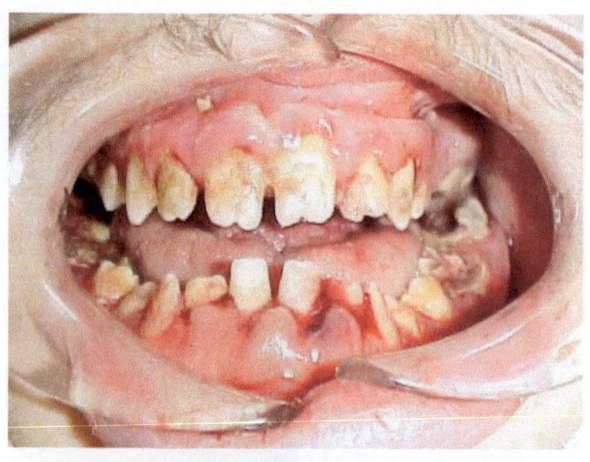

Fig. 4.15 Patient with congenital syphilis

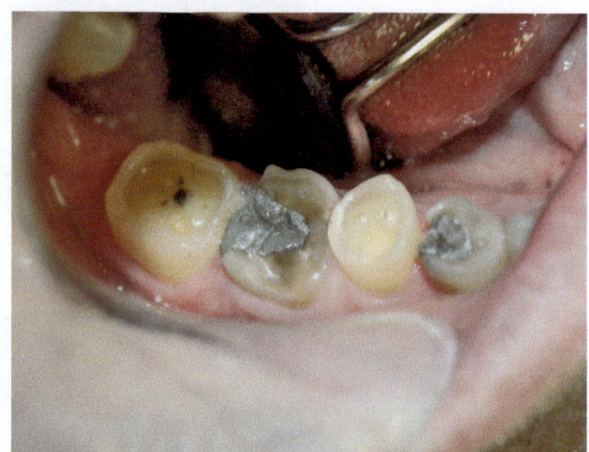

Fig. 4.16 GERD-related erosion of enamel and dentinal tissues

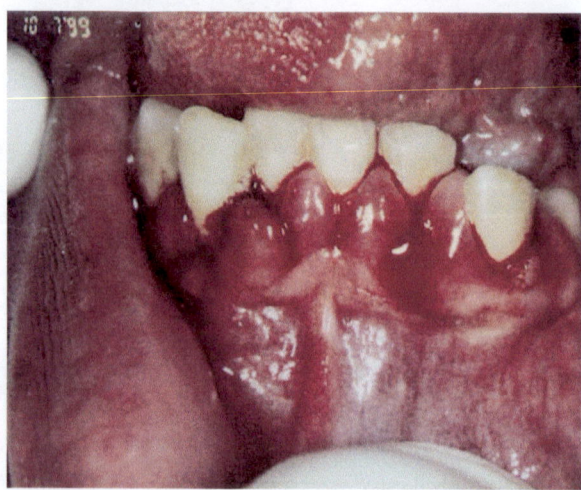

Fig. 4.17 Patient on phenytoin

The diagnosis and management of these secondary health consequences provide dentists and physicians with a unique opportunity to work together to improve the quality of health and quality of life for their patients by implementing a team approach, which crosses the traditional interdisciplinary lines of communication, and which expands each clinician's ability to make meaningful treatment options available. Indeed, it is often the case that quality primary care provided in one discipline will provide potentially valuable information to an attending clinician from another discipline. Such is the case with the patients featured in Figs. 4.16 and 4.17.

4.2.6.3 The Adult Patient with ND/ID and Undiagnosed Syphilis

The patient whose intraoral photograph is featured in Fig. 4.14 is a 19 year-old male patient who presented to a special needs dental clinic accompanied by his mother. The mother indicated that her son was exhibiting hand-mouthing behaviors that she believed suggested he was experiencing mouth pain. A comprehensive radiographic and intraoral exam revealed, among other maladies, notched incisors, multiple diastemas, grossly decayed mulberry molars, and advanced periodontal disease. The patient also exhibited moderate to severe intellectual disability.

These findings were all consistent with a diagnosis of congenital syphilis.[6] However, in developing the medical history with the mother, it was learned that no previous diagnosis of syphilis had been discussed with the mother, nor was it included in the health history.

In cases like this, a comprehensive dental treatment plan should always include consultation with the primary care physician for purposes of moving forward with confirmation of the clinical diagnosis by serologic testing, and consultation with a cardiologist to assist in the management of potential cardiovascular sequelae.

As the dental treatment plan is being developed, consideration should also be given to Human Immunodeficiency Virus (HIV) testing for this patient, as coinfection is a common finding[7]. This issue could easily be attended to by a primary care physician, an internist or an infectious disease specialist. In the absence of any of these team members, the dentist should feel entirely comfortable ordering HIV testing.

The primary care physician and the developmental dentist should continue to advise each other and their respective consultant specialists of any significant developments or new information, which could in any way impact either the medical or the dental treatment plan. As treatment progresses, both the physician and the dentist should expect improvement in the patient's periodontal status, which will likely be reflected in a decrease in the frequency of immune-related illnesses, and in the maladaptive behaviors produced by chronic oral pain.

It is quite often the case in this patient population that, with a reduction in maladaptive behaviors, comes a reduction of the use of psychotropic medications prescribed in a frequently futile attempt to manage behaviors that were born of an undiagnosed medical or dental illness.

4.2.6.4 The Adult Patient with ND/ID and Undiagnosed GERD

GERD is defined as the reflux of gastric contents into the esophagus. GERD is primarily associated with incompetence of the lower esophageal sphincter; however there are numerous co-contributors, which may predispose a patient to GERD or exacerbate an existing reflux problem. These co-contributors include a diet high in fat, neuromotor impairment associated with functional abnormalities such as dysphagia, neuromotor impairment associated with impaired ambulation and prolonged periods of recumbence, and the use of multiple medications including anxiolytics, calcium channel blockers, and anticholinergics. GERD is thought to affect approximately 25–35% of the general US population.

It has been established in the literature that the incidence of GERD in patients with intellectual disabilities is significantly higher than in the neurotypical population, and that the relative number of unreported cases of GERD is much higher in patients with a neurodevelopmental diagnosis, as well.

Patients who have gastric reflux as a function of a neurodevelopmentally-derived neuromotor impairment and a coexisting intellectual disability are impaired in their ability to voice the complaint that would, in the neurotypical patient, commonly lead to an encounter with either a family physician or a gastroenterologist and, ultimately, to a diagnosis. This inability to voice a complaint can be problematic in that, left untreated, GERD can produce maladaptive and sometimes aggressive behaviors in this population. And, of even greater concern, is the fact that undiagnosed esophageal reflux can lead to more complex conditions that can produce significant morbidity or even mortality – maladies such as Barrett's esophagus or adenocarcinoma of the esophagus.

Chronic GERD can also produce an acidic intraoral environment, which can lead to the chemical erosion of the enamel and dentinal tissues of the teeth. Ali et al. have established a link between erosion of the enamel and dentinal tissues of the teeth and GERD. There is additional anecdotal evidence suggesting a link between tooth enamel erosion and GERD, and related maladies. A special needs dental clinic in the eastern United States serving 1,000 patients with ND/ID, has reported that, of nine patients referred to gastroenterology who presented for dental exam with a finding of either tooth enamel erosion or ubiquitous caries, two cases were diagnosed with GERD, two with Barrett's esophagus, three with gastritis, and one with duodenitis. In all cases, medical treatment was required.

In light of all that is known about the incidence of GERD and of the GERD-related risks unique to this patient population; and in light of the link between tooth enamel erosion and GERD, it is incumbent upon any dentist encountering tooth enamel erosion in a patient with an intellectual disability to immediately refer that patient to gastroenterology for a work up, which should include esophagogastroduodenoscopy (EGD) and pH monitoring.

A dentist encountering GERD in a patient with an intellectual disability must be aware that he or she may be the first and only link between that patient and the diagnosis of a potentially life-threatening illness.

4.2.6.5 The Adult Patient with ND/ID and Phenytoin-Induced Gingival Enlargement

Phenytoin-induced gingival enlargement can appear as either an inflammatory lesion or a more dense, fibrotic hyperplastic lesion. The inflammatory lesion is one in which the gingival tissues are swollen and bleeding, and in which pain is often a component. This type of gingival enlargement is the more acute lesion, frequently seen in patients who are currently taking Phenytoin. In advanced cases of inflammatory gingival enlargement, the tissues can appear botryoid, with a characteristic grape-cluster appearance. In advanced cases of Phenytoin-induced gingival enlargement, the lesion can sometimes shroud entire sections of the dentition.

Phenytoin has long been a common medication used to treat seizure disorders in patients with neurodevelopmental disorders and intellectual disabilities. However, the gingival enlargement it produces, and the obstacle this lesion can pose to effective oral hygiene – especially in a population in which oral hygiene is typically compromised – can, over time, lead to periodontal disease, edentulism, and in advanced cases, systemic bacteremias. Gingivectomy performed to reduce Phenytoin-induced gingival enlargement will typically fail unless the patient is weaned off the offending medication, and another anti-seizure medication is titrated to effect. Multiple alternative anti-seizure medications are currently available, which do not have the side effect profile of Phenytoin, and most patients who are weaned off Phenytoin will demonstrate a virtual 100% resolution of the inflammatory lesion within a matter of 3 or 4 months.

The image in Fig. 4.18 is of a 22 year-old, microcephalic African-American male with intellectual disability, neuromotor impairment, and a seizure disorder. Figure 4.17 illustrates the appearance of this patient's gingival tissues while he was currently on Phenytoin. Figure 4.18 features the same patient 4 months after being weaned off Phenytoin and placed on Topiramate.

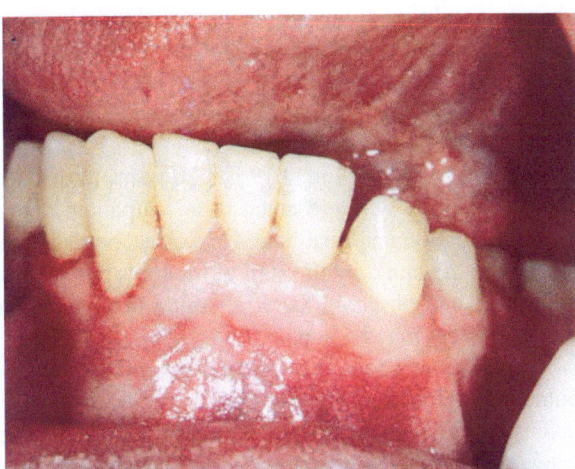

Fig. 4.18 Patient 4 months post-weaning

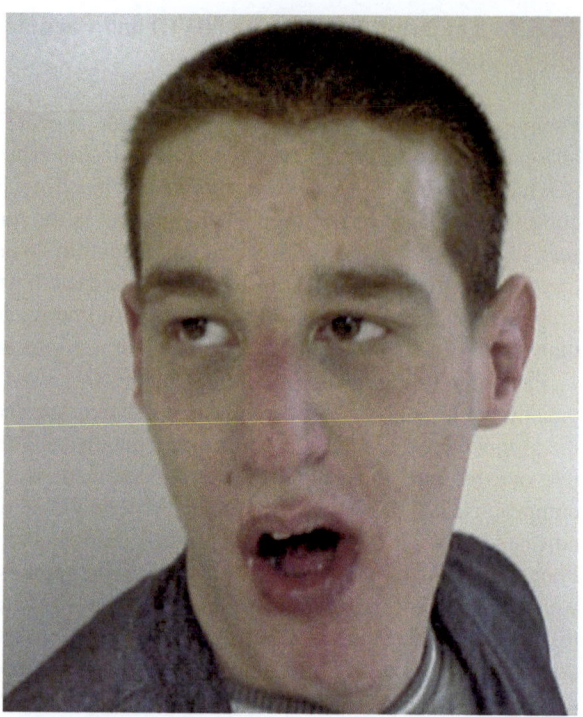

Fig. 4.19 The adult patient suspected of having Fragile X syndrome

These images illustrate the dramatic result that can be achieved when a dentist and a physician work in collaboration in the best interests of the patient. It is worth noting that this particular collaboration required only one intervention to achieve this result: The patient was weaned off Phenytoin and was placed on a safer alternate anti-seizure medication.

Any dentist caring for a patient with an intellectual disability who presents with Phenytoin induced gingival enlargement should immediately contact either the primary care physician or neurologist managing the patient's seizure disorder, and strongly urge that the patient be weaned off Phenytoin and placed on a safer alternative anti-seizure medication. Edentulism and bacteremia need not be a side-effect of a seizure management protocol.

The patient seen in Fig. 4.19 is a 20 year old male patient with idiopathic intellectual disability who presented to an outpatient dental clinic for comprehensive dental evaluation and treatment. He was accompanied by his father. His father was referred to the clinic by the staff at his son's day program workshop. The day program staff had observed hand-mouthing behaviors, and they had voiced concern that the patient may be in pain.

In the waiting room, the patient exhibited behaviors consistent with neurodevelopmental dysfunction. He was non-communicative, and his gaze aversion and tactile defensiveness were suggestive of autism. He was resistant and somewhat combative when directed to the dental chair, and effective behavior management in both the waiting room and operatory required the combined efforts of his father and two staff

4   Broader Considerations of Medical and Dental Data Integration

Fig. 4.20 Pectus excavatum

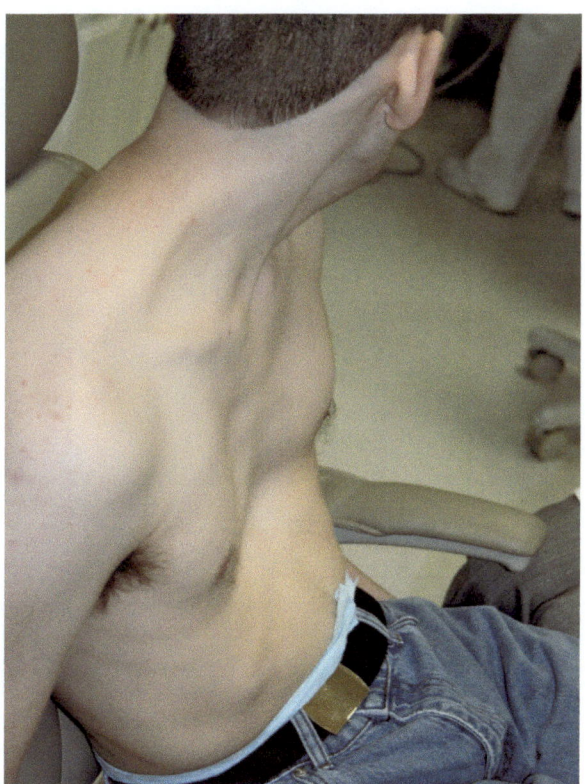

members. The patient's health history was positive for attention deficit hyperactivity disorder (ADHD), and there was no history of seizure or neuromotor impairment.

The father indicated that, at age ten, the patient was admitted to an inpatient psychiatric unit for evaluation of his uncontrollable behavior. The following day, the parents were told that managing the patient's behavior was beyond the ability of the psychiatric unit staff, and the parents were asked to take the child home. The father also indicated that the psychiatric unit staff described the child's behavior as overwhelming.

The patient was last seen by a dentist 12 years prior to presentation; examination and treatment at that time were carried out in the operating room under general anesthesia.

Effective oral examination of this patient required utilization of papoose board and Molt mouth prop. Multiple options for behavior management, including utilization of general anesthesia in the operating room, were discussed with the father, and informed consent to utilize medical immobilization techniques for purposes of this examination was obtained and documented prior to taking the patient into the operatory. In the operatory a dental examination was performed, and a baseline panel of digital radiographs was obtained.

The head and facial features of this patient were suggestive of Fragile X syndrome (See: Fig. 4.20). The body of the mandible was somewhat elongated; the

Fig. 4.21 Joint laxity observed in patient with Fragile X syndrome

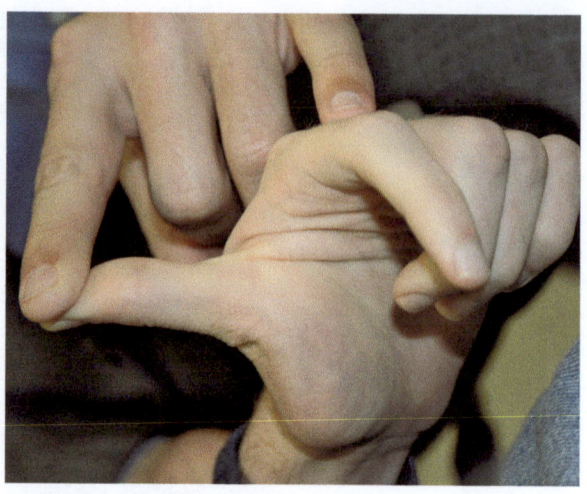

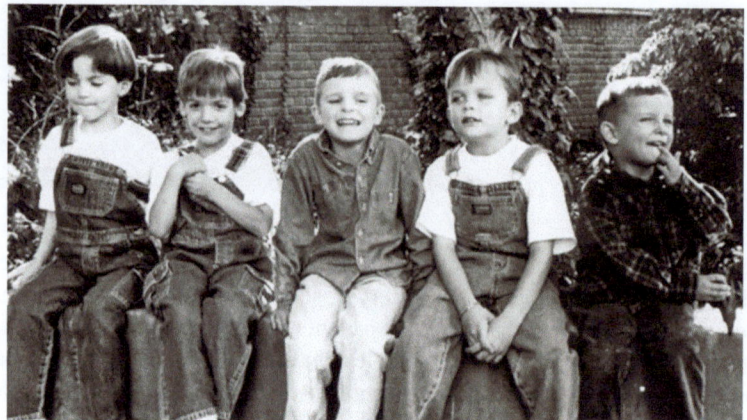

Fig. 4.22 Four children with autism and one neurotypical child

nose was prominent; the head had somewhat of a triangular shape, and the patient readily averted his gaze. Upon further inquiry, the father reported that the patient also exhibited macroorchidism, although he indicated that no physician or dentist had ever suggested a work up for Fragile X.

Fragile X syndrome is a disorder with which many clinicians are unfamiliar. Yet it is the second leading genetic cause of intellectual disability in the United States, and it is the leading known cause of autism in the U.S. In addition to the phenotypic findings noted in this case, there are other frequently-encountered physical characteristics consistent with Fragile X that may move a clinician toward this diagnosis. They include pectus excavatum or funnel chest (see Fig. 4.21) and joint laxity (see Fig. 4.22).

Gaze aversion, as previously mentioned, is a typical finding in autism and in Fragile X syndrome. Indeed, in conjunction with non-verbal behaviors, gaze aversion is often the finding that initially alerts the clinician to the possibility of a neurodevelopmental diagnosis featuring autism as a complication. Figure 4.22 features a photograph of five children at a school for children with special needs. Four of the children have been diagnosed with autism, and a fifth child is a neurotypical child who was visiting his brother on the day the photograph was taken. The reader is left to decide which child is the neurotypical child.

Any physician or dentist who encounters a patient with an obvious intellectual disability, who does not have an established underlying neurodevelopmental diagnosis, and who presents with additional findings, which may include gaze aversion, shyness, a prominent chin, pectus excavatum, a large nose or large ears, should suspect a possible Fragile X diagnosis.

The primary care clinician – physician or dentist – should discuss with the guardian or family member the importance of establishing a neurodevelopmental diagnosis. The family member or guardian should be informed that genetic counseling should be made available to all members of the extended family, since Fragile X syndrome is a genetic disorder that can be passed from parents to offspring. Once this discussion has taken place, a referral to a geneticist for a complete genetic work up is indicated. Both the dentist and physician should feel entirely comfortable making this referral. In remote areas where the services of a geneticist may not be available, the attending physician or dentist may order a high resolution chromosomal analysis and a Fragile X DNA test, and have those results sent to a remote location for interpretation by a geneticist. Consultation with a psychiatrist or a clinical psychologist may also be advisable, as patients with Fragile X can sometimes experience enhanced social integration as a benefit of behavioral therapy.

4.2.6.6 Interdisciplinary Solutions for Interdisciplinary Problems

The healthcare access problem for Americans with neurodevelopmental disorders and intellectual disabilities is, at its core, a healthcare education problem – an education problem resulting from a long-standing deficiency in professional training focused on the care of this patient population. And it is clear that the medical and dental professions share equally in responsibility for these deficiencies.

Eighty-one percent of America's medical students will graduate without ever having rendered clinical care to a single patient with a neurodevelopmental disorder or intellectual disability; and the graduates of 90% of America's medical residency programs will graduate from those residencies having had no formal training whatsoever – didactic or clinical – in the care of this patient population.[1] Additionally, 50% of graduating dentists have never treated a single patient with a disability.[2]

It is no wonder that patients like those whose cases were discussed in earlier sections of this chapter have such difficulty accessing quality health care. As Robert Uchin, Dean of Nova Southeastern University College of Dental Medicine observed in a speech in 2003 to his faculty, "Not only do we not have enough doctors to care for these patients; we don't have enough teachers to teach them how to care for them."

As a result of these deficiencies in professional education, few clinicians with any expertise in developmental medicine or developmental dentistry are to be found in communities across America. The experts in developmental medicine and dentistry, for the most part, tend to be physicians and dentists who work at the few remaining intermediate care facilities, and at special needs outpatient clinics, psychiatric hospitals, and nursing homes. These physicians and dentists possess the knowledge and expertise in these disciplines because they are the physicians and dentists with the clinical experience. Unfortunately for the patients with neurodevelopmental disorders who are clamoring for quality care, there are too few of these clinicians.

National experts in developmental medicine and dentistry, however, have begun to collaborate in the creation of patient care protocols; and they have produced multidisciplinary curricula in both DVD and online format.

The AADMD has made available 9 hours of online curriculum in developmental medicine, developmental dentistry, and developmental psychiatry (See: List of URLs). The curriculum program is entitled, *The Continuum of Quality Care*, and it teaches collaborative patient care in three disciplines through an interdisciplinary format.

The AADMD, through a grant from the Wal Mart Foundation and the North Carolina Developmental Disabilities Council, and in collaboration with the North Carolina Mountain Area Health Education Center and the Family Medicine Education Consortium, has also established the National Curriculum Initiative in Developmental Medicine. This initiative, which is scheduled for completion in 2012, will develop curriculum standards for physicians in the primary care of adults with ND/ID. The curriculum stresses the importance of a collaborative approach, which includes medicine, dentistry, podiatry, optometry, and multiple ancillary health professions.

If the disparities in access to healthcare for Americans with ND/ID are to be resolved, physicians and dentists must be willing to cross professional boundaries and work together to plan and deliver whole-person healthcare to their patients with ND/ID. Interdisciplinary protocols in the diagnosis of neurodevelopmental disorders and in the management of the secondary health consequences associated with these disorders must be established. Additionally, clinicians with expertise in these arenas must be willing to work and teach in our nation's medical and dental schools. The clinicians with expertise must be willing to develop predoctoral and postdoctoral curricula, and the deans of America's professional schools must be willing to include these curricula as part of their larger programs in primary and specialized care.

The clinicians with expertise in developmental medicine and dentistry must also be willing to conduct patient-focused, interdisciplinary, clinical research in an effort to solve the myriad problems that create obstacles to the delivery of the standard of care for patients with ND/ID. They must be willing to obtain Institutional Review Board approval for this research, and they must be willing to make this research available to their colleagues through publication in peer-reviewed journals and text books, and in professional lecture forums.

The patient featured in Figs. 4.23 and 4.24 is a man named James. He is a 48 year old patient with idiopathic intellectual disability who presented to a dental clinic for

Fig. 4.23 Patient upon initial examination

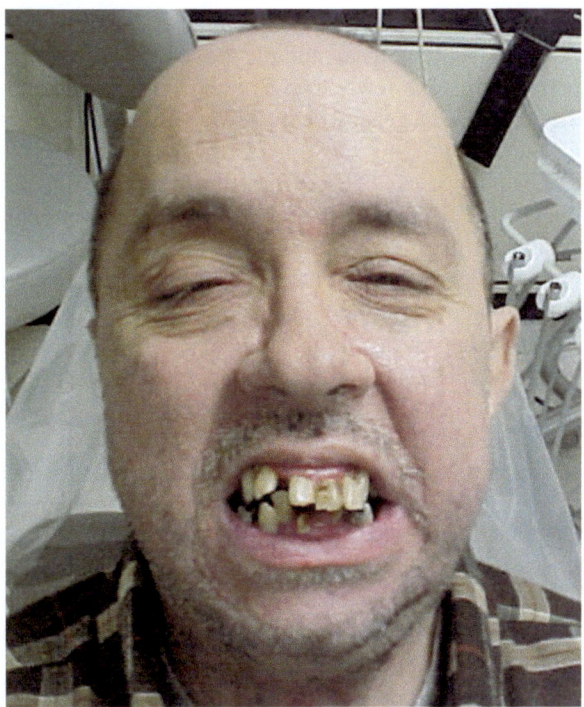

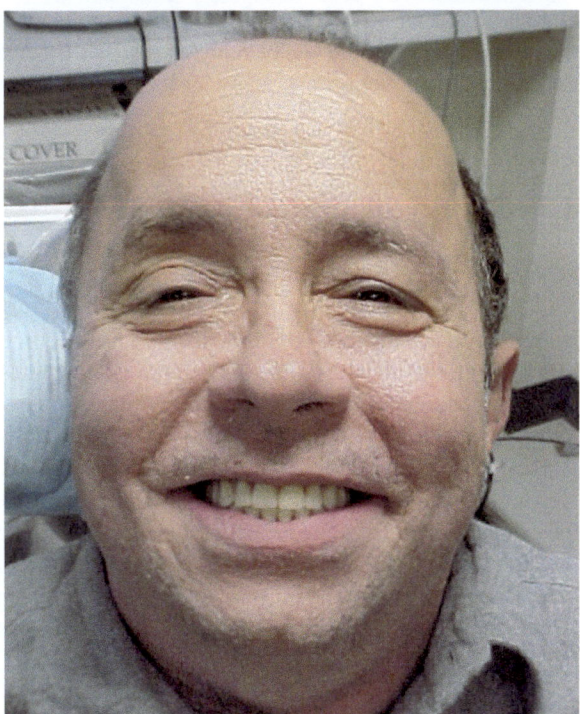

Fig. 4.24 Patient after comprehensive treatment

evaluation of a painful facial swelling. A comprehensive intraoral exam revealed a cellulitis resulting from multiple grossly decayed teeth, and a generalized advanced periodontitis. No fewer than five clinicians became involved in this patient's care. They included a general dentist, two oral surgeons, a family practice physician, and a geneticist.

Over the course of several months, as the treatment plan was completed, and as the chronic dental and periodontal infections were eliminated, James experienced significant improvement in his overall state of health. A comparison of these two photographs reveals not only significant improvement in his aesthetic appearance, but also in his skin turgor and color.

These improvements in the patient's health translated to improvements in his daily life. He found gainful employment, and his caregivers now report that he smiles constantly – at work and at home.

These photographs were entered into evidence in 2007 before a Congressional subcommittee investigating the death of a young African-American boy who died as a result of an untreated dental abscess. The photographs were intended to make the point that patients with intellectual disabilities need not die as a result of medical illnesses derived from untreated dental disease.

This patient's case illustrates that, when physicians and dentists are willing to work together toward a common goal of whole-person health for their patients, profoundly positive outcomes can be achieved.

In a larger context, if our nation's medical and dental professions are willing to commit to a shared agenda, one which promotes the idea of collaborative, interdisciplinary care as a foundational concept, significant improvements in quality of health and quality of life can be realized, not just for Americans with neurodevelopmental disorders, but for every patient seeking quality care.

4.3 Biosurveillance and Dentistry

Miguel Humberto Torres-Urquidy

In light of the events of 2001, bioterrorism has become subject of increased attention from all members of society. Government agencies, professional associations, academia, etc. have expressed their determination to wage war on such threats by all means available. Dentists can also participate in this effort by providing assistance at interested groups and the general public (Flores et al. 2003). In this chapter we will examine the elements and components that may play a role in the establishment of an electronic network for the dental profession for supporting the fight against bioterrorism. In this section we review the threats, the public health system, current electronic surveillance systems, regulations and ethical issues, the computerization of dentistry, and how dentistry can serve in improving biosurveillance efforts.

4.3.1 Background

The aftermath of September 11 and the anthrax incidents in October 2001 (Lane and Fauci 2003), made the US government reorganize its priorities and reform its current structure (White House Office of the Press Secretary 2003). In response to these incidents, President Bush proposed the "Health Security Initiative" (White House Letter 2002) in February 2nd of 2003. This effort labeled the "Bioshield Initiative," (White House Letter 2002) has the purpose to stimulate research and development of medical countermeasures against bioterrorism attacks. However, despite all these efforts, terrorist attacks are likely to happen in the future and even the best work from intelligence and security agencies will be unable to prevent such events (Betts and Richard 2002; Council on Foreign Relations 2003; Baker and Koplan 2002). To cope with this threat, a report published by an independent task force sponsored by the Council on Foreign Relations "America-Still Unprepared, Still in Danger" (Council on Foreign Relations 2003), suggested a series of steps to assist the government in preparing to better protect the country. One of these suggestions is the bolstering of the "Public Health Systems".

4.3.2 Public Health Systems

Baker et al. define the U.S. public health system as a system that consists of a broad range of organizations and partnerships needed to carry out the essential public health services, such as hospitals, voluntary health organizations, other non-governmental organizations and the business community (Baker and Koplan 2002) which can collaborate with local, state and federal public health entities. After the unfortunate incidents in 2001 the public health system was revisited and the realization that "the nation's public health infrastructure is not fully prepared to meet this growing challenge" (Frist 2002) became clear. To address this need, Congress and President Bush enacted the Public Law (P.L.) 107–188 titled "Public Health Security and Bioterrorism Preparedness and Response Act of 2002" (Frist 2002; 107th Congress 2002). The main purpose of this law was to improve the public health capacity by means of increasing funding and fostering other measures. Frist (2002), described the law as a "good start" and that "to be prepared for bioterrorism, it is imperative that we develop a cohesive and comprehensive system of ongoing surveillance and case investigations for early detection". In this way, several early detection systems have been implemented with different levels of success among different geographic regions in the US.

One of the most important initiatives over the years has been the establishment of the National Electronic Disease Surveillance System (NEDSS) (Baker and Koplan 2002; NEDSS 2001). The National Electronic Disease Surveillance Working Group establishes that the "NEDSS is a broad initiative focused on the use of data and information systems standards to advance the development of efficient, integrated, and interoperable surveillance systems at the state and local levels. The long-term objectives for NEDSS are the ongoing automatic capture and analyses of data needed for public health surveillance". The purpose of this system is to take into consideration and integrate the information of current public health systems implemented at different health department levels: county, state and finally at the Centers for Disease Control and Prevention (CDC).

Another initiative spearheaded by the CDC is Biosense (Looks 2004). The purpose of this program is to develop advance detection capabilities of health related events including disease outbreaks. In addition, its emphasis is to improve situational awareness by integrating advanced analytics to process data generated by different health providers and other entities in the US.

Now that we have examined the general aspects, we will continue our background review focusing on the aspects that pertain to the specifics of the dental profession.

4.3.3 Dentistry in the US

This section will provide some perspective of the structure of the dental profession in comparison with its medical counterpart. "There are approximately 150,000 active dentists in the United States" (Mertz and O'Neil 2002). In 1990 the dentist-to-population ratio was of 60–100,000. And it is expected that by the year 2020 the ratio will be 52.7, which translates into one dentist for every 1,898 people. "In contrast, the physician-to-population ratio has been increasing for the past 40 years and now stands at 286 per 100,000, about one physician for every 349 people." Eighty percent of the dentists are in general practice.

4.3.4 Dentistry and Bioterrorism

During March 27 and 28 of 2003, the American Dental Association and the US Public Health Service sponsored the conference "Dentistry's Role in Responding to Bioterrorism and Other Catastrophic Events" (Palmer 2003; National Institute of Dental and Craniofacial Research 2004). This meeting reviewed several aspects of bioterrorism and the dental profession: the nature of biological pathogens and its oral manifestations, what needed to be communicated, how dentists should participate, etc. Dr. Michael C. Alfano described the difficulties that biological pathogens create for clinicians because "they are so insidious." While discussing the anthrax mailings after September 11th he pointed out that: "… early symptoms appeared so they resembled the aches, fever, and malaise of flu so those affected delayed seeking treatment, a delay that has proven fatal in some cases". Lieutenant Colonel Ross H. Pastel of the US Army Medical Research Institute of Infectious Disease (USAMRIID) listed the "Category A" pathogens as defined by the Centers for Disease Control and Prevention, and those are: smallpox, anthrax, plague, botulinum toxin, tularemia and viral hemorrhagic fever. He also described an outbreak of smallpox in Yugoslavia in 1972 and the measure that had to be taken to control it. Dr. Michael Glick described the oral manifestations of smallpox showing "signs 24 hours before skin rash. These oral signs include tongue swelling, multiple mucosa vesicles, ulceration, and mucosal hemorrhaging. Oral signs are also evident in inhalation and gastro-intestinal anthrax. In oropharyngeal anthrax the mucosa appears edematous and congested; there may be neck swelling, fever, and sore throat".

Dr. Ed Thompson, Deputy Director of the Centers for Disease Control and Prevention mentioned that "None of the new counter-bioterrorism measures can be effective unless local health practitioners are vigilant in observing and reporting a possible disease outbreak. Such surveillance–knowing what to look for and whom to report to–is critical and applies not only to suspected bioterrorist agents, but to a list of reportable diseases which has grown to include such entities as West Nile virus and Sever Acute Respiratory Syndrome (SARS)." Dr. Sigurs O. Krolls presented the response at the local level and he "stressed the importance of communication and the need for redundant systems", "to keep all the parties informed". He also posed the question "Can dentists recognize signs and systems of contagious diseases?", and emphasized that education can be essential. Dr. Louis DePaola made several connotations that can be key in the scope of this paper by saying "dentists can contribute to bioterrorism surveillance by being alert to clues that might indicate a bioterrorism attack. Such surveillance would note if there is an influx of people seeking medical attention with non-traumatic conditions and flu-like or possibly neurological or paralytic symptoms… or even specific signs of a bioterrorist agent. Patterns of school of work absence, appointment cancellations or failures to appear, could also be indicators." Dr. DePaola made clear that in cases of limited release of bioterrorist agents, dentists "have little to offer" but "a widespread attack can certainly tap into dental professional skills in recognition, isolation and management". In addition, Dr. Guay (2002) lists all the possible roles in which dentists can participate including "education, risk communication, diagnosis, surveillance and notification, treatment, distribution of medications, decontamination, sample collection and forensic dentistry."

Dental Informatics must pay attention to these and other recommendations, in order to develop integrated systems that take these recommendations into consideration. It is also important to understand that informatics has to work with technologies already in place like the Computer-Based Oral Health Record and current standards. The final recommendation from the meeting stated that to play an important role in biodefense, a serious amount of coordination and preparation will be required, not only from dentists but from other groups, most likely requiring medical and dental data integration.

4.3.5 The Computer-Based Oral Health Record (COHR) and Computer Ownership

The COHR as described by Rhodes (1996) "can provide a structure for documentation that goes beyond the concept of a blank form on a page, it includes a glossary of dental terminology for the entire content of the form as well as knowledge bases and expert systems that can enhance the practitioner's diagnostic and treatment planning decisions". He also acknowledges that one of the advantages of this type of documentation is that it "is much more transportable". He also recognizes the need for standardized methods for collecting information from dentists. Schleyer and Eisner (1997) defined several scenarios where the COHR is used in a "shared" environment where several healthcare providers interact and information is seamless communicated, improving the decisions made by clinicians. Delrose and Steinberg (2000) discuss how the "Digital Patient Record" enhances clinical practice by providing "better quality information" to the clinician. Although all of these benefits sound promising and encouraging some still express concern of the lack of standards among different information systems, which translates in communication breakdowns (Schleyer 2003). On the other hand, Heid and colleagues (2002) mention a list all the steps that are currently being taken by different organizations such as the ADA in order to produce a standardized COHR. Other examples of standardization can be found in a paper presented by Narcisi (1996) where ADA's participation as a voting member in the American National Standards Institute has allowed EDI or the COHR to be discussed and improved at a national level.

Additional influences in the standardization of the COHR are the security regulations mandated by HIPAA, the Health Insurance Portability and Accountability Act of 1996. Dentists are required to "adopt practices necessary for compliance" (Sfikas 2003; Chasteen et al. 2003). These and other regulations (Szekely et al. 1996) will encourage the homogeny among different system vendors. Computer ownership, on the other hand, has increased steadily during the last 25 years. According to Schleyer et al. (2003) in 1976 only 1% of dental professionals used computers in their practices compared to 85% in the year 2000. Additionally similar trends in Internet connectivity where described.

4.3.6 Dentists, Source of Information Against Bioterrorism

The issues mentioned above describe the issues that have to be considered in order to create surveillance system against bioterrorism for the dental profession. This review has tried to be inclusive by covering different aspects starting with the current state of affairs and environment, treats, technology, law, etc. Next we present a blueprint for developing a biosurveillance system.

4.3.7 Proposed System

The purpose of developing an electronic health surveillance system is to gather information from patients directly (Wagner et al. 2006) by detecting signs and/or symptoms, or indirectly by obtaining other types of information such as over the counter medication sales, patients' no-shows, usage of Internet search engines keywords, etc. In this particular case, the proximity of contact between the dentist and the patient is equivalent to a medical inspection in terms of immediacy and/or closeness. Such signs and symptoms can be easily detected if the dentist is properly prompted to search for them. This is just one example of ways how a system could provide assistance in the detection of a bioterrorism incident.

But, before describing our proposed system, it would be important to address the fact that current syndromic surveillance systems have certain advantages in terms of its particular technological implementation (Tsui et al. 2003). The RODS laboratory obtains data directly from chief complains in the emergency departments from hospitals. The advantage of this surveillance system is that the implementation has to be made with only a limited number of parties (hospitals, clinics, health systems, etc.). On the other hand, our system would have to deal with thousands of different implementations (one in each dental office). This and other challenges have to be considered when designing the proposed system:

The proposed system should work at multiple levels:

- The system would have to provide a mechanism to alert the dentist if there is suspicion that a bioterrorist attack may be happening. The mechanism would increase the dentist's awareness in case of finding suspicious signs or symptoms in a patient. This can be triggered by the patient's characteristics such as geographic location of residence, etc.
- Automated collection of information from the patient's oral health record. The system would report to a central database signs or symptoms of interest. The aggregation of this data could generate information that would eventually identify the presence of patterns that may lead to the early detection of such events.
- Collection of additional information, which combined with other sources, can be useful in terms of detecting or tracing some incident. Patients' "no-shows" is the primary example, that, if combined with others such as work or school absenteeism can provide a relevant pattern for public health officials.

4.3.8 Example of a Hypothetical Case

Dr. X, who practices in a community 20 min away from Capitol City, installed a new clinical management system 2 months ago. Among the features that were included in this new clinical management system (CMS), a bioterrorism detection module was added. She felt curious because of recent news she read in the newspaper about possible attacks against the US and decided to install such feature. He read about how the module would work in combination with the CMS she just bought. The educational information provided with the software instructed Dr. X, that in case that a patient victim of a bioterrorism attack happens to be seen in her practice, the software would collect information and would send it to public health officials. When installing the software, Dr. X was asked if she agreed to share such information with authorities. She was provided the option to receive notification in case some information was sent but she decided not to enforce it.

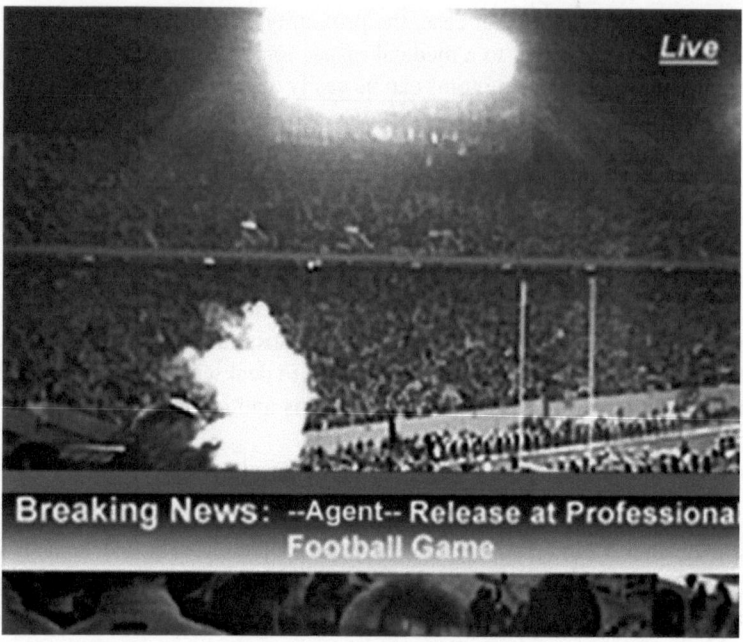

Fig. 4.25 Biosurveillance systems should be cognizant of different kinds of events since this can be linked to issues of public health concern

During the last week a patient walked into Dr. X's dental office. The patient presented some signs that indicated the presence of a disease; still its origin was not clear. An epidemiologic study later would show that the patient was present at the football stadium when an infectious agent was released (Fig. 4.25). Although, at that time his medical history showed no indication of a systemic disease, the presence of multiple oral vesicles prompted the dentist to make an annotation into the COHR. The system, by using a natural language processing engine, detected such sign and sent this information to a central database. The patient was discharged and instructed to take some support medication to treat the oral ulcers. The next day, the central database pinpointed the presence of an out of the ordinary increase in the number of cases with the same signs and symptoms around that region. When the presence of this peak was detected, the central server sent a request to the dentist computer for additional information. One of the requested elements was if there was any use of medication for treating oral ulcers. Fortunately this information was available. The central database crossed this with the information of other surveillance systems together with the information from other patients that happen to have similar clinical signs and/or symptoms. Dr. X received an email from a public health official asking her to communicate to the local health department to discuss information about one her patients.

The case depicted above simulates the release of smallpox during a football game. In the case of smallpox oral symptoms include tongue swelling, multiple oral mucosal vesicles, ulceration, and mucosal hemorrhaging (National Institute of Dental and Craniofacial Research 2004). Dentists could be alerted by an electronic system to search for such signs or they can be detected automatically. In case of a high incidence within a group of patients, in a confined area, public health officials get to be notified.

In our hypothetical case there are issues that need to be addressed in order to make such detection system feasible:

4.3.9 System Design

As described by Schleyer et al. (2006), 85% of dentists in the US use a computer in their practices. This figure would generate an estimate of 127,500 computers in dental practices. This prevalence of computers represents an opportunity for public health data collection.

The creation of a software application for surveillance purposes must rely on existing technology. Currently there are approximately 20 major clinical management software packages in the market (Dentistry Today 2003). Out of these 20, 17 clearly permit direct database manipulation. This characteristic can easily allow the creation of a "querying" application that would look for specific information within the data stored by those packages. Additionally, a natural language processing engine could be embedded into the application in order to detect variations in data input on the computer oral health record. Nevertheless, it is necessary to obtain a detailed list of the oral manifestations of diseases that are likely to be found on patients. Successful implementations of similar systems have been shown to work successfully (Chapman et al. 2001; Ivanov et al. 2002) and using the same approach for our system seems technically feasible.

This collected information later would be send to a central server in order to be analyzed and interpreted.

4.3.10 Software Architecture

The components of our system would be as follows (Fig. 4.26):

- Thin client: a software application distributed for data collection. It would be conformed of a "querying" mechanism, combined with a natural language processing engine and a communication module. This software client should be as thin as possible to reduce the work load on the dentist's equipment and should be embedded as a plug-in for current clinical management systems. Vendors should be contacted to ask for their collaboration in the development of such application to ensure maximum compatibility and integrity of data collection.

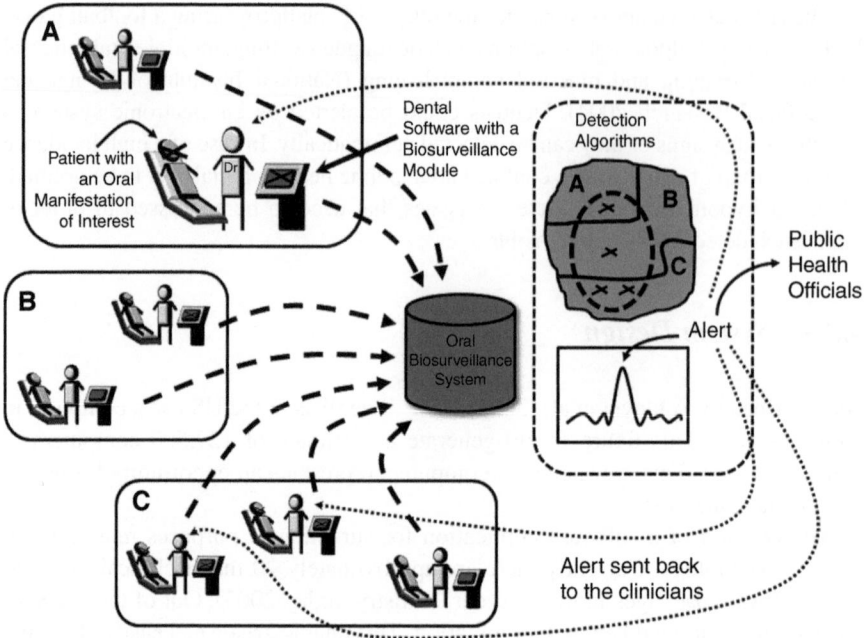

Fig. 4.26 Biosurveillance system architecture

- Central servers: server software in charge of integrating all the data collected from dental offices. It has to be capable of handling simultaneous requests from multiple users. This server would integrate all the data and would perform an analysis with the intention of detecting anomalies. It would be recommended that redundant servers should be located in different data centers with mirroring capabilities to guarantee their survivability in case of technical difficulties.
- Communication network: the transmission of information should be done using the Internet. This, of course, would essentially depend on the practitioner's current connectivity. If that is not available, backup connection to the central servers should be established.

4.3.11 Standards

Dentistry uses several standards for transmission of health related information. Clinical management systems use standard-based technology to transmit information (Narcisi 1996; Chasteen et al. 2003; Szekely et al. 1996; Dentrix Dental Systems 2011). Dentists are aware of these standards and use them in a day-to-day basis to transmit information to insurers. Additionally, in order to interact with other surveillance systems such as the NEDSS, our application should rely on the same standards.

4.3.12 Security and Redundancy

The software both client and server should be thoroughly verified to be secure in terms of being safe against hacker attacks. On the server side, redundancy should be provided so downtime is reduced from design. The system should be developed so mirrored servers are always up and running. Data integrity mechanism should also be considered.

4.3.13 Privacy and Confidentiality

Privacy and Confidentiality are important issues that need to be incorporated as part of a robust biosurveillance system and distinct regulations such as HIPAA require protecting patient information (Frist 2002; Chasteen et al. 2003; Bayer and Colgrove 2002; Etzioni 2002; Ivanov et al. 2002). In our hypothetical case we describe the use of several sources of information for detecting a bioterrorist attack. We described how syndromic information is transmitted to a central database which initially should be de-identified. Later, after the suspicion a bioterrorist attack more information is requested (medications) and more inferences are made. This, although technically possible, would require changing our processes and also the will to share clinical information. This leads to the discussion mentioned in the background section about "individual rights" vs. "common good". Although HIPAA addresses public health (Gesteland et al. 2003), some other implications may arise and the health professionals including dentists, physicians, public health officials and patients should discuss and address such issues.

As discussed earlier, legislators face a difficult task in terms of determining what is best on behalf of the individuals they were asked to represent. Legislation may have to be passed in order to guarantee the functioning of such a system. Individual freedom and privacy are important values which may pose a conflict when collecting individuals' information even for their own good.

In any case, careful consideration has to be given to which information is required to detect a bioterrorist attack and also, by keeping in mind that it is always important to reduce, as much as possible, the collection and transmission of patients' information over the Internet or any other network.

4.3.14 Detection Algorithms and Evaluation

A detection algorithm has to be created or adapted in order to determine the presence of a bioterrorist attack. Some algorithms have proven their effectiveness (Wong et al. 2003a, b) and it is likely that from these, a new analysis should be done in order to select or create one that addresses the particular needs of our system.

A study was conducted to assess the feasibility of using oral manifestations in order to detect disease outbreaks (Torres-Urquidy et al. 2009). It was found that for diseases such as Botulism and Smallpox it would be feasible to gather data that contains oral manifestations that would allow creating a detection signal using natural language processing followed by the use of statistical methods such as Moving Average to serve as part of a detection algorithm.

The system should also be thoroughly evaluated, before and after implementation. To perform the evaluation before the system implementation computer simulation can be used to assess the effectiveness and likelihood of detection. Simulation and modeling techniques (Reshetin and Regens 2003) have been used to estimate the effects of a bioterrorist attack. The same techniques can be used to evaluate our system. In case of the study by Torres-Urquidy (2009), the investigators utilized synthetic outbreaks to test the performance of different signals. From their evaluation process, they learned, for instance, how many cases would be necessary to occur for the system to reach certain detection thresholds.

4.3.15 Organizations Interested in Participating in Our Efforts

Several dental organizations have shown publicly their support of measures against bioterrorism. The American Dental Association and the National Institute of Dental and Craniofacial Research are two organizations who could play an important role in the development, deployment and ongoing support for our system. Local dental societies also would also play an important role in the deployment of the proposed system. Similarly, local, state and federal public health agencies should engage in activities that could make these mechanisms for health surveillance feasible.

If dentists want to play an active role in the fight against bioterrorism, they should commit to collaborate with public health entities as well as to seek a way to integrate their information with the rest of electronic biosurveillance systems. Professional organizations such as the American Dental Association can also participate by endorsing such efforts and by collaborating in the educational process of the dental professionals and their patients.

4.3.16 Conclusion

As mentioned by Dr. DePaola (National Institute of Dental and Craniofacial Research 2004) dentists "have little to offer" in the current biosurveillance state of affairs. However, the integration of different technologies can change this perception. Goldenberg et al. (2002) described over-the-counter medication sales as a technique for discovering disease outbreaks and stated that their approach may be "more timely" than traditional medical or public health approaches. Medical cases that result from bioterrorism attacks do not produce symptoms until they have fully developed, so it is likely that different patterns can be detected before the patients start reaching the Emergency Department. As stated earlier (Torres-Urquidy et al. 2009), it may be possible to have dentists participating of biosurveillance efforts, if we solve the proper organizational and technical challenges.

Dr. John R. Lumpkin (2001) states that "Hippocrates noted the health of the community was dependent on characteristics of a community and the habits of the people who lived there." Dr. Krolls (NIDCR 2003) in his final remarks during his presentation at the Dentistry's Role Conference Against Bioterrorism, said, "dentists may pick up telltale information about what is happening in the community. After all, dentists spend more time with their patients than any other health specialty".

Further Reading

Kass-Hout T, Zhang X. Biosurveillance: methods and case studies. Boca Raton: Chapman and Hall/CRC; 2010.
Lombardo JS, Buckeridge DL. Disease surveillance: a public health informatics approach. Hoboken: Wiley; 2007.
Wagner MM, Moore AW, Aryel RM. Handbook of biosurveillance. Burlington: Elsevier Academic Press; 2006.

4.4 Integration of Patient Records and Clinical Research: Lack of Integration as a Barrier to Needed Research; Integration as a Prerequisite to Research

Muhammad F. Walji

4.4.1 Introduction

Maintaining patient records are essential for both clinical care and research. Clinical research often occurs in the context of also providing patient care, yet the systems that are used for each are different and often cannot exchange data. The lack of data exchange between systems pose significant barriers to efficiently treating patient and conducting clinical research in dentistry. The purpose of this section is to review the benefits and challenges of integrating electronic health record (EHR) used for patient care and electronic data capture (EDC) which is used for clinical research such as clinical trials.

An increasing number of dentists routinely use EHRs (Schleyer et al. 2006). Most dental schools in North America also use EHRs. Benefits of using EHRs include increased legibility, portability, and improved patient safety (Buntin et al. 2011). Recent federal incentives, although not directly beneficial to dentists, will also likely spur the adoption of EHR (Blumenthal and Tavenner 2010).

Clinical researchers, especially those conducting clinical trials, are also discovering benefits of using electronic data capture compared to paper. A clinical trial is a process in which new treatments, medications and other innovations are tested to evaluate safety and efficacy. A standard part of health care, clinical trials are often lengthy and costly due to myriads of regulatory oversight. Recent estimates set the cost of drug development in excess of $800 million (Grabowski et al. 2002).

4.4.2 Electronic Health Records and Electronic Data Capture

Accurately documenting data with sufficient detail is critical for providing patient care and conducting clinical research. While the medical record is the foundation for patient care, the case report form is the foundation in a clinical trial. Not all clinical research is clinical trials. Clinical trials whose data will be submitted to the FDA as a new therapy or device have additional requirements relating to the collection and transmission of the data. Similarly for patient care data, EHRs need to meet the privacy and security requirements of HIPAA.

Case report forms (CRF) are a medium in which research study sites collect subject data in pre-defined formats for communication with clinical trial sponsors (Rondel and Webb 2000) Many clinical trials data are collected on paper (Rondel and Webb 2000). Data measurement, collection, and recording are considered the "most crucial stage" in the data management process (Hosking et al. 1995).

Traditionally, study coordinators often record information in a case report form and subsequently mail or fax the CRF to the centralized coordinating center. There, data entry staff, sometimes with the aid of optical character recognition systems, input CRF data into a computer. Errors made during this second data entry process are difficult to detect and correct (Hosking et al. 1995). Lengthy guidelines in literature discuss methods for developing paper case report forms to reduce data entry mistakes (Hosking 1995). A well-designed CRF may allow a user to efficiently collect and record pertinent data. However, forms are often revised and redesigned during a clinical trial due to changes in protocol, unforeseen outcomes, or oversight (Singer and Meinert 1995).

There has been a recent drive to use electronic case report forms (eCRF). Direct data entry at a study site shortens time to analysis and provides opportunities to audit data at time of entry. This could reduce data errors that might otherwise be caught weeks after submission. For quality control purposes, some studies require double data entry using computers and paper (Day et al. 1998), though alternative solutions have been explored including the use of data sampling (King and Lashley 2000) and probability statistics to select only those forms likely to contain errors (Kleinman 2001).

ECRFs may also facilitate data collection from existing electronic information systems such as lab systems. However, eCRFs are almost always reside in a separate system that is not linked to a patients record.

Although many clinical research studies are still being conducted using paper, an increasing number of studies are using eCRFS and electronic data capture (EDC). For example, a review of Canadian clinical trials found that 40% use EDC (El Emam et al. 2009). Studies that are sponsored by a pharmaceutical company and are multi-center appear to use EDC at a higher rate than those sponsored by government or a university. The cost of a commercial EDC is substantial. Recently a freely available EDC has become popular amongst universities called REDCap. A tool originally developed at Vanderbilt University, it is now being used at over a 100 institutions worldwide (Harris et al. 2009). However, such tools are generally not integrated with the institutions EHR. Although moving from paper to electronic will afford benefits there is a great need to allow data exchange between the patient care and clinical research components of information systems.

Although EHR and EDC are similar, several challenges remain unresolved that prevent integration. One of the major barriers is likely to be different workflows for patient care purposes and to collect data for research. Research is needed in defining an optimal workflow that can streamline the tasks associated with patient care and research, while at the same time providing a unified information system that support these activities. Also, the data that are collected for care and research are likely to differ. A researcher may require far more granularity of an oral health measurement than a clinician seeking to provide care. In cases when conducting a double blind placebo controlled clinical trial, the investigator may not even know the type of treatment that has been delivered to the patient. Due to complexities of each domain, and large differences in goals, to date mutually exclusive workflows have arisen. A clinician investigator who sees a patient for both care and research, will likely need to enter data on this same patient twice; once in the EHR and once in the EDC system.

4.4.3 Need for a Common Language

Despite the availability of electronic systems, a major barrier is the integration and compatibility of disparate health information systems to converse with one another. The languages are important because they can help data sharing. Clinical trials are not usually conducted in isolation, but are part of conventional medical care. Therefore sharing data by clinical trials, patient care and laboratory systems becomes especially important with the adoption of EHRs in dentistry.

In biomedical informatics, standardized terminologies are recognized as a critically important area to help better represent and share data for use in electronic systems (Cimino 2000).

The Systematized Nomenclature of Medicine Clinical Terms (SNOMED-CT), developed by the College of American Pathologists, is the most comprehensive medical terminology (Strang et al. 2002; Chute et al. 1996) and is used in a number of health informatics applications. The US Department of Health and Human Services (2010) has also licensed SNOMED-CT, allowing access throughout the US at no charge. Therefore SNOMED-CT is even more likely to be the vocabulary used in electronic formats of patient records in the future.

The Medical Dictionary for Regulatory Activities (MedDRA) is terminology used by the FDA and drug development industry to classify, retrieve, present, and communicate medical information throughout the medical product regulatory cycle (Brown et al. 1999). In particular it is used to record and report adverse drug event data.

Therefore standard languages are essential in sharing clinical trials data between sites, and also with regulatory agencies. No one single terminology is suited for all tasks. SNOMED-CT is likely to be more comprehensive to code clinical encounters, while MedDRA is more suited to help adverse event reporting. However, it is important that terminologies are widely adopted and used for similar purposes.

Even when standard terminologies are agreed upon, such information needs to be interchanged in standard formats. Health Level 7 (HL7) is an important organization whose standards are widely adopted in healthcare to exchange information between computer systems. The Clinical Data Interchange Standards Consortium (CDISC) is also an important group that helps to define different data standards specifically for clinical trials research, such as clinical trials or regulatory submissions.

One particular challenge in oral health has been the lack of a standardized terminology to describe diagnoses. Although ICD contains oral health concepts, they are often not granular enough to be useful for some patient care or research purposes. Recently a dental diagnostic terminology has been developed by a group of dental schools, and has already been adopted by several institutions and used within dental EHRs (Kalenderian et al. 2010). The American Dental Association (ADA) has also been developing SNODENT, but is not yet publically available for clinical use (Goldberg et al. 2005).

4.4.4 Cohort Selection and Patient Recruitment

Another link between EHR data and clinical research is the potential to find human subjects. Recruiting sufficient numbers of patients that meet eligibility requirements within an allotted time frame for clinical trials is challenging. As EHRs contain detailed information about patients, they can be used to find patients that meet specific inclusion and exclusion criteria. Informatics for Integrating Biology and the Bedside (i2b2), an open source data warehousing platform, has been found to be a useful tool for cohort selection especially if the source data from an EHR is represented in a structured format (Deshmukh et al. 2009).

Further, with health information increasingly available to patients through the Internet, it is possible interested patients will be more effective in finding clinical trials than investigators looking for patients. Many clinical trial registers are now available online. The National Institutes of Health (NIH) have made available their database of NIH funded research (McCray 2000). There is currently no single repository for patients to find all trials studying a health condition. A recent study assessed the comprehensiveness of online trial databases concerning prostate and colon cancer and found that online trial registries are incomplete, especially for industry-sponsored trials (Manheimer and Anderson 2002). A more collaborative effort between government and industry-sponsored research groups to compile and standardize information may be a mutually beneficial effort. It is not clear how many patients now enroll in clinical trials through online discovery.

4.4.5 Secondary Use of EHR Data

EHR data originally collected for patient purposes can be potentially used for research. Aggregating data from multiple sources can provide a large dataset that could otherwise not be available.

Electronic health records (EHR) contain a wealth of information and are a promising source to conduct research. Data extracted from EHRs differ from other sources such as population surveys or data obtained from payers, as they provide a more detailed and longitudinal view of patients, symptoms, diseases, treatments, outcomes, and differences among providers. Therefore EHR data in dentistry can potentially provide valuable insight into oral health diseases, and treatments performed on a large cohort of subjects. EHRs also play an important role in enhancing evidence-based decision-making in dentistry (EBD) and improving clinical effectiveness through decision support (Atkinson et al. 2002; Walji et al. 2007; Valenza and Walji 2007; Taylor et al. 2007; Spence et al. 2007; Chambers et al. 2007; Langabeer 2nd et al. 2008; Walji MF et al. 2009).

The Consortium of Oral Health Related Informatics (COHRI) provides an example of how dental EHRs are used for research purposes (Schleyer et al. 2006; Stark et al. 2010). COHRI was formed in 2007 by a group of dental schools who used the same EHR platform and who are interested in sharing clinical and education data. Through funding from the National Library of Medicine, four dental schools are participating in a pilot project to develop an inter-university oral health research database by extracting and integrating data from EHRs.

One promising area where data repositories derived from EHR data can be used for new discoveries is in the area of comparative effectiveness research. Comparative effectiveness research is defined as "a rigorous evaluation of the impact of different options that are available for treating a given medical condition for a particular set of patients." (Congressional Budget Office 2007) Further, such research includes focusing on the clinical benefits and risks of each option (clinical effectiveness), and an analysis on the costs and benefits (cost effectiveness analysis).

Comparative effectiveness research (CER) is also likely to reduce costs of dental care and increase access to the majority of the population who currently receive no dental care. Unfortunately many recent systematic reviews focusing on CER questions in dentistry have been inconclusive due to the lack of existing evidence in the scientific literature. Secondary analysis of the data that reside in dental electronic health records (EHR) is a particularly appealing approach to facilitate CER and generate new knowledge. EHR data has the potential to provide a comprehensive picture of patients' histories, treatments, and outcomes, and if integrated with similar data from other dental clinics can include a large and diverse set of patients.

However, numerous challenges must be solved before EHRs can be used for CER. First, data suitable for CER must actually be collected from EHR systems. Second, this data, which often resides in proprietary systems, must be accessible and retrievable. And lastly, this data should be structured in a format that can be integrated with data from other sources or institutions.

4.4.6 *Practice-Based Research Networks*

Practice-based Research Networks (PBRN) are groups of primary care clinicians and practices working together to answer community-based health care questions and translate research findings into practice. PBRNs engage clinicians in quality improvement activities and an evidence-based culture in primary care practice to improve the health of all Americans. In 2005, the National Institute of Dental Craniofacial Research funded three such research networks. The dental PBRN's to date have been conducting both prospective and retrospective research. For example, Barasch et al. conducted a case controlled study to investigate risk factors associated with osteonecrosis of the jaws (Barasch A et al. 2011). Many prospective studies conducted as part of PBRNs still require separate data collection systems for the research data.

EHR data contained in practices as part of PBRNs are beginning to be used for secondary purposes. For example Fellows et al. conducted a retrospective analysis of data contained in electronic health records to estimate incidence rates of osteonecrosis of the jaws (Fellows et al. 2011). PBRNs provide great promise of how EHR and clinical research data can be used effectively to promote both patient care and new discoveries.

4.4.7 Patient Registries

Another area that intersects both the patient care and research realm are patient registries. Patient registries are ways to track groups of patients who have had specific diseases or have had certain treatments. While EHR data would contain information on all types of patients, their diseases, and treatments, registries would allow focus on specific diseases or treatments of interest. Registries would not be as costly in terms of resource requirements like a traditional clinical trial, but would require specific eligibility criteria, informed consents, and collection addition to that collected as part of routing care. Dentistry has lagged far behind in forming data registries, primarily because dentistry is practiced in small offices and not in large hospitals making the process of integrating data very difficulty. However, dental schools which themselves house large clinical operations are ideally positioned to create disease specific registries that can potentially use data collected for patient care and extend for research purposes.

4.4.8 Future Directions

There is great potential for providing new insight in oral health by the integration of patient records and clinical research from both a workflow and information systems perspective. The technology challenges of developing systems that can exchange data, and use standardized terminologies appear solvable. However, the socio-technical issues such as determining how to incorporate optimal workflows for conducing both patient care and research with minimal additional overhead appear to be the greatest challenge before widespread adoption. Similarly, there appears to be great potential in using EHR data originally collected for patient care for the secondary use of research and discovery. This will require collaboration between patients, providers and researchers from all healthcare disciples, and institutions with friendly policies for sharing data to improve both patient care and drive new discoveries.

4.5 State of Health Information Technology and Informatics Within the Dental School in the United States

Amit Acharya, Andrea Mahnke, Po-Huang Chyou, and Franklin M. Din

4.5.1 Introduction

More recently there has been a strong push from the United States federal government for the adoption of the Electronic Health Record (EHR) within the healthcare industry. As a result, $19.2 Billion is made available to incentivize the physicians, dentists and hospitals for the adoption of the EHR through the Health Information Technology for Economic and Clinical Health (HITECH) Act. As the nation head towards adoption of the EHRs, there has also been a growing interest with the majority of the U.S. dental schools to implement EHRs within the educational setting. Fifty of the fifty-six U.S. dental schools, as well as dental schools in Canada and Europe, are either using or in the process of adopting some aspects of a common dental EHR framework (White et al. 2011). A group of dental schools known as Consortium for Oral Health-Related Informatics (COHRI) was formed in 2007 which used this common dental EHR framework – axiUm (Stark et al. 2010). Currently there are about 20 dental schools within COHRI. The EHR will not only support clinical care, but will also result in training the next generation dental students and to conduct innovative research that was not possible earlier. However, not much is known about how many of these dental schools' electronic dental records are integrated with their respective university's electronic medical record. A common medical-dental EHR model at healthcare universities would enable a holistic approach to providing patient care and provide the much needed electronic infrastructure to study interrelationship between the various oral-systemic diseases.

4.5.2 United States Dental School EHR Adoption Survey

Recently a group of researchers from Marshfield Clinic in Wisconsin, US conducted a survey to investigate the current states of Health Information Technology and Informatics within the dental school in the US. List of US dental schools were identified through the American Dental Education Association (ADEA) web site. Dental schools were contacted to determine who the most appropriate person to take the survey would be.

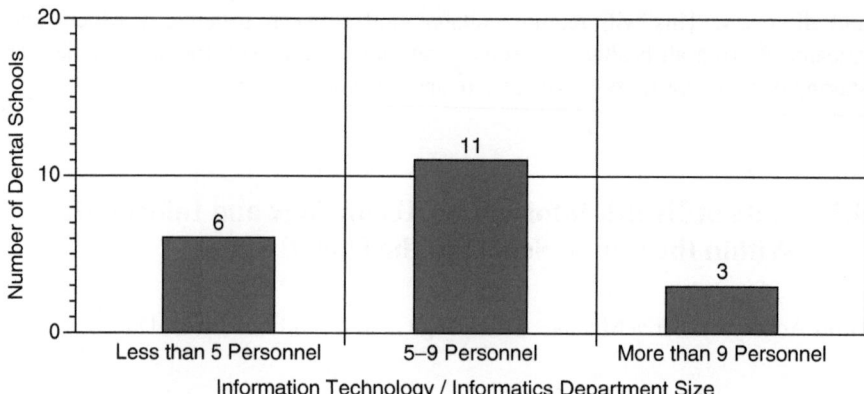

Fig. 4.27 Information technology – informatics department size at Dental Schools in US

Once the list of contact was developed from each dental school, an email was sent to 55 US dental schools with a link to a survey created in SurveyMonkey. The survey was administered on Tuesday March 1, 2011. Reminder survey emails were sent to all recipients on March 9 and March 17. The survey was closed on March 31.

The anonymous survey was at most 23 questions, depending on how questions were answered. The survey focused on topics such as presence of dental informaticians within the dental schools, use of financial and clinical information systems, interest in federal stimulus support for EHR adoption provided through American Recovery and Reinvestment Act and Meaningful Use of EHR, relationships with health care entities and bidirectional nature of the dental and medical EHRs. The study was approved as exempt from the Marshfield Clinic Institutional Review Board under section 45 CFR 46.101(b) and waived requirement for an authorization.

Thirty out of the fifty five dental schools responded to the survey (response rate of 55%). However, five of the thirty dental schools representative did not complete the survey and hence their response was not included in the analysis.

4.5.3 Key Findings of the Survey

4.5.3.1 Section 1: Dedicated Department/Center for Information Technology/Informatics

Regarding the question about the presence of a dedicated department or a center for information technology (IT) or informatics within the dental school in US, 80% (n = 20) of the responding dental schools had a dedicated IT/Informatics department or center (p-value of 0.0027). The IT or the informatics department size (in terms of the number of personnel) at the 20 dental schools is illustrated in Fig. 4.27.

Thirty five percent (n = 7) of the US dental schools that housed an IT / Informatics departments had personnel with not only IT training but also dental informatics training.

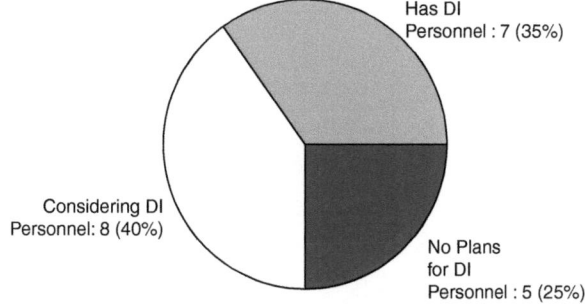

Fig. 4.28 US Dental School IT/informatics department personnel with and without dental informatics (DI) training

Table 4.6 Partial responses to additional question in Sect. 1 of the survey

	N	%
Do you know the ratio between numbers of employees in this department to the number of employees in your entire school? If yes can you provide the ratio?		
4%	1	7.14
50-1 excluding students, 100-1 including	1	7.14
5:1100	1	7.14
No	9	64.29
About 39:1, about 74:1 if you include students	1	7.14
Two/very many	1	7.14
What percentage of the school's operating budget is devoted to this department?		
1%	2	11.11
2%	1	5.56
5%	2	11.11
Don't know	10	55.60
By department, contract for services	1	5.56
It's high, but not sure how high	1	5.56
Small	1	5.56

While 40% (n = 8) of the dental schools were considering integration of dental informatics personnel within their department or center. Twenty five percent (n = 5) of the dental schools did not have any plans of integrating personnel with dental informatics personnel within their department or center (see Fig. 4.28). Partial responses to additional questions in the Section 1 of the survey is provided under Table 4.6.

4.5.3.2 Section 2: Current Use of Electronic Financial Systems and Electronic Dental Records

The majority of the responding dental schools were currently using Financial Electronic Systems (FES) (p-value of <0.0001) and Electronic Dental Records (EDR) (p-value of 0.0001). The use of FES outnumbered the use of EDRs in the dental

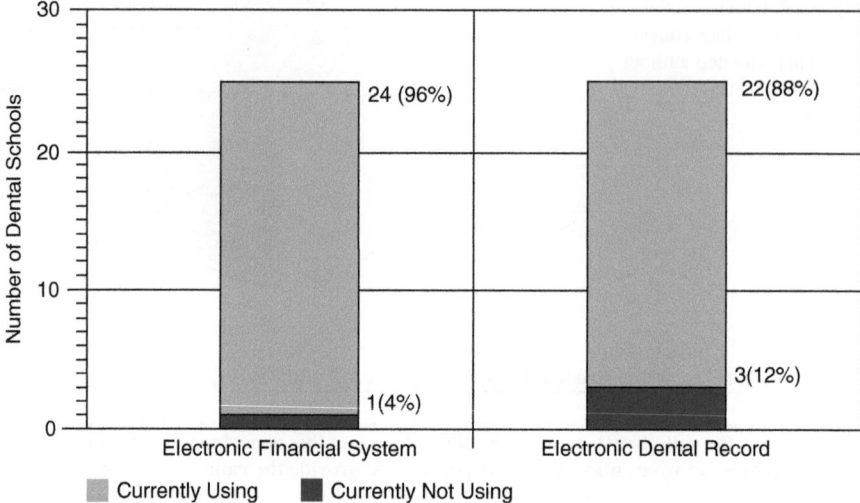

Fig. 4.29 Current usage of electronic financial systems and electronic dental records among the responded Dental Schools

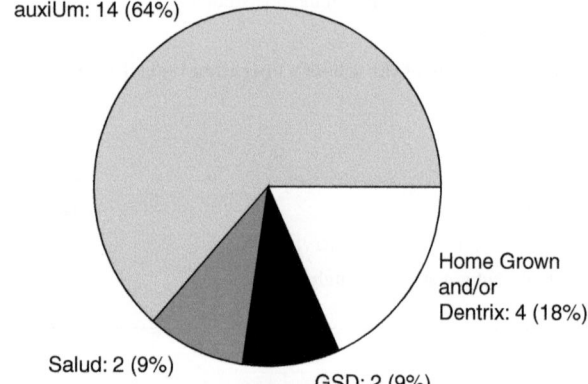

Fig. 4.30 Commercial electronic dental records used in the US Dental Schools

schools (see Fig 4.29). About 77% of the dental schools that were currently utilizing the EDRs used it in all the clinical modules (p-value of 0.0105), while 23% of the dental schools used the EDRs in some of the clinical modules.

When asked about the commercial EDR system that the dental schools were using, axiUm (Exan Group, Canada) was by far the most implemented EDR system. Two dental schools had Salud (Two-Ten Health Limited, Ireland) implemented and two dental schools had GSD Academic (General Systems Design Group, Iowa, US) implemented. Combinations of two EHR systems (Home Grown and Dentrix) were implemented at two dental schools. One school had a Dentrix only implementation, while another had developed its own EDR system (Home Grown) (see Fig. 4.30). There were 13 dental schools which had implemented an EDR five or more years

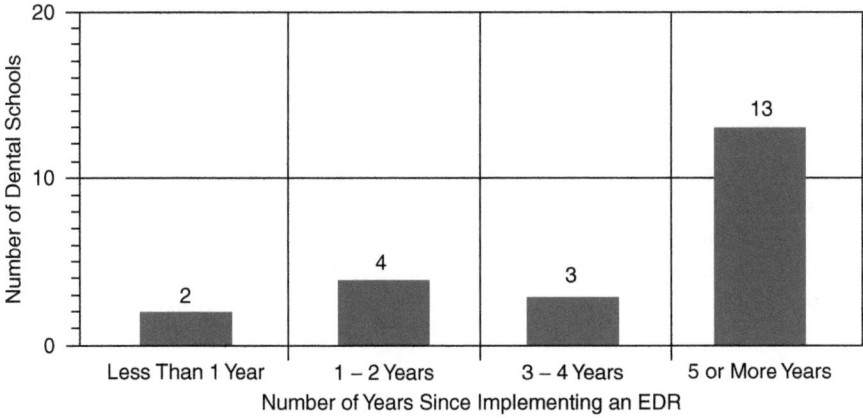

Fig. 4.31 Number of years since implementing an EDR at the US Dental Schools

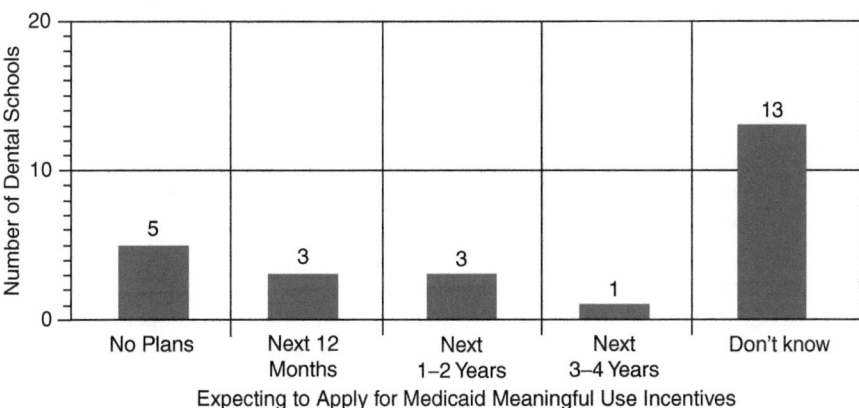

Fig. 4.32 US Dental Schools' plan for applying to medicaid meaningful use incentive program

ago, 3 dental schools 3–4 years ago, 4 dental schools 1–2 years ago and 2 dental schools less than a year ago (see Fig. 4.31) (p value of 0.0029).

4.5.3.3 Section 3: Medicaid Meaningful Use of EHR Incentives

When the dental schools were asked the question as to whether they were expecting to apply for the Medicaid Meaningful Use incentive program, majority (52%) of the dental schools did not know and only 28% of the dental schools were expecting to apply within the next 4 years (Fig. 4.32) (p-value of 0.0044). Challenges or barriers identified by some of the dental schools in complying with the Meaningful Use objectives were (a). lack of certified EDR and information regarding it, (b). issues with getting auxiUm certified and (c). qualifications of the EDR as many of the Meaningful Use objectives do not apply to dentistry and lack of specific information about it.

4.5.3.4 Section 4: Dental School and Health System Relationship

Only 44% of the responded dental schools were part of a health system. Fifty two percent (n = 13) of the responded dental schools had a formal relationship with other health care delivery entities in terms of sharing facilities, patient transfer, training programs. Some of the types of relationship mentioned by the dental schools that had a formal relationship with other health care delivery entities included: (a). a GPR program and an emergency dental unit in the hospital, (b). affiliated hospital, (c). affiliation agreements, (d). oral and maxillofacial surgery (OMFS), anesthesia and pedodontics all have some portion of education in medical health center, (e). OMFS residents are also residents of medical health center, (f). residents providing care under contract with area hospitals, (g). sharing patients wand facilities with the health center, (h). students rotating in the community health centers and (i) collaborative grand programs. Eighty five percent of the dental schools that had a formal relationship with the health care delivery entities had routine interaction with them because of their existing relationship (p-value of 0.0015). Their usual method for exchanging information was through informal medium such as phones, emails and faxes and formal medium such as memorandums, letters and contracts.

4.5.3.5 Section 5: Communication Between Health System's Electronic Medical Record (EMR) and Dental School's Electronic Dental Record (EDR)

When the dental schools were asked about the communication between the health systems' EMR and the school's EDR, majority of the dental schools did not have any communication (60%) or did not know is such a communication existed (25%) (p-value of <0.0001) (see Fig. 4.33).

Out of the 60% (n = 15) of the responded dental schools who's EDR did not communicate with the health system's EMR, 47% (n = 7) of the dental schools stated that they did not need to exchange patient information electronically as a reason for the non-communication, while 33% (n = 5) dental schools states that they would like to exchange patient information electronically but there were barriers that prevent them from doing so. Some of the barriers identified by these dental schools were (a). the hospitals and the dental school are not part of the same medial system and HIPAA concerns prevent sharing data, (b). the dental school currently neither did have an EDR nor the infrastructure to support one and (c). hospital is not interested and has high and perhaps unrealistic security standards. The remaining 20% (n = 3) of the dental schools expected to exchange patient information electronically in the near future (next 5 years). Some of the information categories that were shared between the EDR and EMR in the small number of dental schools are illustrated in Fig 4.34. Finally when asked about any research projects under way in their dental school to investigate discrepancies between medical and dental records for the same patient, only 1 (4%) dental school was currently undertaking such project.

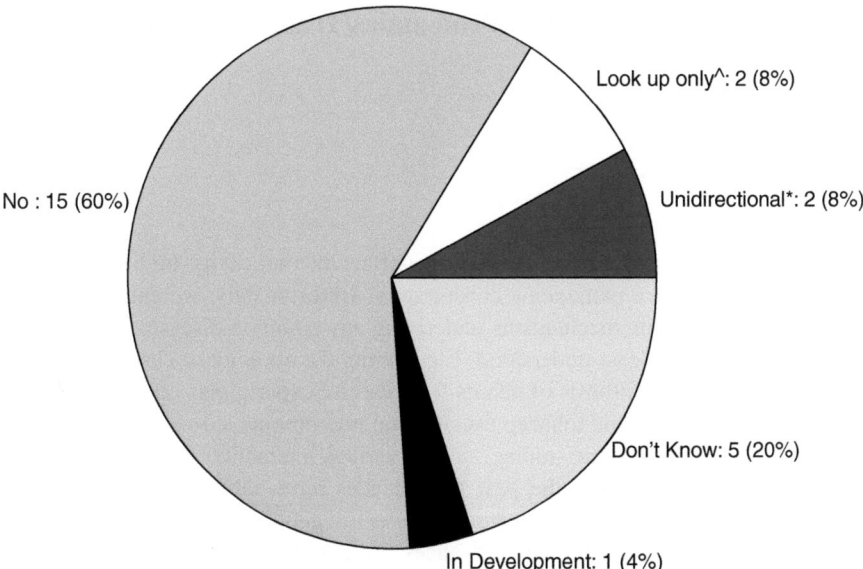

^ Look up only in both directions
* Unidirectional - Information moves in only one direction, look up only in other direction

Fig. 4.33 Communication between EMR and EDR among the responding US Dental Schools

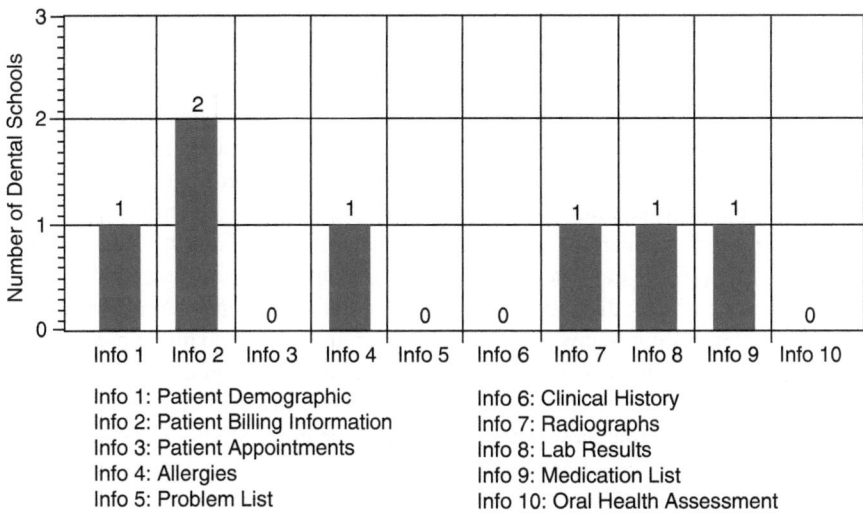

Fig. 4.34 Information categories shared between EDR and EMR in some of the US Dental Schools

4.6 Genomics/Phenomics/Proteomics/Translational Research

Steven J. Schrodi

4.6.1 Introduction

In all common diseases, including those that affect the oral cavity, both the environment and genetics are pathogenic conspirators. Unfortunately, we currently know little about the specific mechanisms underlying any common disease; and oral diseases are among the least understood. Elucidating the etiology of chronic oral diseases will involve a synthesis of results from careful experiments of environmental exposures such as diet and tobacco use, the oral microbiome, co-morbidities, large-scale, well-designed genetic studies, and the various interaction effects.

With regard to genetics, the past few decades have witnessed transformative developments in our ability to interrogate the entire genome for genes that contribute to disease. While dramatic advances in experimental designs, statistical approaches, and clinical insights have greatly aided this scientific campaign, the central driver of this progress has been the development of high-throughput, inexpensive genetic technologies. Following initial molecular studies using variant forms of enzymes, or allozymes, a major breakthrough was the use of highly informative DNA-based markers throughout the genome (Botstein et al. 1980). This idea of directly assaying existing DNA variation to conduct linkage and association studies in genetics began a revolution in disease gene mapping. Recent interest from commercial entities has produced a feverish pace of technological innovation, markedly reducing cost and expanding the depth of inquiry. Previously unfathomable, the testing of over one million single nucleotide polymorphisms (SNPs) in thousands of patients and controls is now commonplace (Wellcome Trust Case Control Consortium 2007; Schaefer et al. 2010); and very recently, next generation sequencing technologies have progressed to the point where sequencing of the entire protein-coding portion of the genome (exome) or even the entire genome is a cost-effective method to examine disease traits across the entire spectrum of genetic variants in small numbers of affected individuals (Ng et al. 2010). There is little doubt that soon whole genome sequencing will be applied to nuclear family-based designs, studies among distantly-related affected individuals in extended pedigrees, and case/control studies involving thousands of individuals. This unprecedented scope of inquiry made possible by large-scale genetics, has begun to yield fascinating resulting into predisposition to oral cancers, caries, and periodontal disease that will molecularly redefine these pathologies, explicate unique biological connections with related diseases, give impetus to the development of directed therapeutics, and indeed personalize medicine. Still, much more genetic focus on oral disease phenotypes is required if we are to realize this medical impact in a timely fashion.

As genetic technologies have allowed the progression of interrogating single protein variants to single DNA markers to entire genes to markers across the genome, and now to the entire genome sequence, the promises of these large-scale genetic studies have understandably undergone monumental expansion. It may be reasonable to expect the results from whole genome sequencing to decidedly revolutionize medicine within the next two decades. However, this new scientific capacity comes at a cost. As genetics, and biology in general, transitions to a data-rich science, practitioners have found themselves woefully unprepared to store and analyze the volume of data generated. Once analyzed, interpretation and integration of these abundant and multifaceted results into medical practice will also be an appreciable challenge. Insufficient assimilation of genetic findings into merged dental and medical records will severely limit the ability of clinicians to appropriately treat patients. Inadequately addressing these informatics issues will severely derail efforts in the basic sciences efforts as well as the translational and clinical sciences.

This chapter explores the current state of genomics studies, what we have learned from genetic investigations into oral diseases, and where we may be headed. Genetic studies have much to offer investigations of disease etiology. Why do some acquire diseases and others do not? For those affected, why do some progress more rapidly than others? What causes some patients to respond to therapies, while others suffer from adverse reactions? These are all fundamental questions in both biology and medicine, whether the focus is on the gastrointestinal tract, the hippocampus, the lymphatic system, metabolic disorders, or oral diseases. Speaking generally across disease areas, a portion of the answers to these questions often lies in described environmental effects. In numerous chronic diseases, infectious agents are likely contributors to the disease process – periodontitis, for example, is initiated by gram negative anaerobes in susceptible individuals (Holt and Ebersole 2005). Surely, unique and latent environmental exposures provide a random component to common disease susceptibility and progression. Through twin studies, studies of risk in close relatives, and quantitative traits experiments, it is well-understood that heritable factors, including but not limited to DNA variation, are typically responsible for 30–90% of the phenotype variability for common diseases. This section will attempt to cover, at least at a cursory level, the major salient developments affecting genetic insights into chronic and aggressive periodontitis, with some comment on genetic factors influencing susceptibility to caries and oral cancers. While it would be extremely naïve to view genetic studies as an immediate panacea for our ills, the discovery of disease-causing genes does illuminate hitherto unknown biological pathways and molecular mechanisms, draws unforeseen connections with other traits, may improve prognostic models applicable for individuals, and suggests specific therapeutics.

4.6.2 Oral Disease Phenotypes

4.6.2.1 Chronic Inflammation, Metabolic Dysfunction, and Infection

Industrialization has brought forth increased lifespan and wellness through vaccination, modern sanitation practices, public health policies, and advances in medical science translated into practice. However, the accompanying physical inactivity coupled with a high calorie diet are probable contributors to an extremely common, chronically inflamed metabolic syndrome (Hotamisligil 2006) that is thought to give rise to a multitude of intimately related disease traits: insulin resistance, compromised insulin signaling, hyperglycemia, obesity, dyslipidemia, hypertension, impaired kidney function, elevated liver enzymes and steatohepatitis, poor wound healing, neurodegeneration, vascular disease, pregnancy complications, accelerated immunosenescence, and periodontal disease (Ford et al. 2002; Ferrannini et al. 1991; Eaton et al. 1994; Holvoet et al. 2008; Speliotes et al. 2010; Eckel et al. 2005; D'Aiuto et al. 2008). These diseases often co-occur within the same patient and could be considered variable expression complications arising from a state of aberrant caloric flux that induces metabolic dysfunction and chronic, systemic inflammation. These features constitute a disruption in a fundamental homeostatic mechanism with intensifying pathogenic consequences. The rapidly increasing incidence and decreasing age of onset for this pathophysiological state have generated a major source of mortality and morbidity in modern cultures (Ford et al. 2002; Ferrannini et al. 1991; Weiss et al. 2004).

It is becoming increasing clear that many chronic diseases have an infectious component. There is relatively convincing evidence that many systemic, T-cell mediated autoimmune disorders may be initiated by infections. For example, from archaeological data, it is believed that an infectious agent – currently unknown – is necessary for rheumatoid arthritis (Firestein 2003), and both Guillain-Barre syndrome and rheumatic fever have well-described pathogeneses triggered by specific infections in susceptible individuals (Bach 2005). In many instances, oncogenesis and tumor progression can be traced to pro-inflammatory responses at the site of chronic infection (Coussens and Werb 2002), although it is not known whether these effects are mediated through the actions of the immune system, the infectious agents, or a combination thereof. Several cancers fall into this category including gastric adenocarcinoma (Uemura et al. 2001), cervical cancer (Walboomers et al. 1999), hepatocellular carcinoma (Saito et al. 1990), and Kaposi's sarcoma (Dictor 1997), all having unequivocal infectious agent etiologies. Recent findings of anti-inflammatory pharmaceuticals, particularly those that inhibit COX-1 and COX-2, reduce the incidence of certain classes of cancers are consistent with this view (Dannenberg and Subbaramaiah 2003, Rothwell Rothwell et al. 2010). In addition, there is moderate evidence that several bacteria – the most studied is *Chlamydia pneumoniae* – play a role in atherosclerosis and myocardial infarction (Saikku et al. 1988; Watson and Alp 2008), however the studies are not conclusive and antibiotic treatment does not appear to be effective (Andraws et al. 2005).

4.6.2.2 Periodontitis

Chronic periodontal disease is firmly footed at the intersection of infection, chronic inflammation, and metabolic dysfunction. Chronic periodontitis is characterized by inflammation of the periodontal membrane, slowly causing gingival recession and eventual bone loss. The proximate cause of periodontitis is the virulent oral microbiome. The involvement of gram negative anaerobes has been firmly established for the disease. Aside from the known oral pathogenic species *P. gingivalis*, *T. denticola*, and *T. forsythensis*, the so-called "red complex" (Holt and Ebersole 2005), new bacterial species associated with chronic periodontitis have also been described (Kumar et al. 2003). The advent of an extensive database covering the oral microbiome will surely propel such investigations (Chen et al. 2010).

Numerous studies have shown that periodontal disease covaries with many diseases, presumably due to overlapping molecular etiologies. Compelling meta-analyses demonstrate a highly significant synchronicity of obesity and periodontal disease (Chaffee and Weston 2010). In addition, the correlation between periodontal diseases/alveolar bone loss and frank metabolic syndrome is repetitively observed (Nesbitt et al. 2010; Andriankaja et al. 2010). Extensive work has also shown a strong role for both inflammation-related genes and circulating inflammatory markers in periodontal disease (Nikolopoulos et al. 2008; Bretz et al. 2005a, b). Treatment studies further support the link between periodontal disease and immuno-metabolic syndrome. These experiments have demonstrated a significant improvement in intermediate molecular markers of inflammation when chronic periodontitis in the presence of metabolic syndrome (Acharya et al. 2010) or type 2 diabetes (Iwamoto et al. 2001) was treated. Conversely, treatment of periodontal disease with reduction of bacterial load leads to greater glycemic control among diabetic patients (Simpson et al. 2010; Stewart et al. 2001). Given the high prevalence of periodontitis and the co-morbidity of metabolic syndrome with periodontal disease, these treatment experiments appear to suggest that the virulent oral microbiome could play an important role in the pathogenesis of systemic inflammatory metabolic syndrome, and is exacerbated by the syndrome. Certainly, further studies are needed to definitively answer this question.

As chronic periodontal disease seems to be a critical feature of sustained, systemic dysfunction of both metabolic and inflammatory networks, uncovering the genetic variants carried by susceptible individuals would not only provide much needed insight into the molecular pathogenesis of chronic periodontal disease, but would also markedly aid our understanding of the inflammatory metabolic syndrome and how it drives related co-morbidities. Such genetic studies may also shed light on the specific mechanisms that appear to improve cardiovascular, inflammatory, and diabetic outcomes when periodontal disease is treated, potentially leading to therapies and medical/dental intervention with greater effectiveness. Such studies may also provide clues to which subsets of individuals respond more effectively than others and why they do so.

Periodontal disease can also present in a rapid manner with aggressive bone loss and early-onset. This is termed aggressive periodontitis (Lang et al. 1999). In contrast to chronic periodontitis, there is often a greater degree of familial aggregation with aggressive periodontitis, and it is hypothesized that most aggressive cases may afflict individuals with one or more defective immune genes (Zhang et al. 2003; Amer et al. 1988; Machulla et al. 2002; Carvalho et al. 2010; Toomes et al. 1999; Hart et al. 2000; Hewitt et al. 2004). Mutations in the lysosomal protease, cathepsin C, have been shown to be responsible for some forms of aggressive periodontitis, along with complications associated with other inflammatory diseases (Laine and

Busch-Petersen 2010). The specific HLA variants thought to play a role in aggressive periodontitis, are also involved in infectious disease susceptibility and autoimmunity; and, interestingly, two of the non-MHC-linked regions, *FAM5C* and a locus on chromosome 9p21, have been implicated in myocardial infarction (Connelly et al. 2008) and may have action as a tumor suppressor in tongue squamous cell carcinoma (Kuroiwa et al. 2009). As with chronic periodontal disease, an infectious microbiome is heavily involved. However, in general, microbiome differences could not explain the presence of chronic versus aggressive forms of the disease, although in some aggressive periodontitis patients, a highly leukotoxic *A. actinomycetemcomitans* strain may contribute to the disease process (Mombelli et al. 2002). We currently do not fully know the differences between the genetic susceptibility factors for the chronic and aggressive forms of the disease.

4.6.2.3 Caries

The most prevalent chronic disease in both children and adults is dental caries (National Institute of Dental and Craniofacial Research). Caries formation is a complex disease with several interacting components form the environment and host genetics. Similar to gingivitis and periodontitis, caries have an infection-initiating etiology with acidification leading to localized demineralization. Epidemiological studies have long shown that diet is a strong predictor of caries formation; and the reduction in pH is exacerbated by high consumption of carbohydrates. The principal pathobacterial species are *Streptococcus mutans* and *Lactobacillus* (van Houte 1994). There are also several reports of positive correlations of caries with inflammatory diseases, although the association is not always repeatable. It is also not clear what proportion of the putative association with inflammatory disease is due to innate upregulation of immune networks in contrast to the immuno-modulating pharmaceuticals prescribed to those with inflammatory disease (Steinbacher and Glick 2001). Much of the effect is reported to result from lack of saliva volume (Steinbacher and Glick 2001). Interestingly, the presence of epilepsy may be associated with higher caries rates (Anjomshoaa et al. 2009). Fluoride is an effective antimicrobial agent that interferes with bacterial growth and metabolism (Wiegand et al. 2007). Hence, topical fluoride administration as well as ingestion of fluoridated water inhibits cariogenesis and caries progression (Ripa 1993). Amelogenesis is a key process involved in modifying the rate of caries formation. Both common variation and rare mutations in enamel formation genes such as amelogenin and enamelin are involved in caries rates (Patir et al. 2008; Kim et al. 2004; Crawford et al. 2007), the molecular actions of which are beginning to be revealed (Lakshminarayanan et al. 2010).

4.6.2.4 Oral Cancers

Over 35,000 new cases of cancers affecting the oral cavity and pharynx were expected in the United States for 2009, with deaths numbering 11,000 (Jemal et al.

2009). The majority of these malignancies involved solid tumors originating from cancerous changes in squamous cells of the mouth. Again, oral cancers have a complex etiology existing of entangled genetic, epigenetic, infectious, and dietary causes, further modified by tobacco, alcohol and other environmental exposures. As with most cancers, it is reasonable to expect that both germline and somatic genetic changes will be involved in carcinogenesis, tumor growth, and metastasis. Promoter hypermethylation of genes central to cellular growth, differentiation, DNA fidelity, apoptosis, and metabolic stability is an important facet of these cancers (Poage et al. 2010). Indeed, methylation-mediated silencing of genes involved in tumor suppression (e.g. the cyclin-dependent kinase inhibitor 2A), detoxification (e.g. *MGMT*), and apoptosis (e.g. the death-associated protein kinase-1) are commonly found in oral squamous cell carcinoma samples (Ha and Califano 2006).

4.6.3 Modern Genetics

4.6.3.1 Heritability

To quantify the proportion of the variance in a phenotypic trait that is due to variance in genetic factors, population geneticists defined the concept of heritability (Visscher et al. 2008; Falconer and MacKay 1996). Researchers subsequently developed several methods for estimating heritabilities using the measure of a trait (e.g. occurrence of disease/not-disease) in combinations of relatives (e.g. parent-offspring, or monozygotic-dizygotic twins). In general, the higher the measured heritability of a variable phenotype, the larger the contribution of genetic factors is in comparison to environmental effects. It is fallacious to assume that the heritable variation is composed entirely of alleles residing in the DNA sequence, for heritability studies simply examine the covariance between relatives without comment on specific molecular mechanisms. Hence, any heritable variation such as methylation patterns, vertically-transmitted infectious agents, as well as DNA variation can contribute to the heritability measure. Heritability results are important because they not only give a rough estimate of the collective effects of heritable factors, but also can provide a measure to quantify how much of the total genetic effect is accounted for by specific loci examined.

For periodontal disease, four twin-based studies of heritability have been performed (Michalowicz et al. 1991; Corey et al. 1993; Michalowicz et al. 2000; Mucci et al. 2005). Although varying in sample size and methodological details, all four arrived at consistent results, with 30–50% of the variance in periodontal disease being attributed to genetic variability for chronic periodontitis. Given the segregation patterns described in the literature, it is reasonable to assume that aggressive periodontal disease exhibits a higher heritability. Therefore, given the prevalence of periodontal disease, heritable factors within the population at large are likely appreciable. Using 314 twin pairs, Bretz and colleagues reported substantial heritability values for multiple traits related to caries ranging from 30% to 56% (Bretz et al. 2005a, b). Lastly, mutagen sensitivity studies of head and neck cancer patients suggest a significant effect of genetic factors for the carcinogenesis of oral cancers (Cloos et al. 1996). Hence, there is every reason to believe that a sizable pool of genetic and/or epigenetic factors await discovery for oral diseases.

4.6.3.2 Genetic Technologies and Disease Gene Mapping

Once the development of PCR (Saiki et al. 1985) was applied to the idea of using naturally-occurring DNA variation (Botstein et al. 1980), large-scale DNA-based studies of disease underwent a substantial acceleration (Schlotterer 2004). Genotyping of short, tandem repeated sequences (Weber and May 1989) – microsatellites – spurred on a wave of genome-wide linkage studies, which evaluate the co-segregation of disease state with microsatellite markers, for both rare Mendelian disorders as well as more common diseases with complex inheritance patterns. While the rarer traits with more coherent transmission patterns generally relinquished their genetic secrets to linkage analysis, more common diseases did not. In the mid- to late 1990s, several theoretical studies had shown that the power to detect disease-causing alleles is higher with association-based designs such as a case/control experiment or association in the presence of a linkage signal as in the transmission/disequilibrium test if the frequency of those alleles is high and the effects are moderate (Kaplan et al. 1995; Risch and Merikangas 1996; Jones 1998; Long and Langley 1999). However, to conduct genome-wide association studies presented an ominous obstacle for the genetic technologies at the time. The number of markers required to effectively cover the genome was prohibitively large as the chromosomal blocks in population-based samples used in association designs were expected to be small. Even within large extended families, the limited number of recombination events generates substantial chromosomal blocks passed through the pedigree, but researchers had both theoretical and empirical evidence that the blocks in population-based samples were on the order of 50 K base pairs for most large human populations. As the reader can imagine, the mean length of blocks that are shared by descent is inversely related to the product of recombination rate, the number of affected individuals and the number of meioses separating the affected individuals. In practice, even very large extended families segregate regions shared by affected members on the order of several million base pairs in length. However, once geneticists seriously considered large-scale studies using a case/control design where individuals are separated by say 5,000 meioses, it became clear that to adequately cover the much smaller shared regions across the entire genome, hundreds of thousands of markers would be required (Kruglyak 1999). Utilizing the human genome sequence (Venter et al. 2001; Lander et al. 2001), a number of studies at Celera Diagnostics provided an intermediate solution, where approximately 30,000 putative functional SNPs primarily located in genes were assayed through allele-specific PCR in a number of common diseases using a staged case/control design. These studies were successful in identifying several gene-centric polymorphisms associated with common diseases (Begovich et al. 2004; Cargill et al. 2007) (Fig. 4.35).

Concurrently, several groups had performed extensive sequencing and genotyping across the genome to produce a genome-wide map of haplotype structure (Hinds

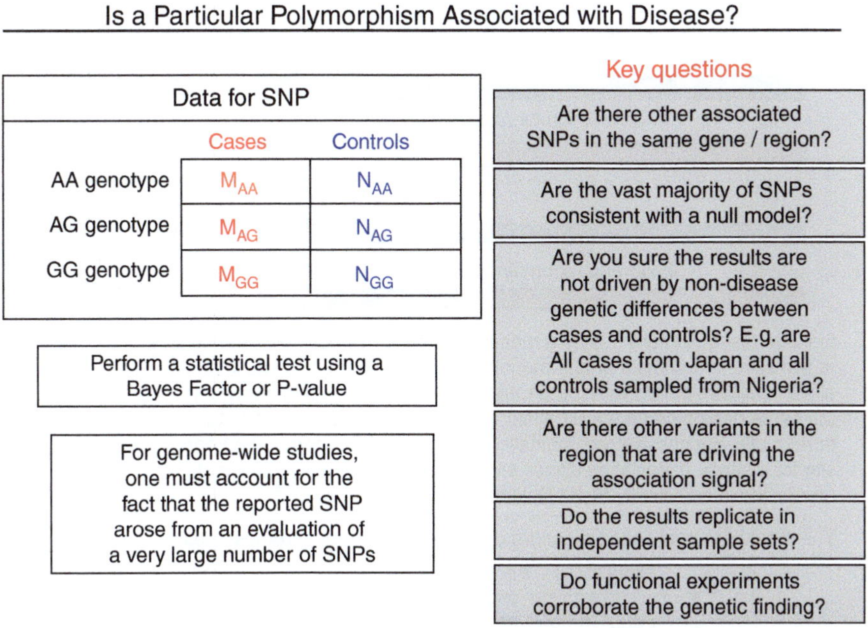

Is a Particular Polymorphism Associated with Disease?

Data for SNP		
	Cases	Controls
AA genotype	M_{AA}	N_{AA}
AG genotype	M_{AG}	N_{AG}
GG genotype	M_{GG}	N_{GG}

Perform a statistical test using a Bayes Factor or P-value

For genome-wide studies, one must account for the fact that the reported SNP arose from an evaluation of a very large number of SNPs

Key questions

Are there other associated SNPs in the same gene / region?

Are the vast majority of SNPs consistent with a null model?

Are you sure the results are not driven by non-disease genetic differences between cases and controls? E.g. are All cases from Japan and all controls sampled from Nigeria?

Are there other variants in the region that are driving the association signal?

Do the results replicate in independent sample sets?

Do functional experiments corroborate the genetic finding?

Fig. 4.35 Is a polymorphism associated with disease?

et al. 2005), useful in linkage disequilibrium mapping. Within 2 years, technology for SNP hybridization arrays had advanced so as to enable genome-wide association studies capable of capturing most of the common genetic variation in the genome either through direct genotyping or indirect interrogation using linkage disequilibrium – the term linkage disequilibrium is a measure of the correlation of alleles at closely-linked sites (see Fig. 4.36).

These investigations were met with numerous successes (Klein et al. 2005; Kathiresan et al. 2008; Graham et al. 2008; Gudmundsson et al. 2009). Inexpensive genotyping platforms and urging from theoreticians ensured that these genome-wide association studies were, in general, highly powered to detect all but very mild effects from high frequency alleles. These efforts, led by large academic consortia such as the Wellcome Trust, The International Multiple Sclerosis Genetics Consortium, and the Broad Institute and commercial entities such as deCODE genetics and Perlegen have greatly expanded our understanding of the basic biology of common diseases: we now know, for example, that (i) autophagy-related genes are involved in Crohn's disease (Rioux et al. 2007), (ii) there are a number of genes such as the protein tyrosine phosphatase, *PTPN22* and the interleukin-23 receptor, *IL23R*, that exhibit ample pleiotropic effects among autoimmune conditions (Lopez-Escamez 2010; Safrany and Melegh 2009), (iii) in the case of age-related macular degeneration, predictive models using the genetic results enable fairly accurate prognosis of individuals who are at high risk of disease (Seddon et al. 2008), (iv) Wnt signaling through the

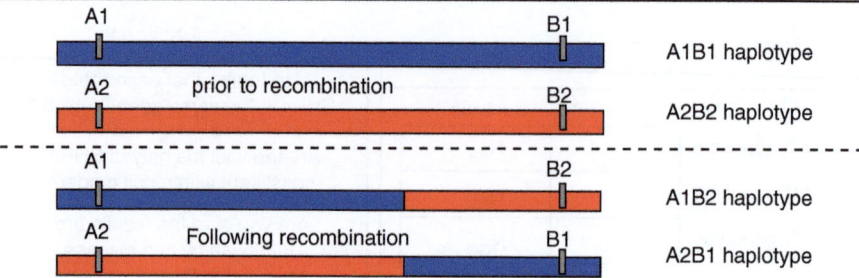

Fig. 4.36 The concept of linkage disequilibrium

transcription factor *TCF7L2* plays a role in type 2 diabetes (Grant et al. 2006), and (v) aberrant IL-7 signaling likely contributes to multiple sclerosis susceptibility (Gregory et al. 2007).

The plot shows the tremendous progress in genotyping technology where, a decade ago, very little of the genome was accessible for disease studies using association designs through the current wave of viable sequencing-based whole exome studies (2010–2011) and whole genome studies (2012–2013). In Fig. 4.37, the average distance between adjacent genetic markers is plotted as a function of year of introduction to the disease mapping community. Impressively, the total number of genetic markers has increased a million-fold over the past decade.

Although successful in uncovering numerous pathogenic pathways for common diseases, results from the current wave of genome-wide association studies, with a few exceptions, explain little of existing disease heritability. The reasons for this are cryptic and the subject of heavy debate (Manolio et al. 2009). Multiple rare sequence variants generating high levels of allelic heterogeneity, functional *de novo* mutations, structural mutations such as copy number variants and large deletions, and epigenetic effects constitute four of several possible disease models that could account for the heritability discrepancy. The answer will almost certainly consist of a conglomeration of these and other effects. Bringing forth the new genome-wide technologies that illuminate these previously non- or under-interrogated properties of the genome to bear on this enigma is a reasonable next step for all complex traits including oral diseases.

Fig. 4.37 Technological progress in genomics

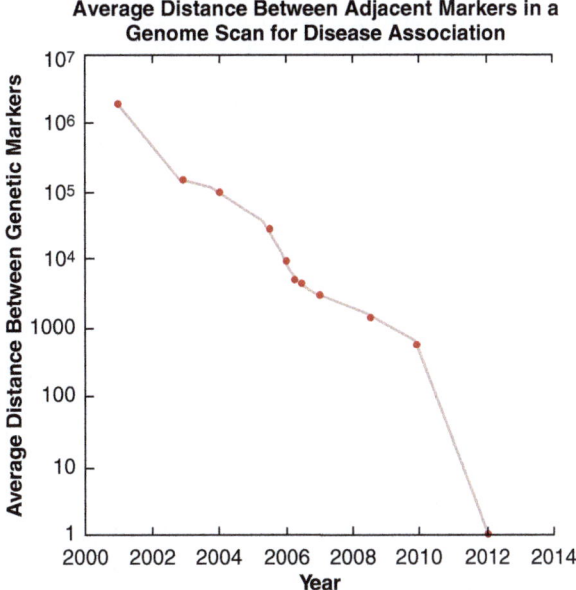

4.6.3.3 Structural Variants, Rare Variants, De Novo Mutations, and the Site Frequency Spectrum

A key feature explicitly studied in molecular population genetics and implicitly used in disease gene mapping studies is the site frequency spectrum; that is, the distribution of allele frequencies at single sites in the genome that vary in the human population studied. From both diffusion models (Kimura 1970) and coalescent theory (Hudson 1991) in theoretical population genetics, we know that the vast majority of realistic models generate many more rare variants compared to common polymorphisms. This is particularly true for expanding populations. Are these rare variants the source of much of the missing heritability? Recently, with the application of high-throughput sequencing technology to human studies over the past decade, empirical studies have clearly verified these predictions – the large majority of variants have low frequencies (The International HapMap 3 Consortium 2010). The distribution of deletions appears to be skewed toward more rare frequencies, presumably due to the deleterious effects of such variants. Individual mutations appearing *de novo* typically are extremely rare events per locus, but collectively are numerous. Other types of genetic variability, such as copy number repeats, span both ends of the frequency spectrum with the preponderance of the markers being rare. Thus, there is a sizable pool of low-frequency variants in human populations that have yet to be thoroughly investigated.

Over the past few years it has become increasingly clear that structural variants exist in the human genome at a far higher rate than previously thought. Structural variants can exist in a multitude of forms including deletions, copy number variants, and inversions among others. Due to the nature of these genetic changes, many are considered to be highly disruptive of molecular function if they lie in functional motifs. Indeed, there are several Mendelian diseases are caused by fully-penetrant structural variants impacting a chromosomal region (Lupski 2007). Numerous structural variants have recently been reported to be associated with common diseases, particularly in the neurological field (Sebat et al. 2007; Stefansson et al. 2008; Elia et al. 2010), infectious disease susceptibility (Gonzalez et al. 2005), and drug metabolism (Zackrisson et al. 2010). Although they have improved dramatically over the past few years, algorithms using SNP-based data from hybridization arrays to infer copy number variants have had high error rates, perhaps explaining the rather low rates of replication of structural variation association results for common diseases. Nevertheless, given the high frequency of structural variants, their pathogenic potential, and that we are on the precipice of a sequencing revolution in genome-wide studies, examination of these variants should be a high priority for new sequencing-based studies in oral disease susceptibility, progression, and related pharmacogenetic applications.

As different technologies examine different portions of the site frequency spectrum (i.e. genome-wide SNP scans interrogate variation that is common in the HapMap populations, whereas sequencing-based studies typically interrogate the entire frequency spectrum), where one believes genetic causation is harbored should influence the selection of genotyping technology. If common genetic variation contains the vast majority of heritable effects on disease phenotypes, then an investigator would be wise to employ a SNP-based experimental design. If, however, there is reason to believe that a significant portion of the genetic load of the disease studied exists in the highly populated portion of the distribution – the rare variants – then a sequencing-based study may be better suited to unravel causative alleles.

4.6.3.4 Epigenetics

The studies of heritability discussed previously show that there is heritable variation underlying a substantial portion of the variance observed in oral diseases. As discussed above, sequencing technologies may address many aspects of DNA variation including copy number loci, rare haplotypes, inversions, and insertions/deletions, but it is also worthwhile to repeat that the molecular mechanisms for disease heritability are not necessarily limited to variation at the DNA level. For a disease state, the covariance between relatives could be driven by co-inherited chromosomal regions or other phenomena. Chief alternative heritable mechanisms include DNA methylation (Hammoud et al. 2009), modifications to the histones (Bestor 2000), complex RNA zygotic transfer (Rassoulzadegan et al. 2006), and vertical transmission of infectious agents. Additionally, transgenerational effects offer an intriguing class of epigenetic mechanisms (Nadeau 2009). In a thorough review on epigenetics and periodontitis, Gomez et al. make a strong argument for consideration of both CpG dinucleotide methylation and deacetylation actions on cytokine expression as a credible avenue for further investigation in periodontal disease etiology (Gomez et al. 2009). Genome-wide epigenetic studies have been successfully conducted for oral cancers (Poage et al. 2010). The scale of this study on head and neck squamous cell carcinomas allowed these researchers to show a global pattern of tumor copy number changes significantly correlated with methylation profiles that was not detectable at the individual gene promoter level. With advanced chromatin immunoprecipitation and new methods to study DNA methylation, efforts to apply high-throughput epigenetic methods to oral diseases should be accelerated.

4.6.4 Genetics of Oral Diseases

4.6.4.1 Candidate Gene Studies

Numerous studies have been conducted in oral disease traits using a candidate gene approach. There are two large reviews of the existing candidate gene results (Nikolopoulos et al. 2008; Laine et al. 2010). Laine and colleagues have recently put together a comprehensive review article covering gene polymorphisms. There are some suggestive findings for cyclooxygenase-2 gene, *COX-2*, the cytokine-encoding genes, *IL6* and *IL1B*, the vitamin D receptor, *VDR*, a polymorphism immediately upstream of *CD14*, and the matrix metalloproteinase-1 gene, *MMP1*. However, these initial results will require further confirmation, for the association patterns are inconsistent across independent studies, the statistical significance is moderate, and the posterior probability of disease is decidedly bland. The striking pattern that emerges from the Laine et al. summary data is the lack of coherent replication of genetic association for the vast majority of polymorphisms examined. The situation is reminiscent of genetic association studies prior to large-scale SNP studies where poor repeatability of results plagued the field. In a pivotal study from 2002, Hirschhorn and colleagues (Hirschhorn et al. 2002) examined the state of genetic association studies, finding that "of the 166 putative associations that had been studied three or more times, only six have been consistently replicated." The dearth of robust results was largely remedied when large-scale genetic studies were applied to very substantial numbers of well-characterized patients and genetically-matched controls and stringent statistical criteria enforced. One can only suspect that a similar state of affairs is operating in genetic studies of chronic periodontitis. Perhaps efforts to (1) reduce the heterogeneity of the disease state through detailed clinical and laboratory assessments, (2) drastically increase sample sizes, and (3) expand the scope of inquiry to larger numbers of genes/regions, and examine a more comprehensive set of variants/epigenetic effects will improve the current situation.

The second large study is a meta-analysis of 53 studies, where Nikolopoulos and colleagues analyzed six cytokine polymorphisms linked to *IL1A*, *IL1B*, *IL6*, and TNF-alpha (Nikolopoulos et al. 2008). Two of these, an upstream SNP in *IL1A* and a SNP in *IL1B*, exhibited significant association with chronic periodontal disease risk. Although the results were not particularly strong, as is typical with complex diseases, the results do suggest the importance of inflammation-response variability in chronic periodontitis predisposition.

Perhaps the strongest, most replicable genetic association finding with coronary heart disease and myocardial infarction is centered on the short arm of chromosome 9 (9p21.3) (McPherson et al. 2007; Helgadottir et al. 2007). Two studies of periodontal disease showed that the same alleles at the 9p21.3 locus confer risk for aggressive periodontitis (Schaefer et al. 2009; Ernst et al. 2010). The discovery of such a pleiotropic locus may explain a portion of the aggregation of periodontal disease with other co-morbid conditions. Further studies investigating overlapping genetic susceptibility factors between periodontitis and cardiovascular disease, diabetes mellitus, metabolic syndrome, rheumatoid arthritis, and other related diseases may be a fruitful strategy for honing in on shared genes affecting these immuno-metabolic disorders.

4.6.4.2 Linkage Studies

Using patients from 46 families from the Philippines, the first genome-wide linkage study for caries was completed in 2008 (Vieira et al. 2008). The study identified five loci which exhibit suggestive statistical evidence (LOD scores exceeding 2.0): 5q13.3, 14q11.2, Xq27.1, 13q31.1, and 14q24.3. The latter of which overlapped with a quantitative trait locus discovered from mapping work in the mouse. Further work is necessary to refine these signals and localize the variants that may be driving these linkage signals.

Aggressive periodontal disease and rarer dental diseases have also been subjected to linkage analysis. Results from linkage studies for dentinogenesis imperfecta type I, for example, have gone on to produce the novel gene findings of the dentin sialophosphoprotein-encoding gene on 4q21.3 being responsible (Song et al. 2008; Crosby et al. 1995). A linkage study in African American families examining localized aggressive periodontitis found a strong linkage signal in a region covering approximately 26 megabases on chromosome 1 (Li et al. 2004). Several interesting genes are in this region. In a study earlier this year further mapping from Carvalho et al. in Brazilian families identified haplotypes in this region on 1q in *FAM5C* which were associated with aggressive periodontitis (Carvalho et al. 2010). The function of the FAM5C protein is not fully understood. FAM5C is localized in the mitochondria and it appears to play a role in vascular plaque dynamics and risk of myocardial infarction (Laass et al. 1997).

It should also be noted here that other types of mapping analyses such as homozygosity mapping to identify have yielded gene discoveries. For example, the lysosomal protease cathepsin C gene for the recessively-inherited Papillon-Lefevre syndrome which is characterized by aggressive and progressive periodontitis was effectively mapped using homozygosity mapping (Fischer et al. 1997; Connelly et al. 2008). Cathepsin C is highly expressed in leukocytes and macrophages and is a key coordinating molecule in natural killer cells (Rao et al. 1997; Meade et al. 2006). Although sparse, these linkage results are undoubtedly encouraging. Employing very large extended families subjected to genome-wide genotyping or sequencing will surely shed much needed light on chromosomal regions and genes relevant to oral disease research (Fig. 4.38).

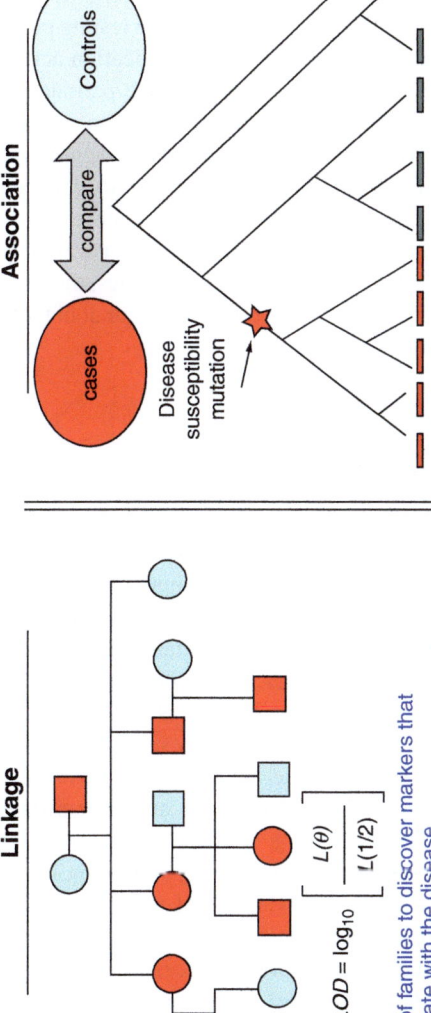

Fig. 4.38 Linkage studies vs. association studies to discover disease genes

4.6.4.3 Genome-Wide Association Studies

For periodontitis, a single study has employed a genome-wide association design in an effort to uncover aggressive periodontal variants (Schaefer et al. 2010). This study by Schaefer and colleagues discovered and replicated an intronic SNP, rs1537415, in the glycosyltransferase *GLT6D1* which is significantly correlated with aggressive periodontal disease in both German and Dutch samples. Often, seemingly significant results from large studies are due to the effect of reporting the top result from a great many statistical tests – this is called the multiple testing problem. In this situation, the strength of the finding, along with the replication across three case/control studies, argues for true association with aggressive periodontal susceptibility. The SNP may modulate the binding affinity of GATA-3. The association with *GLT6D1* is currently one of strongest genetic associations for aggressive periodontal disease, testifying to the power of genome-wide studies to generate novel, relevant molecular pathophysiology for complex diseases. It seems unlikely that *GLT6D1* would be extremely high on a candidate gene list, and it was only through a genome-wide scan that it appeared. Like many excellent studies, the finding by Schaefer et al. raises more questions than it answers and will undoubtedly provide fertile ground for ensuing molecular work.

4.6.5 *The Future of Oral Disease Genetics*

After a somewhat sluggish start, due to a lack of critical mass of investigators aiming to collect large numbers of patient samples and bring high throughput genetic technologies to caries susceptibility, gingivitis, and periodontal disease traits, the future of genetic studies in oral health is bright. Scientific progress in revealing the molecular pathogenesis of oral diseases is dependent on genome-wide genetic studies; and I have argued that progress in related immuno-metabolic diseases is also dependent on these large-scale genetic studies in periodontal disease. To study sporadic disease, substantial patient collection efforts are required for the application of these technologies. This may involve a combination of new recruitment and consortium-relationships with existing collections. The beginning of such a collection for sporadic aggressive periodontitis in Europe has shown extremely intriguing initial results, but more patients are needed to examine rare variants of moderate effect. Both the German/Dutch collection of aggressive periodontitis and the Brazilian collection have begun to revolutionize the study of periodontal disease susceptibility with the discovery of *GLT6D1* SNPs and *FAM5C*-linked haplotypes. There is little doubt that subsequent molecular work on these two genes will uncover novel mechanisms for the predisposition to aggressive periodontal disease. Focus should also be placed on the collection of extended families segregating these diseases. Applying sequencing technologies to large pedigrees can be an effective method of identifying rare variants and structural variants in a highly-refined phenotype. Furthermore, applying these methods to the entire genome would make for a comprehensive genetic study.

Several trends in large-scale genomics science hold promise to significantly advance our understanding of oral disease pathogenesis:

- The sociology of biological sciences has changed over the past 15 years so as to become more collaborative. Essential for association-based designs, consortium-based genetic research has blossomed over that time period, increasing sample sizes and therefore the power to detect disease-causing variants. There currently is consortium-based research in periodontal disease and oral cancer. Further expanding these efforts will enhance subsequent studies, particularly those investigating rare alleles and/or rare epigenetic effects.
- Through over a century of laboratory work, the collective knowledge of biochemical pathways, signal transduction, cell physiology, regulatory mechanisms, and structural biochemistry is weighty. Incorporation of this information into etiological models may substantially advance oral disease work as well as the field of complex disease genetics in general. Sophisticated analysis techniques are needed to perform this task. Recent advances merging results from network science with probability theory within the context of computer science have produced the field of machine learning. This rigorous framework can be used to identify those factors responsible for disease status and can also be used to develop robust predictive models using known biological networks and genetic data. The output from such models, typically the probability of disease, an estimate of disease progression rate, or a probability of adverse reaction, can be used by physicians and dentists to personalize medical care.
- Until relatively recently, population genetics did not contribute a great deal to human genetics research. That has changed in the past decade where effort spent on association studies surpassed that spent on family-based studies. Those investigating disease gene mapping began to collaborate with population geneticists and population geneticists took up a wide-spread interest in finding disease alleles. Incorporation of population genetics theory into such studies markedly improved association studies on several levels: confounding by population stratification was effectively treated using population genetics, linkage disequilibrium patterns. Use of population genetics theory in large-scale oral disease mapping studies may accelerate discoveries.
- Sequencing technology has rapidly progressed over the past decade. Currently, sequencing studies across the exome can be accomplished at reasonable cost and yield data for all known genes in the genome. Within the next few years, sequencing costs will depreciate to a point where whole-genome sequencing studies will be commonplace, using both family-based and population designs. Application of these technologies to oral disease studies is imperative for comprehensive studies of etiology.
- High-throughput DNA methylation and chromatin immunoprecipitation studies will enable large-scale epigenetic studies in oral diseases (Meade et al. 2006; Ehrich et al. 2005; Bibikova et al. 2006; Ren et al. 2000; Pokholok et al. 2005). These have already started to play an important role in delineating mechanisms responsible for oral cancers (Poage et al. 2010). Additional application of these techniques to studies of gingivitis, caries, and periodontal diseases may generate novel findings.

- Molecular biologists and pharmacologists have increasingly become able to develop and evaluate highly targeted pharmaceuticals based on genetic discoveries. The use of such genetic information may improve the chances of developing efficacious therapies.
- Geneticists and disease researchers are beginning to realize that oral diseases both impact and are intrinsically tied to susceptibility and progression of other common diseases. A synthesis of genetic findings from immuno-metabolic-linked disorders would seem to greatly increase the knowledge of these diseases and better pinpoint their respective etiologies.
- As the new high-throughput genomics and epigenomics technologies become implemented in oral disease research, the storage, management, analysis, and interpretation of the ensuing colossal amounts of data will be critical to enable clinicians to use these results in daily practice. Advances in dental and medical informatics will facilitate these steps.

We are in exciting times where advances in genetic technologies will uncover the genetic causes of diseases, including those that affect the oral cavity. With more focus in the area of oral disease genomics and the harnessing of new high-throughput sequencing and epigenetic technologies, novel insights into the pathways driving these diseases are imminent. These discoveries will, in turn, motivate directed therapies, aid in illuminating the molecular etiology of related disorders such as diabetes, and increase the level of personalized medicine.

4.7 Education – When You Come to a Fork in the Road, Take It

Joseph Kilsdonk

4.7.1 Introduction

The title of this section reinforces a 1995 Institute of Medicine (IOM) report titled "Dental Education: at the Crossroads." To quote Yogi Berra, a baseball sage: "When you come to a fork in the road, take it." The implication being that dental education must take action and move beyond its crossroads. These crossroads are described in the first third of the section. It includes a summary and recommendations of the IOM report and three transitional reports that followed: the 2000 Surgeon General's report identifying oral health as a silent epidemic, the Josiah Macy Foundation report, and a "Pipeline" study funded by both the Robert Wood Johnson and the California foundations. Having been at the crossroads for a decade or so, the middle portion of the section highlights educational models that may lead to a more promising future. The later third of this section describes an alternative path of action for dental education which emphasizes the central roles of clinic-based education and dental informatics in dental education curriculum. It is unknown how traditional dental educators may view this model; however, it is effectively a logical conclusion and responsive to the reports.

4.7.2 Where We Were

In 1995 the Institute of Medicine (IOM) published "Dental Education at the Crossroads" (Field 1995). The title was apropos as the authors' analysis concluded: (1) economics surrounding dental education were unsustainable ; (2) student service learning opportunities and access to care for patients were limited; and (3) new dental schools were not replacing those forced to close due to the economic climate. The IOM report additionally proposed key recommendations to reform dental education and service delivery. Fifteen years later, we remain at "the crossroads" as these issues remain largely unresolved. Furthermore, these recommendations have retained their validity. Their implementation would directly impact structures and services for contemporary models of dental education in the future.

The following IOM recommendations (Field 1995) are intrinsic to the proposed dental education reform:

Recommendation 2: To increase access to care and improve the oral health status of underserved populations…

Recommendation 3: To improve the availability of dental care in underserved areas and to limit the negative effects of high student debt…

Recommendation 5: To prepare future practitioners for more medically based modes of oral health care and more medically complicated patients, dental educators should work with their colleagues in medical schools and academic health centers to:

- Move toward integrated basic science education for dental and medical students;
- Require and provide for dental students at least one rotation, clerkship or equivalent experience in relevant areas of medicine and offer opportunities for additional elective experience in hospitals, nursing homes, ambulatory care clinics and other settings;
- Continue and expand experiments with combined MD-DDS programs and similar programs for interested students and residents;
- Increase the experience of dental faculty in clinical medicine so that they, and not just physicians, can impart medical knowledge to dental students and serve as role models for them.

Recommendation 6: To prepare students and faculty for an environment that will demand increasing efficiency, accountability, and evidence of effectiveness, the committee recommends that dental students and faculty participate in efficiently managed clinics and faculty practices in which the following occurs:

- Patient-centered, comprehensive care is the norm;
- Patients' preferences and their social, economic, and emotional circumstances are sensitively considered;
- Teamwork and cost-effective use of well-trained allied dental personnel are stressed;
- Evaluations of practice patterns and of the outcomes of care guide actions to improve both the quality and the efficiency of such care;
- General dentists serve as role models in the appropriate treatment and referral of patients needing advanced therapies;
- Larger numbers of patients, including those with more diverse characteristics and clinical problems, are served.

Recommendation 17: Because no single financing strategy exists, the committee recommends that dental schools individually and, when appropriate collectively evaluate and implement a mix of actions to reduce costs and increase revenues. Potential strategies, each of which needs to be guided by solid financial information and projections as well as educational and other considerations, include the following:

- Increasing the productivity, quality, efficiency, and profitability of faculty practice plans, student clinics, and other patient care activities;
- Pursuing financial support at the federal, state, and local levels for patient-centered predoctoral and postdoctoral dental education, including adequate reimbursement of services for Medicaid and indigent populations and contractual or other arrangements for states without dental schools to support the education of some of their students in states with dental schools;
- Rethinking basic models of dental education and experimenting with less costly alternatives;
- Raising tuition for in or out-of-state students if current tuition and fees are low compared to similar schools;
- Developing high-quality, competitive research and continuing education programs;
- Consolidating or merging courses, departments, programs, and even entire schools.

In summary, the IOM report identified that: (1) an outdated curriculum continues to be retained which reflects past dental practice rather than current and emerging practice and knowledge; (2) clinical education does not sufficiently incorporate the goal of comprehensive care, with instruction focusing too heavily on procedures; (3) medical care and dentistry are not integrated; and (4) the curriculum is crowded with redundant material, often taught in disciplinary silos.

The 1995 IOM's Report was followed by the Surgeon General's Report on Oral Health in 2000 and a subsequent supplement by the Surgeon General in 2003 called "The National Call to Action" (U.S. Department of Health and Human Services

2003). Five significant findings and recommendations from the Surgeon General's Report(s) that have implications pertaining to the envisioned structure and services of new models for dental education include:

- Changing the perception of oral health so that it will no longer be considered separate from general health;
- Improving oral health care delivery by reducing disparities associated with populations whose access to dental treatment is compromised by poverty, limited education or language skills, geographic isolation, age, gender, disability, or an existing medical condition;
- Encouraging oral health research, expanding preventive and early detection programs, and facilitating the transfer of knowledge about them to the general population;
- Increasing oral health workforce diversity, capacity, and flexibility to overcome the underrepresentation of specific racial and ethnic groups in the dental profession. In this regard, the National Call to Action urged the development of dental school recruitment programs to correct these disparities and to encourage part-time dental service in community clinics in areas of oral health shortage;
- Increasing collaboration between the private sector and the public sector to create the kind of cross-disciplinary, culturally sensitive, community-based, and community-wide efforts to expand initiatives for oral health promotion and dental disease prevention.

Spurred by the 1995 IOM report and the 2000 Surgeon General's report, the Josiah Macy Foundation (2004) conducted a study entitled "New Models of Dental Education." The study was prompted by concerns about declines in dental school budgets and the difficulties experienced by schools in meeting their educational, research, and service missions. The Macy study concluded that:

- Financial problems of dental schools are real and certain to increase.
- Current responses of schools to these economic challenges are not adequate.
- Most promising solutions require new models of clinical dental education.

Macy study lead researcher Dr Howard Bailit, and his team recently concluded in reference to points one and two above, that: "If current trends (to aforementioned) continue for the next 10 years, there is little doubt that the term *crisis* will describe the situation faced by dental schools. Further, assuming that it will take at least ten or even more years to address and resolve these financial problems, now is the time for dental educators, practitioners, and other interested parties from the private and public sectors to come to a consensus on how to deal with the coming crisis. Clearly, these financial problems will not be solved by minor adjustments to the curriculum, modest improvements in the clinical productivity of students or faculty, or even significant increases in contributions from alumni. The solutions 'must involve basic structural changes in the way dental education is financed and organized' (Bailit et al. 2008)." This statement is supported by the fact that in the past 25 years more dental schools have closed than opened. Specifically eight schools have closed, whereas to date a couple has opened and a handful is pending.

Curriculum relevance was also a focus of the study. Findings concluded that "changing the curriculums in dental schools to allow students to spend more time in community venues would be highly beneficial to both society and student. Society benefited from having underserved patients cared for while students were assessed as being five to ten times more productive, more proficient, more confident, more technically skilled and more competent in treating and interacting with minority patients" (Brodeur 2008).

Macy study (Formicola et al. 2005) outcomes represented significant and foundational guideposts for assessing and planning any future models for dental education. Their report led to the Robert Wood Johnson Foundation Pipeline Study (2007), a major research study funded by the Robert Wood Johnson Foundation and The California Endowment (TCE). The goal of the Dental Pipeline Program was to reduce disparities in access to dental care. The Pipeline study provided over $30 million for the start up or expansion of 15 schools and student clinical programs that incorporated services to underserved extramural clinical settings (primarily community health centers).

- The following recommendations from the Surgeon General's report structured the goals of the Pipeline's initiative: Increase the number of under-represented minority and low-income students enrolled in the dental schools participating in the Pipeline Program so that there would be a voice of minority and low-income students at all the funded schools.
- Provide dental students with courses and clinical experience that would prepare them for treating disadvantaged patients in community sites.
- Have senior dental students spend an average of 60 days in community clinics and practices treating underserved patients. Increasing the community experience of dental students was expected to have an immediate impact on increasing care to underserved patients (Brodeur 2008). This third point is pivotal to future success of dental curricula and dental education economics.

Recently published in a supplemental volume to the *Journal of Dental Education*, February, 2009, the Pipeline study reported the following outcomes:

- Minority recruitment of low-income students increased by 27%;
- The rate of recruitment for under-represented populations was almost twice that of non-pipeline schools;
- The length of time dental students spent in extramural rotations increased from a mean of 16 days to a mean of 39 days over a period of 4 years.
- Procedural proficiency increased compared to that of their non-extramural peers.
- Of the 15 Pipeline-funded programs, only four schools achieved the goal of 60 days of extramural rotations; Through extra funding from TCE, the four schools extended extramural rotations to an average of 198 days;
- Based on this publication, it appears that only a handful of pipeline schools definitely plan to sustain their extended extramural rotations. Financial concerns were highlighted as the major problem in sustaining future recruitment and placement of students beyond the timeframe of the study;

- A survey of program seniors indicated a mean of 26% [range of 14–60% by school] were planning to devote ≥25% of their practice to serving minority patients. Only 9% [range of 3–22% by school] were planning to practice at community clinics.

In the context of these outcomes, discussion indicated that the unwillingness of students to practice in underserved settings was based on several factors:

- Students that participated were already enrolled in traditional programs and were not necessarily seeking a pipeline experience or a future in community service.
- Concern over future reimbursement as a provider in a community setting;
- Limited time spent in underserved settings;
- Limited loan forgiveness scholarship opportunities.

The fact that the large majority of pipelines were unsustainable was attributed to lack of productivity in the school clinics while the students were on rotation at community based clinics. Schools generate meager, yet necessary revenue streams on intramural student clinical activity to support the costly clinical and faculty infrastructure. Currently, similar economic constraints involved with outsourcing students to serving rural and underserved populations impacts the ability of tradition dental schools to participate in sustained outreach programs.

Most recently, the Pew Center on the States National Academy for Health Policy (2009) released "Help Wanted: A Policy Makers Guide to New Dental Providers". This report provided an excellent summary outlining workforce needs, access issues, and strategies for dental-related services to help states and institutions develop creative ways to solve oral health access and care issues. The Guide proposes the following relevant components and trends for consideration in development of future sustainable school models:

- Dental colleges are willing to bear a large and disproportionate share of the burden in terms of access to care, particularly during a time of incredibly scarce resources.
- Expanded, extensive, and/or creative extramural rotations have been developed in recent years under the conceptual umbrella of service-learning. These often involve clinics providing direct or indirect payment to dental schools or clinics managed in some way by dental schools.

4.7.3 Where We Are: Economics, Equity, and Education Converge

Dental education has certain obligations. First, education must adhere to accreditation standards with the goal of producing competent practitioners. Second, education must remain responsive and impact the societal need for care. Lastly, the delivery of dental education must be economically sustainable. The Macy, RWJF, and IOM reports note that improved oral health, sustainable dental education economic models, and competent workforce pipelines converge around Community Health Centers (CHC). University of Michigan researchers Fitzgerald and

Fig. 4.39 The synergy between access to care, student competency, and financially sustainable dental education converge around CHC/FQHCs

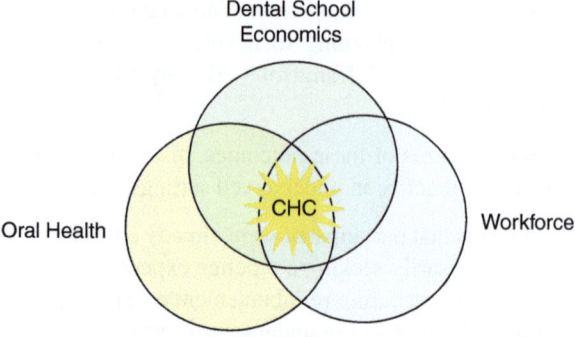

Piskorowski (2009) reaffirm this conclusion in an evaluation of an ongoing 7-year program, stating that:

> (the CHC model) is self-sustaining and can be used to increase service to the underserved and increase the value of students' clinical educational experiences without requiring grant or school funding, thus improving the value of dental education without increased cost. Self-sustaining contracts with seven Federally Qualified Health Centers (FQHCs) have resulted in win-win-win-win outcomes: win for the underserved communities, which experienced increased access to care; win for the FQHCs, which experienced increased and more consistent productivity; win for the students, who increased their clinical skills and broadened their experience base; and win for the school in the form of predictable and continuing full coverage of all program costs (Fitzgerald and Piskorowski 2009) (Fig. 4.39).

However, unlike medicine that outsources their students to clinical sites, dental education programs retain the majority of the student time within their own "clinical laboratories." As documented by the aforementioned studies, this limits students' exposure to extramural experiences. Costs to operate such intramural clinical programs are ever increasing and many schools' clinical operations run deficits. If that component can be outsourced to community-based resources such as a CHC, then the burden of cost is shifted away from the school.

An example would be A.T. Still University's Arizona School of Dentistry and Oral Health (ASDOH) which matriculated its first class in 2003. At the prompting of the State's community based clinics, ASDOH designed a program that placed students into community-based settings for up to 6 months, an unprecedented length of time for an extramural rotation. They also saw this as an opportunity to use an adjunct centric faculty that significantly reduced traditional education overhead. Through this innovation, the school was able to develop a program that was sustained by "fair market" value tuition and trained students where community needs were greatest for up to 6 months (which was then unprecedented). Conversely, if the CHC can rely on student service-learning to care for patients, the cost of care is reduced.

Other schools are also advancing with innovative education and care delivery. ADEA's Charting Progress (Valachovic 2009) identified several schools that are in planning stages and two in progress. They include Western University in Pomona, California; East Carolina University in North Carolina; Midwestern University in Glendale, Arizona; University of New England in Portland, Maine; Texas Tech University Health Sciences Center in El Paso, Texas; the University of Arkansas in

Little Rock, Arkansas; and the University of Southern Nevada in South Jordan, Utah. Western University is planning placement of 50% of their fourth year class in community health centers, while East Carolina is seeking to set up rural clinical campuses as well as clinical partnerships with the State's FQHC. At the time of this publication, several existing schools are expanding or looking to expand including the University of North Carolina, Marquette University, Midwestern University in Downer's Grove, IL. Such expansions will contribute to solving the existent access supply and demand issues. However, it was observed even with all the start ups and expansions, graduation numbers will not approach the output of schools in the late 1970s and early 1980s.

These creative models establish the foundation for a sustainable clinic structure by generating self-sustaining revenue through student service-learning, which, unlike medical student services, are billable. Simultaneously these new models provide access to care for the needy while student exposure to clinical experiences that are often not available in academic patient pools. These models also shift some of the cost of providing clinical education from the dental college to community-based clinics.

However, this innovation is not without criticism. Schools are dependent on the success of their clinics and clinic partnerships. One author cautions: "However, these creative models also may present potential political strategic risk or conflict: private practitioners may organize and protest higher than normal reimbursement schemes. Potentially, such protests could even jeopardize the very existence of such models (Dunning et al. 2009)." Notably, community health centers have historically received strong bipartisan support. For example, during the Bush administration, FQHC funding was doubled and most recently expanded through health reform legislation by the Obama administration.

4.7.4 A Road to the Future

According to the Institute for Oral Health, "The group practice of the future is the dentist working with the physician" (Ryan 2007). The ADA reported "multidisciplinary education must become the norm and represent the meaning and purposes of primary care as it applies to dentistry. Educational sequences should include rotation strategies across discipline specialties in medicine and dentistry, clerkships and hospital rotations, and experience in faculty and residency clinics." (Barnett and Brown 2000) The models alluded to, were school-based attempts at improving educational outcomes. Perhaps the proverbial fork in the road regarding the future of dental education leaves two paths for consideration. Is it better to travel down a road that leads a school to develop and operate a clinic? Or is the road less traveled, where a clinic becomes a school, the better of the two options? The answer, perhaps, is that a combination of both will accomplish the desired outcome. For example, didactic knowledge is measured by examination whereas competency as a practitioner is measured by clinical demonstration. At a minimum, the result must achieve learner competency, quality, and sustainability. However, the road less traveled has not been taken yet. William Gies, in his revered report written 85 years ago on the state of American dental education, wrote "Dental faculties should show the need.... for integrated instruction in the general principles of clinical dentistry and in its correlations with clinical medicine" (Gies 1926). Basic sciences aside, could a clinical-based educational training center have an advantage over a school-based clinical center? Soon-to-be-implemented new Commission on Dental Accreditation (CODA) standards will require schools to demonstrate competency in patient-centered care (Valachovic 2010). Might an enterprise proficient at running a successful clinical business model have an advantage running a professional, patient-centered clinical training program as compared to a pedagogical business model attempting to run a clinical training model? These questions should challenge us to reexamine why our thinking about educational models should be limited to schools being the starting point for the development of a profession that demands clinical competency, patient-centeredness, and integration as outcomes. The clinic based model may serve as an equivalent starting point and, have some distinct advantages for achieving responsiveness to recommendations and directions cited in this section.

4.7.5 A FQHC Model

Beginning in November 2002 through August 2010, the Family Health Center (FHC) of Marshfield, Inc, Marshfield, Wisconsin, launched of a broad network of developing dental clinics, targeting dental professional shortage areas with the provision of dental services to the underserved communities whose dental needs were not being adequately met by the existing infrastructure. FHC-Marshfield is a Federally Qualified Health Center (FQHC). As an FQHC, FHC receives cost-based reimbursement for its dental services to Medicaid populations. Along with the cost- based reimbursement, FQHCs are obligated to provide care to anyone regardless of their ability to pay. Presently, FHC is the nation's largest federally qualified dental health center. To date, this network of dental clinics has served over 58,000 unique patients, 85% of whom were under 200% of poverty. Notably, service was provided to a significant number of cognitively and developmentally disabled patients in special stations developed for serving patients with special needs. These patients frequently travel the furthest to get to our dental centers for care. Beginning in 2008, FHC stepped up the pace of dental clinic expansion, constructing two new dental centers in 2009, two in 2010, and two more are slated to open in 2011. When fully operational, this will establish capacity to serve 66,000 patients annually. Each site has proactively included dedicated clinical and classroom training space for dental residents or students, thus laying the framework for clinic-based training of new dental professionals. The plan is to continue to stand up new dental centers until they have the capacity to serve 158,000 patients annually or approximately 50% of the 300,000 underserved patients in the rural service area. In addition to the capacity for training residents and students, a dental post-baccalaureate program is being considered in partnership with regional 4 year under graduate campuses. The post-baccalaureate program is aimed at preparing students from rural and underserved areas who desire to practice in rural and underserved areas for acceptance and success in dental schools.

Presently FHC in partnership with Marshfield Clinic is moving forward with plans to develop dental residencies at these sites and a dental post baccalaureate training program to better prepare pre-doctoral students from rural and/or underserved backgrounds to be successful in dental school as a means to create a dental academic infrastructure responsive to rural environments which have been classically underserved. Marshfield Clinic has a long-standing history in medical student education and multiple medical residency programs.

4.7.6 Train Where the Need Is

Creating access for the underserved population was the major motivational force driving the establishment of the dental clinic network back in 2002. The findings of the IOM, Macy, and RWJF reports became the foundational framework for developing the vision of a dental education model that would realize the major recommendations found in the reports. By establishing clinical campuses in regional underserved dental health professional shortage areas, access to care where care is needed most was provided. Sustainment of a work force for provision of care across the dental clinic network is accomplished by schools contracting with FQHC's for service learning, thus circumventing challenges associated with releasing dental students at traditional dental schools to distant extramural training sites as discussed previously. This model is however not without its own set of challenges including calibration of faculty, supervision and evaluation of students in training, and achieving accreditation acceptance. However, through video connectivity and iEHR technology curriculum, learning plans, competency assessment, progression, performance, faculty development, and learner evaluations can be centrally calibrated. Additionally, this dental service-learning model based in a community health center setting offers students unique state-of-the-art exposures to alternative access models, cutting-edge informatics (including access to a combined dental-medical record) and a quality-based outcomes-driven practice.

Given the novelty of such an extended extramural dental clinical training model, there is limited data on the success of rural placement leading to retention to practice in a rural setting. The Pipeline study piloted a model for getting students into underserved communities. However, that experiment was limited to 60 day rotations. Outcome driven programs may provide a predictive surrogate for purposes of comparative analysis. For example, the Rural Medical Education "RMED" program of the University of Illinois medical school at Rockford, has sustained a longstanding program in Illinois. Over 17 years in duration with over 200 student participants of whom 70% have been retained as primary care medicine practitioners in rural Illinois. Rabinowitz et al. (2008a) further reinforced that medical school rural programs have been highly successful in increasing the supply of rural physicians, with an average of 53–64% of graduates choosing to practice in rural areas. They also noted rural retention rates of 79–87% among the programs (Rabinowitz et al. 2008a).

Recently, the University of Wisconsin School of Medicine and Public Health (UWSMPH) launched the Wisconsin Academy for Rural Medicine (WARM program). The WARM program places medical students in rural academic medical centers during their third and fourth years in medical school. Marshfield Clinic is one of those sites. WARM students affiliating with Marshfield Clinic's system would ultimately share learning experiences with dental students, clinical rotations, team-based rounding, lectures, and exposure to a combined medical-dental patient record. In an analogous manner, the Marshfield Clinic dental education model will incorporate a curriculum that embeds students in rural clinical practice for up to 2 years.

A secondary but not insignificant outcome of placing residents and students in clinical campuses focused on developing competency and providing care where needs are often greatest is the cost savings to taxpayers associated with the public care of patients. These savings are accomplished through the "service-learning" of the student. For example, in the model described where clinical training is embedded within the FHC clinics, the stipend resident or unpaid student learner provides the patient care as part of their service learning training while requiring oversight from one paid faculty per four to six learners. As a result, an academic based clinical partnership creates a model that reduces the cost for care provided to underserved patients. An additional benefit to the community based clinic might be realized through tuition assistance by the academic program to help support patient procedures that develop learner competencies.

> In educational quality and influence, dental schools should equal medical schools, for their responsibilities are similar and their tasks analogous (William Gies 1926).

The Commission on Dental Accreditation (CODA) notes that one of the learning objectives of an Advanced Education General Dentistry (AEGD) Residency is to have the graduate function as a "primary care provider". To function competently in this role, the graduate needs to have a strong academic linkage to primary care medicine. At a 2010 dental deans forum, 84 years after the Gies report, Dr Polverini made the statement "Dentistry has never been linked to the medical network but unless dentistry becomes part of the solution to the challenge of providing comprehensive patient care, it will be looked on as part of the problem, and ultimately, all dental schools will be called into question." (Polverini 2010) The use of dental informatics and an integrated record are elements essential to this competency. On April 1, 2010, FHC and Marshfield Clinic successfully transitioned all of their dental centers to a new practice management and electronic health record system that fully integrates medical and dental; one of the first such systems in the nation. Along with the benefits derived in Fig. 4.39, CHC placement also exposes students to an integrated medical-dental care setting where learners can develop skills in system-based practice to include the interdependence of health professionals, systems, and the coordination of care. On the administrative side, dental and medical appointments can be coordinated to enhance convenience for patients and improve compliance with preventive dental visits. In 2009, Marshfield Clinic's Research Foundation Biomedical Informatics Research Center hired their first Dental Informatician, Dr. Amit Acharya, BDS, MS, PhD. With dedicated biomedical informatics and research resource centers, the Marshfield Clinic has laid the groundwork for true medical/dental integration with appropriate electronic health record decision support and is positioned to develop a dental education curriculum capable of implementing the IOM recommendations. Downstream benefits of using such a curriculum are the ability of future practitioners to use informatics to improve quality of care and reduce the burden of disease.

According to an Institute of Oral Health Report (2010) it is widely accepted across the dental profession that oral health has a direct impact on systemic health, and increasingly, medical and dental care providers are building to bridge relationships to create treatment solutions. As early as 1926, William Gies recognized that "the frequency of periodic examination gives dentists exceptional opportunity to note early signs of many types of illnesses outside the domain of dentistry" (Gies 1926). The following examples show how integration of dental and medical care can impact patient outcomes, underlining the importance of this concept in dental curriculum design.

A 2009 study of 21,000 Blue Cross Blue Shield of Michigan (BCBS) members with diabetes, who had access to dental care lead researchers, and BCBS executives to conclude that treatment of periodontal disease significantly impacts outcomes related to diabetes care and related costs (Blue Cross Blue Shield of Michigan 2009). Another example is found in the context of preterm delivery and miscarriage. According to research cited by CIGNA (2006), expecting mothers with chronic periodontal disease during the second trimester are seven times more likely to deliver preterm (before 37th week), and have dramatically more healthcare challenges throughout their life. CIGNA also cites the correlation between periodontal disease and low birth weights, pre-eclampsia, gestational diabetes.

Equally important is the opportunity to develop and implement the team-based curriculum that trains future dentists and physicians in the management of chronic disease as an Accountable Care Organization (ACO) in a patient-centered environment. As an example, Joseph Errante, D.D.S., Vice President, Blue Cross Blue Shield of MA, reported that medical costs for diabetics who accessed dental care for prevention and periodontal services were significantly lower than those who didn't get dental care (Errante 2007).

These data suggest that team based case management of prevalent chronic health conditions have considerable cost savings opportunities for government payers, third party payers, employers and employees (Errante 2007). These economic benefits to integration as it relates to the iEHR are discussed elsewhere in this book, but begin with the ability of providers to function in a team based environment and as such, underscore the importance of training in such an environment.

Dentists trained in a FQHC iEHR integrated educational model will be well positioned to function successfully within an ACO model. An ACO is a system where providers are accountable for the outcomes and expenditures of the insured population of patients they serve. The providers within the system are charged with collectively improving care around cost and quality targets set by the payor.

Within this system, care must be delivered in a patient-centered environment. The patient-centered environment according to the National Committee for Quality Assurance (NCQA), is a health care setting that cultivates partnerships between individual patients and their personal physicians and, when appropriate, the patient's family. Care is facilitated by registries, information technology, health information exchange and other means to assure that patients receive defined, timely and appropriate care while remaining cognizant of cultural, linguistic and literacy needs of the patient being served. The model includes the opportunity to deliver patient care that is patient-centric, incorporates the patient in the care planning, considers the patient's beliefs and views, and incorporates the patient's families as needed. The model allows providers to deliver care that is inclusive of needs, attentive, and accessible. The model equips payers to purchase high quality and coordinated care among teams of providers across healthcare settings. While this describes the medical home, most dental practices also follow this process. Many dental practices function in this regard with insured populations and reflect elements of the model that medicine is creating. William Gies would be proud.

Training in the delivery of accountable and patient-centered medical–dental care must be done purposefully. Commenting on the inadequate training relative to the integration of medical and dental education, Baum (2007) stated that "we need to design new curricula with meaningful core competencies for the next generation of dentists rather than apply patches to our existing ones." While this statement was made in reference to the basic sciences, the same holds true for patient-centered system-based practice competencies. Utilizing state-of-the-art electronic medical records as a tool and the FHC infrastructure as the service venue, meaningful patient-centered system-based practice core competencies achievement becomes possible in a manner highly responsive to societal needs. By definition, FQHCs must provide primary medical care, dental care, and behavioral health. FQHC have also historically been utilized as healthcare workforce training centers and the Affordable Care Act of 2010 reinforced their role as healthcare training centers. Specifically, this legislation serves to promote FQHCs as the entity through which the primary care workforce (including dental) will be developed and expanded. In combination, FQHCs and primary care centers are positioned to be the front runners in a medical/-dental home training model which will be essential to preparing future practitioners for practice in an ACO. Critical to this success is the ability to train these practitioners on an integrated medical-dental record and informatics platform. Use of this platform imprints most strongly during the learner's formative years of training; instructing and guiding disease management, decision making, patient care coordination, prevention, and both outcome-based and comprehensive care. Training in this hybrid academically orientated clinically integrated setting moves dental education off its crossroads and creates the highway to its future.

4.7.7 Concerns

Concerns with the new models extend to their ability to integrate medical and dental disciplines at the clinical and informatics level. While the 1995 IOM report identified the need to integrate medical and dental curriculum, success at the curricular and technological level within schools, has been limited. Three major factors have contributed to the limited progress:

- Access priorities. Creating access to care has outranked the need to integrate care. In part, this reflects societal need for care and public demand to reduce the burden of the "silent epidemic." Schools play an important role as a safety net to care for the uninsured and underinsured through intramural clinical service learning. Even though "dental colleges seem to be willing to bearing a large and disproportionate share of the burden in terms of access to care" (Dunning et al. 2009), schools were challenged as part of IOM, Surgeon General, and Macy reports, to expand that role. While these reports have prompted creative educational solutions to increase access, the reports understate the tremendous opportunity, quality and cost benefits that could result from an integration of medicine and dentistry.
- It is difficult to change the culture and structure of existing schools. This is not unique to dentistry. However, the 1995 IOM report specifically recommended that schools "eliminate marginally useful and redundant courses and design an integrated basic and clinical science curriculum". The challenges with this are many. Examples include:
  - Some schools may not have other disciplines to draw from to create an integrated curriculum;
  - A number of schools use a faculty senate to determine curriculum. This can result in curriculum that preserves the current faculty structure;
  - Changing curriculum is associated with expense and can be financially prohibitive to some schools
  - Physical changes may be needed and represent an expense and/or may, in some instances, may not be practicable based on structure of existing facilities.
  - Public school programs may direct the final curriculum, as boards or regent's one or two steps removed from the curriculum often have final authority conversely, private schools may specify business or mission objectives that determine final design.
- Perhaps most germane to this text is the lack of a common technology platform between disciplines in a learning environment. An integrated curriculum requires an integrated platform to accomplish delivery and evaluation. This is particularly essential to clinical management of the patient by professionals in training as part of a healthcare delivery team. Some progress in establishing shared basic sciences curricula has been documented in the literature. To date, no single integrated electronic health (medical-dental) record has been meaningfully adapted for educational purposes, including incorporation of assessment of the learner relative to integrated competencies, integrated case-based and problem-based curriculum, and integrated evaluation and assessment.

Another concern with new educational programs emerging in response to these reports and relative to creating a transformational integrated curriculum is that some of the programs are focusing primarily on creating clinicians with no value or emphasis on integrating training with research and/or scholarly activity. Integrated training models counter such concerns. Research will be fundamental to measuring the relative benefits and outcomes associated with treatment of patients in a shared curriculum setting and will be the catalyst for the development of integrated medical-dental informatics incorporating educational capabilities.

Additionally, accreditation will also need to evaluate its response to such models. Presently it is unclear how accrediting bodies will view an integrated cross-disciplinary curriculum. Further, due to its integrated nature, such a curriculum would lie outside of the expertise of a single traditional accrediting body focused on one particular discipline. It has yet to be determined how accrediting bodies will review and appraise such cross-disciplinary competencies.

Lastly, it is important to recognize that a successful education model with innovative informatics is only successful if its focus is patient care. Graduating learners with competency only in the use of informatics will be limited unless adapted to training and delivery programs that result in patient centric care.

4.7.8 Conclusions

Research and reports over the past 15 years support the need to reform dental education. First steps have been taken and lead the way for continued innovation around clinic-based education and integrated curriculum. The models identified point to a strong partnership and interrelationship with CHCs for creative, cost saving, effective and sustainable delivery methods. Moreover, CHC's must be more involved in a training curriculum integrated with informatics. CHCs, in turn, benefit from residents and students through service-learning to help meet a societal and workforce need, while the learners benefit from increased competency. In order to train an evidence-based, patient-centered, medical-dental workforce, it is imperative that medical and dental data and record accessibility be incorporated into these training and care delivery initiatives. In order to keep moving away from the crossroads, such integration must become the pathway on which curriculum is developed and implemented.

References

107th Congress. Public Law 107–188. 2002. http://frwebgate.access.gpo.gov/cgi-bin/getdoc.cgi?dbname=107_cong_public_laws&docid=f:publ188.107.pdf. Accessed May 2011.

Acharya A, Bhavsar N, Jadav B, Parikh H. Cardioprotective effect of periodontal therapy in metabolic syndrome: a pilot study in Indian subjects. Metab Syndr Relat Disord. 2010;8(4): 335–41.

Adachi M, Ishihara K, Abe S, Okuda K, Ishikawa T. Effect of professional oral health care on the elderly living in nursing homes. Oral Surg Oral Med Oral Pathol. 2002. doi:10.1067/moe.2002.123493.

Aetna. Study shows preventive dental care may help reduce risk of preterm birth. 2008. http://www.aetna.com/news/newsReleases/2008/1001_DMI_Preterm_Birth_Risk.html. Accessed 26 June 2011.

Aggarwal V, Joughin A, Zakrzewska J, Crawford F, Tickle M. Dentists' and specialists' knowledge of chronic orofacial pain: results from a continuing professional development survey. Prim Dent Care. 2011;18(1):41–4.

Albert DA, Sadowsky D, Papapanou P, Conicella ML, Ward A. An examination of periodontal treatment and per member per month (PMPM) medical costs in an insured population. BMC Health Serv Res. 2006;6(103):1–10. doi:10.1186/1472-6963-6-103.

Albert DA, Begg MD, Andrews HF, Williams SZ, Ward A, Conicella ML, Rauh V, Thomson JL, Papapanou PN. An examination of periodontal treatment, dental care, and pregnancy outcomes in an insured population in the united states. Am J Public Health. 2011. doi:10.2105/AJPH.2009.185884.

Al-Humayed S, Mohamed-Elbagir A, Al-Wabel A, Argobi Y. The changing pattern of upper gastro-intestinal lesions in Southern Saudi Arabia: an endoscopic study. Saudi J Gastroenterol. 2010;16(1):35–7.

Amer A, Singh G, Darke C, Dolby AE. Association between HLA antigens and periodontal disease. Tissue Antigens. 1988;31(2):53–8.

Anderson G. Chronic care: making the case for ongoing care. Princeton: Robert Wood Johnson Foundation; 2010.

Andraws R, Berger JS, Brown DL. Effects of antibiotic therapy on outcomes of patients with coronary artery disease: a meta-analysis of randomized controlled trials. JAMA. 2005;293(21):2641–7.

Andriankaja OM, Sreenivasa S, Dunford R, DeNardin E. Association between metabolic syndrome and periodontal disease. Aust Dent J. 2010;55(3):252–9.

Anjomshoaa I, Cooper ME, Vieira AR. Caries is associated with asthma and epilepsy. Eur J Dent. 2009;3:297–303.

Ashkenazy R, Abrahamson M. Medicare coverage for patients with diabetes. J Gen Intern Med. 2006;21:386–94.

Bach J-F. Infections and autoimmune diseases. J Autoimmun. 2005;25(1):74–80.

Bailit HL, Beazoglou TJ, Formicola AJ, Tedesco LA, Brown LJ, Weaver RG. U.S. state-supported dental schools: financial projections and implications. J Dent Educ. 2008;72(2 Suppl):98–109.

Baker EL, Koplan JP. Strengthening the Nation's public health infrastructure: historic challenge, unprecedented opportunity. Health Aff. 2002;21(6):15–27.

Barnett WS, Brown KC. Dental health policy analysis series: issues in children's access to dental care under Medicaid. Chicago: American Dental Association; 2000.

Baum BJ. Inadequate training in the biological sciences and medicine for dental students. J Am Dent Assoc. 2007;138:16–25.

Bayer R, Colgrove J. Bioterrorism, public health and the law. Health Aff. 2002;21(6):98–101.

Begovich AB, Carlton VEH, Honigberg LA, Schrodi SJ, et al. A missense single-nucleotide polymorphism in a gene encoding a protein tyrosine phosphatase (*PTPN22*) is associated with rheumatoid arthritis. Am J Hum Genet. 2004;75(2):330–7.

Bestor TH. The DNA methyltransferases of mammals. Hum Mol Genet. 2000;9(16):2395–402.

Betts RK. Fixing intelligence, foreign affairs, January/February. 2002. URL: http://www.foreignaffairs.org/20020101faessay6556/richard-k-betts/fixing-intelligence.html?mode=print. Accessed May 2011.

Bibikova M, Lin Z, Zhou L, Chudin E, et al. High-throughput DNA methylation profiling using universal bead arrays. Genome Res. 2006;16(3):383–93.

Blue Cross Blue Shield of Michigan. Study links good oral care to lower diabetes care costs. 2009. http://www.bcbsm.com/pr/pr_08-27-2009_71090.shtml. Accessed 26 June 2011.

Bollen CM, Rompen EH, Demanez JP. Halitosis: a multidisciplinary problem. Rev Med Liege. 1999;54(1):32–6.

Botstein D, White RL, Skolnick M, Davis RW. Construction of a genetic linkage map in man using restriction fragment length polymorphisms. Am J Hum Genet. 1980;32(3):314–31.

Bretz WA, Corby PM, Schork NJ, Robinson MT, et al. Longitudinal analysis of heritability for dental caries traits. J Dent Res. 2005a;84(11):1047–51.

Bretz WA, Weyant RJ, Corby PM, Ren D, et al. Systemic inflammatory markers, periodontal diseases, and periodontal infections in an elderly population. J Am Geriatr Soc. 2005b;53: 1532–7.

Broadwater C. Attention to dental coverage lacking in health-care debate. From St. Petersburg Times. 2009. http://www.tampabay.com/news/health/attention-to-dental-coverage-lacking-in-health-care-debate/1048349. Retrieved Mar 21 2011.

Brodeur P. Community based dental education: the pipeline, profession and practice program. Robert Wood Johnson Foundation . 2008. http://www.rwjf.org/files/research/anthology2009.chapter8.pdf. Accessed 26 June 2011.

Brown GC, Brown MM, Hiller T, Fischer D, Benson W, Magargal L. Cotton-wool spots. Retina. 1985;5(4):206–14.

Cargill M, Schrodi SJ, Chang M, Garcia VE, et al. A large-scale genetic association study confirms IL12B and leads to the identification of IL23R as psoriasis-risk genes. Am J Hum Genet. 2007;80(2):273–90.

Carroll L. Mother's gum disease linked to infant's death. 2010. http://www.msnbc.msn.com/id/34979552/ns/health-oral_health/. Accessed 26 June 2011.

Cartwright-Smith L. Chronic disease management. Health reform GPS: navigating the implementation process. 2011. http://www.healthreformgps.org/resources/chronic-disease-management/. Accessed 25 June 2011.

Carvalho FM, Tinoco EMB, Deeley K, Duarte PM, et al. FAM5C contributes to aggressive periodontitis. PLoS One. 2010;5(4):e10053.

Center for Medicare and Medicaid Services. Data compendium. Washington, D.C.: US Government Printing Office; 2010.

Center for Medicare and Medicaid Services. Medicare physician group practice demonstration. 2010. http://www.cms.gov/DemoProjectsEvalRpts/downloads/PGP_Fact_Sheet.pdf. Accessed 25 June 2011.

Centers for Disease Control. Dental service use and dental insurance coverage-United States, behavioral risk factor surveillance system. MMWR Morb Mortal Wkly Rep. 1997;46(50): 1199–203.

Chaffee BW, Weston SJ. Association between chronic periodontal disease and obesity: a systematic review and meta-analysis. J Periodontol. 2010;81(12):1708–24.

Chapman WW, Bridewell W, Hanbury P, Cooper GF, Buchanan BG. Evaluation of negation phrases in narrative clinical reports. Proc AMIA Symp. 2001;105–9.

Chasteen JE, Murphy G, Forrey A, Heid D. The health insurance and portability and accountability act: practice of dentistry in the united states: privacy and confidentiality. J Contemp Dent Pract. 2003;1(4):059–70.

Chen T, Yu W-H, Izard J, Baranova OV, et al. The human oral microbiome database: a web accessible resource for investigating oral microbiome taxonomic and genomic information. Database (Oxford). 2010;Article ID baq013.

Cheng Y, Hootman J, Murphy L, Langmaid G, Helmick C, Centers for Disease Control and Prevention (CDC). Prevalence of doctor diagnosed arthritis and arthritis attributable activity limitation – United States, 2007–2009. MMWR Morb Mortal Wkly Rep. 2010;59(39): 1–2.

CIGNA. CIGNA dental oral health maternity program. 2006. http://www.cigna.com/our_plans/programs/dental_health/oral_health_maternity_program.html. Accessed 26 June 2011.

Cisternas M, Murphy L, Yelin E, Foreman A, Pasta D, Helmick C. Trends in medical care expenditures of US adults with arthritis and other rheumatic conditions 1997 to 2005. J Rheumatol. 2009;36(11):2531–8.

Cloos J, Spitz MR, Schantz SP, Hsu TC, et al. Genetic susceptibility to head and neck squamous cell carcinoma. J Natl Cancer Inst. 1996;88:530–5.

Connelly JJ, Shah SH, Doss JF, Gadson S, et al. Genetic and functional association of FAM5C with myocardial infarction. BMC Med Genet. 2008;9:33.

Corey LA, Nance WE, Hofstede P, Schenkein HA. Self-reported periodontal disease in a Virginia twin population. J Periodontol. 1993;64:1205–8.

Coussens LM, Werb Z. Inflammation and cancer. Nature. 2002;420:860–7.

Crawford PJM, Aldred M, Bloch-Zupan A. Amelogenesis imperfecta. Orphanet J Rare Dis. 2007;2:17.
Crosby AH, Scherpbier-Heddema T, Wijmenga C, Altherr MR, et al. Genetic mapping of the dentinogenesis imperfecta type II locus. Am J Hum Genet. 1995;57:832–9.
D'Aiuto F, Sabbah W, Netuveli G, Donos N, et al. Association of the metabolic syndrome with severe periodontitis in a large U.S. population-based survey. J Clin Endocrinol Metab. 2008;93(1):3989–94.
Dall T, Zhang Y, Chen J, Quick W, Yang W, Fogli J. The economic burden of diabetes. Health Aff. 2010;29(2):297–304.
Dannenberg AJ, Subbaramaiah K. Targeting cyclooxygenase-2 in human neoplasia: rationale and promise. Cancer Cell. 2003;4(6):431–6.
Delanghe G, Ghyselen J, Bollen C, van Steenberghe D, Vandekerckhove BN, Feenstra L. An inventory of patients' response to treatment at a multidisciplinary breath odor clinic. Quintessence Int. 1999;30(5):307–10.
Delrose DC, Steinberg RW. The clinical significance of the digital patient record. J Am Dent Assoc. 2000;131(sup):57S–60.
Delta Dental of Wisconsin. Evidence-based integrated care plan. 2011. http://www.deltadentalwi.com/EBICP. Accessed 26 June 2011.
Dental, Oral and Craniofacial Data Resource Center of the National Institute of Dental and Craniofacial Research. Oral health US, 2002. Washington, D.C.: US Government Printing Office; 2002.
Dentistry Today. Buyers' guide to dental software. Dent Today. 2003;22(9):126–39.
Dentrix Dental Systems (2011). HIPAA. URL: http://www.dentrix.com/support/hipaa.aspx Accessed May 2011
Dentrix Dental Systems. HIPAA. 2003. URL: http://www.dentrix.com/support/hipaa.aspx. Accessed May 2011.
Department of Veterans Affairs. VA health information technology improves quality of health care while reducing costs. 2010. http://www1.va.gov/opa/pressrel/pressrelease.cfm?id=1881. Accessed 26 June 2011.
DeStefano F, Anda R, Kahn H, Williamson D, Russell C. Dental disease and risk of coronary heart disease and mortality. Br Med J. 1993;306:688–92.
Dictor M. Human herpesvirus 8 and Kaposi's sarcoma. Seim Cutan Med Surg. 1997;16(3):181–7.
Dunning DG, Durham TM, Lange BM, Aksu MN. Strategic management and organizational behavior in dental education: reflections on key issues in an environment of change. J Dent Educ. 2009;73:689–95.
Eaton CB, Feldman HA, Assaf AR, McPhillips JB, et al. Prevalence of hypertension, dyslipidemia, and dyslipidemic hypertension. J Fam Pract. 1994;38(1):17–23.
Eckel RH, Grundy SM, Zimmet PZ. The metabolic syndrome. Lancet. 2005;365(9468):1415–28.
eHow. About Medicaid dental coverage. From Health. 2011. http://www.ehow.com/about_5070293_medicaid-dental-coverage.html. Retrieved Mar 21 2011
Ehrich M, Nelson MR, Stanssens P, Zabeau M, et al. Quantitative high throughput analysis of DNA methylation patterns by base-specific cleavage and mass spectrometry. Proc Natl Acad Sci USA. 2005;102(44):15785–90.
Elia J, Gai X, Xie HM, Perin JC, et al. Rare structural variants found in attention-deficit hyperactivity disorder are preferentially associated with neurodevelopmental genes. Mol Psychiatry. 2010;15:637–46.
Ernst FD, Uhr K, Teumer A, Fanghanel J, et al. Replication of the association of chromosomal region 9p21.3 with generalized aggressive periodontitis (gAgP) using an independent case-control cohort. BMC Genet. 2010;11:119.
Errante JV. Integration of medical and dental benefits for improved overall health. Institute for Oral Health. 2007. http://www.institutefororalhealth.org/2007/ppt/IOH07_Errante.pdf. Accessed 26 June 2011
Etzioni A. Public health Law: a communitarian perspective. Health Aff. 2002;21(6):102–4.
Falconer DS, MacKay TFC. Introduction to quantitative genetics. 4th ed. Essex: Harlow; 1996.

Ferrannini E, Haffner SM, Mitchell BD, Stern MP. Hyperinsulinaemia: the key feature of a cardiovascular and metabolic syndrome. Diabetologia. 1991;34(6):416–22.

Field MJ. Dental education at the crossroads: challenges and change. An Institute of Medicine Report. Washington, D.C.: National Academy Press; 1995.

Firestein GS. Evolving concepts of rheumatoid arthritis. Nature. 2003;423:356–61.

Fischer J, Blanchet-Bardon C, Prud'homme J-F, Pavek S, et al. Mapping of papillon-lefevre syndrome to the chromosome 11q14 region. Eur J Hum Genet. 1997;5:156–60.

Fisher ES. Building a medical neighborhood for the medical home. N Engl J Med. 2008;359(12):1202–5. doi:10.1056/NEJMp0806233.

Fisher MA, Taylor GW, Est BT, McCarthy ET. Bidirectional relationship between chronic kidney and periodontal disease: a study using structural equation modeling. Kidney Int. 2011;79:347–55.

Fitzgerald M, Piskorowski W. Clinical outreach: seven years of a self-sustaining model. J Dent Educ. 2009;73:249.

Flores S, Mills SE, Shackelford L. Dentistry and bioterrorism. Dent Clin North Am. 2003;47(4): 733–44.

Ford ES, Giles WH, Dietz WH. Prevalence of the metabolic syndrome among US adults. JAMA. 2002;287(3):356–9.

Formicola AJ, Bailit H, Beazoglou T, Tedesco LA. The Macy study: a framework for consensus. J Dent Educ. 2005;69:1183–5.

Frieden J. CMS projects focus on chronic illnesses: three demonstration projects seek to improve efficiency and care. Caring for ages. 2006. http://www.caringfortheages.com/news/geriatric-medicine/single-article/cms-projects-focus-on-chronic-illnesses-three-demonstration-projects-seek-to-improve-efficiency-and-care/7be973db97ab1f83fd4473b96d58e48a.html. Accessed 25 June 2011.

Friedenberg FK, Rai J, Vanar V, Bongiorno C, Nelson DB, Parepally M, et al. Prevalence and risk factors for gastroesophageal reflux disease in an impoverished minority population. Obes Res Clin Pract. 2010;4(4):e261–9.

Frist B. Public health and national security: the critical role of increased federal support. Health Aff. 2002;21(6):117–30.

Furr MC, Larkin E, Blakeley R, Albert TW, Tsugawa L, Weber SM. Extending multidisciplinary management of cleft palate to the developing world. J Oral Maxillofac Surg. 2011;69(1): 237–41.

Gesteland PH, Gardner RM, Tsui FC, Espino JU, Rolfs RT, James BC, Chapman WW, Moore AW, Wagner MM. Automated syndromic surveillance for the 2002 winter olympics. J Am Med Inform Assoc. 2003;10(6):547–54.

Ghezzi EM, Ship JA. Systemic diseases and their treatment in the elderly: impact on oral health. J Public Health Dent. 2000;60(4):297–303.

Gies W. Dental education in the United States and Canada. 1926. http://www.adeagiesfoundation.org/about/Pages/AboutWilliamJGiesandtheGiesReport.aspx. Accessed 26 June 2011.

Goldenberg A, Shmueli G, Caruana RA, Fienberg SE. Early statistical detection of anthrax outbreaks by tracking over-the-counter medication sales. Proc Natl Acad Sci USA. 2002;99(8): 5237–40.

Gomez RS, Dutra WO, Moreira PR. Epigenetics and periodontal disease: future perspectives. Inflamm Res. 2009;58:625–9.

Gonzalez E, Kulkarni H, Bolivar H, Mangano A, et al. The influence of CCL3L1 gene-containing segmental duplications on HIV-1/AIDS susceptibility. Science. 2005;307:1434–40.

Graham RR, Cotsapas C, Davies L, Hackett R, et al. Genetic variants near TNFAIP3 on 6q23 are associated with systemic lupus erythematosus. Nat Genet. 2008;40:1059–61.

Grant SFA, Thorleifsson G, Reynisdottir I, Benediktsson R, et al. Variant of transcription factor 7-like 2 (*TCF7L2*) gene confers risk of type 2 diabetes. Nat Genet. 2006;38:320–3.

Gregory SG, Schmidt S, Seth P, Oksenberg JR, et al. Interleukin 7 receptor a chain (*IL7R*) shows allelic and functional association with multiple sclerosis. Nat Genet. 2007;39:1083–91.

Grubbs V, Plantinga LC, Crews DC, Bibbins-Domingo K, Saran R, Heung M, Patel PR, Burrows NR, Ernst KL, Powe NR, for the Centers for Disease Control and Prevention CKD Surveillance

Team. Vulnerable populations and the association between periodontal and chronic kidney disease. Clin J Am Soc Nephrol. 2011;6:711–7.
Guay AH. Dentistry's response to bioterrorism: a report of a consensus workshop. J Am Dent Assoc. 2002;133:1181–1187.
Gudmundsson J, Sulem P, Gudbjartsson DF, Blondal T, et al. Genome-wide association and replication studies identify four variants associated with prostate cancer susceptibility. Nat Genet. 2009;41:1122–6.
Ha PK, Califano JA. Promoter methylation and inactivation of tumour-suppressor genes in oral squamous-cell carcinoma. Lancet Oncol. 2006;7:77–82.
Hammoud SS, Nix DA, Zhang H, Purwar J, et al. Distinctive chromatin in human sperm packages genes for embryo development. Nature. 2009;460:473–8.
Hart TC, Hart PS, Michalec MD, Zhang Y, et al. Localisation of a gene for prepubertal periodontitis to chromosome 11q14 and identification of a cathepsin C gene mutation. J Med Genet. 2000;37(2):95–101.
Heid DW, Chasteen J, Forrey AW. The electronic oral health record. J Contemp Dent Pract. 2002;1(3):043–54.
Helgadottir A, Thorleifsson G, Manolescu A, Gretarsdottir S, et al. A common variant on chromosome 9p21 affects the risk of myocardial infarction. Science. 2007;316(5830):1491–3.
Hewitt C, McCormick D, Linden G, Turk D, et al. The role of cathepsin C in papillon-lefevre syndrome, prepubertal periodontitis, and aggressive periodontitis. Hum Mutat. 2004;23(3): 222–8.
Hinds DA, Stuve LL, Nilsen GB, Halperin E, et al. Whole-genome patterns of common DNA variation in three human populations. Science. 2005;307(5712):1072–9.
Hirschhorn JN, Lohmueller K, Byrne E, Hirschhorn K. A comprehensive review of genetic association studies. Genet Med. 2002;4(2):45–61.
Hogan P, Dall T, Nikolov P. Economic cost of babies in the US in 2002. Alexandria: American Diabetes Association; 2002.
Holder M, Waldman H, Hood H. Preparing health professionals to provide care to individuals with disabilities. Int J Oral Sci. 2009;1(2):54–9.
Holt SC, Ebersole JL. Porphyromonas gingivalis, Treponema denticola, and Tennerella forsythia: the "red complex", a prototype polybacterial pathogenic consortium in periodontitis. Periodontol. 2005;38:72–122.
Holvoet P, Lee DH, Steffes M, Gross M, Jacobs Jr DR. Association between circulating oxidized low-density lipoprotein and incidence of the metabolic syndrome. JAMA. 2008;299(19): 2287–93.
Hotamisligil GS. Inflammation and metabolic disorders. Nature. 2006;444:860–7.
http://www.dentaleconomics.com/index/display/article-display/1177919242/articles/dental-economics/volume-101/issue-4/practice/the-convergence-of-dental-and-medical-care.html. Accessed 25 June 2011.
Hudson RR. Gene genealogies and the coalescent process. In: Futuyma D, Antonovics J, editors. Oxford surveys in evolutionary biology, vol. 7. New York: Oxford University Press; 1991. p. 1–44.
Hund H, Willett W, Merchant A, Rosner B, Ascherio A, Joshipura K. Oral health and a referral arterial disease. Circulation. 2003;107:1152–9.
Ide R, Hoshuyama T, Takakhashi K. The effect of periodontal disease on medical and dental costs in a middle-aged japanese population: a longitudinal worksite study. J Periodontol. 2007;78(11):2120–6. doi:10.1902/jop. 2007.070193.
Independent Task Force. Council on foreign relations "America-still unprepared, still in danger". 2011. URL: http://www.cfr.org/pdf/Homeland_Security_TF.pdf. Accessed May 2011.
Institute for Oral Health. Focus Groups on Oral Health in Healthcare Reform – Focus Group #2. 2010. http://www.institutefororalhealth.org/2010fg/IOH-APR2010-Focus-Group-whitepaper.pdf. Accessed 26 June 2011.
Ivanov O, Wagner MM, Chapman WW, Olszewski RT. Accuracy of three classifiers of acute gastrointestinal syndrome for syndromic surveillance. Proc AMIA Symp. 2002; 345–9.

Iwamoto Y, Nishimura F, Nakagawa M, Sugimoto K, et al. The effect of antimicrobial periodontal treatment on circulating tumor necrosis factor-alpha and glycated hemoglobin level in patients with type 2 diabetes. J Periodontol. 2001;72(6):774–8.

Jemal A, Siegel R, Ward E, Hao Y, et al. Cancer statistics, 2009. CA Cancer J Clin. 2009;59: 225–49.

Jones HB. The relative power of linkage and association studies for the detection of genes involved in hypertension. Kidney Int. 1998;53:1446–8.

Joshipura K, Hung H, Rimm E, Willett W, Ascherio A. Periodontal disease, tooth loss and incidence of ischemic stroke. Stroke. 2003;34:47–54.

Josiah Macy Foundation. New models of dental education. 2004. http://www.josiahmacyfoundation.org/grantees/profile/new-models-for-dental-education. Accessed 26 June 2011.

Kaiser Family Foundation. The uninsured. Washington, D.C.: The Henry J. Kaiser Family Foundation; 2010.

Kaplan NL, Hill WG, Weir BS. Likelihood methods for locating disease genes in nonequilibrium populations. Am J Hum Genet. 1995;56:18–32.

Kathiresan S, Melander O, Guiducci C, Surti A, et al. Six new loci associated with blood low-density lipoprotein cholesterol, high-density lipoprotein cholesterol or triglycerides in humans. Nat Genet. 2008;40:189–97.

Kim JW, Simmer JP, Hu YY, Lin BP, et al. Amelogenin p.M1T and p.W4S mutations underlying hypoplastic X-linked amelogenesis imperfecta. J Dent Res. 2004;83(5):378–83.

Kim DS, Cheang P, Dover S, Drake-Lee AB. Dental otalgia. J Laryngol Otol. 2007;121(12): 1129–34.

Kimura M. Stochastic processes in population genetics, with special reference to distribution of gene frequencies and probability of gene fixation. In: Kojima K, editor. Mathematical topics in population genetics. Berlin/New York: Springer; 1970. p. 178–245.

Klein RJ, Zeiss C, Chew EY, Tsai J-Y, et al. Complement factor H polymorphism in age-related macular degeneration. Science. 2005;308(5720):385–9.

Kruglyak L. Prospects for whole-genome linkage disequilibrium mapping of common disease genes. Nat Genet. 1999;22(2):139–44.

Kshirsagar AV, Craig RG, Moss KL, et al. Periodontal disease adversely affects the survival of patients with end-stage renal disease. Kidney Int. 2009;75:746–51.

Kumar PS, Griffen AL, Barton JA, Paster BJ, et al. New bacterial species associated with chronic periodontitis. J Dent Res. 2003;82(5):338–44.

Kuroiwa T, Yamamoto N, Onda T, Shibahara T. Expression of the FAM5C in tongue squamous cell carcinoma. Oncol Rep. 2009;22(5):1005–11.

Laass MW, Hennies HC, Preis S, Stevens HP, et al. Localisation of a gene for papillon-lefevre syndrome to chromosome 11q14-q21 by homozygosity mapping. Hum Genet. 1997;101: 376–82.

Laine DI, Busch-Petersen J. Inhibitors of cathepsin C (dipeptidyl peptidase I). Expert Opin Ther Pat. 2010;20(4):497–506.

Laine ML, Loos BG, Crielaard W. Gene polymorphisms in chronic periodontitis. Int J Dent. 2010;1–22. Article ID 324719.

Lakshminarayanan R, Bromley KM, Lei Y-P, Snead ML, Moradian-Oldak J. Perturbed amelogenin secondary structure leads to uncontrolled aggregation in amelogenesis imperfecta mutant proteins. J Biol Chem. 2010;285:40593–603.

Lander ES, Linton LM, Birren B, Nusbaum C, et al. Initial sequencing and analysis of the human genome. Nature. 2001;409:860–921.

Lane CH, Fauci AS. Bioterrorism on the home front a new challenge for American medicine. JAMA. 2001;286(20):2595–7.

Lang N, Bartold PM, Cullinan M, Jeffcoat M, et al. Consensus report: aggressive periodontitis. Ann Periodontol. 1999;4(1):53.

Letter from the President. White House. 2002. URL: http://web.archive.org/web/20031224053212/http://www.whitehouse.gov/homeland/book/letterfromthepresident.pdf. Accessed May 2011.

Leung H, Wang JJ, Rochtchina E, Wong TY, Klein R, Mitchell P. Impact of current and past blood pressure on retinal arteriolar diameter in an older population. J Hypertens. 2004;22:1543–9.

Li Y, Xu L, Hasturk H, Kantarci A, et al. Localized aggressive periodontitis is linked to human chromosome 1q25. Hum Genet. 2004;114(3):291–7.

Lloyd-Jones D, Adams R, Brown T, Carnethon M, Dai S, DeSimone G, et al. Heart disease & stroke statistics – 2010 update. Circulation. 2010;121:e46–215.

Long AD, Langley CH. The power of association studies to detect the contribution of candidate genetic loci to variation in complex traits. Genome Res. 1999;9:720–31.

Looks JW. BioSense – a national initiative for early detection and quantification of public health emergencies. MMWR Morb Mortal Wkly Rep. 2004;53(suppl):53–5.

Lopez NJ, Da Silva I, Ipinza J, Gutierrez J. Periodontal therapy reduces the rate of preterm low birth weight in women with pregnancy-associated gingivitis. J Periodontol. 2005;76 Suppl 11:2144–53.

Lopez-Escamez JA. A variant of PTPN22 gene conferring risk to autoimmune diseases may protect against tuberculosis. J Postgrad Med. 2010;56:242–3.

Lumpkin JR. Air, water, places, and data—public health in the information age. J Public Health Manag Pract. 2001;7(6):22–30.

Lukic M, Segec A, Segeca I, Pinotic L, Pinotic K, Atalic B, et al. The role of the nutrition in the pathogenesis of gastroesophageal reflux disease, Barrett's oesophagus and oesophageal adenocarcinoma. Coll Antropol. 2010;34(3):905–9.

Lupski JR. Structural variation in the human genome. N Engl J Med. 2007;356:1169–71.

Machulla HK, Stein J, Gautsch A, Langner J, et al. HLA-A, B, Cw, DRB1, DRB3/4/5, DQB1 in German patients suffering from rapidly progressive periodontitis (RPP) and adult periodontitis (AP). J Clin Periodontol. 2002;29(6):573–9.

Manolio TA, Collins FS, Cox NJ, Goldstein DB, et al. Finding the missing heritability of complex diseases. Nature. 2009;461:747–53.

Manski R. Dental insurance: design, need and public policy. J Am Coll Dent. 2001;69(9):9–13.

Martin JA, Hamilton BE, Sutton PD, Ventura SJ, et al. Births: final data for 2006. National vital statistics reports; vol 57 no 7. Hyattsville: National Center for Health Statistics. 2009.

McBride M. VA uses integrated health informatics to produce $3 billion in savings. Daily break. 2011. http://www.darkdaily.com/va-uses-integrated-health-informatics-to-produce-3-billion-in-savings-12811. Accessed 26 June 2011.

McPherson R, Pertsemlidis A, Kavasalar N, Stewart A, et al. A common allele on chromosome 9 associated with coronary heart disease. Science. 2007;316(5830):1488–91.

Meade JL, de Wynter EA, Brett P, Sharif SM, et al. A family with papillon-lefevre syndrome reveals a requirement for cathepsin C in granzyme B activation and NK cell cytolytic activity. Blood. 2006;107(9):3665–8.

Mealey B, Rose L. Diabetes mellitius and inflammatory periodontal diseases. Curr Opin Endocrinol Diabetes Obes. 2008;15:135–41.

Mertz E, O'Neil E. The growing challenge of providing oral health care services to all Americans. Health Aff. 2002;21(5):65–77.

Michalowicz BS, Aeppli D, Virag JG, Klump DG, et al. Periodontal findings in adult twins. J Periodontol. 1991;62:293–9.

Michalowicz BS, Diehl SR, Gunsolley JC, Sparks BS, et al. Evidence of a substantial genetic basis for risk of adult periodontitis. J Periodontol. 2000;71:1699–707.

Michigan Dental Association. Woman's Death Spotlights Need to Restore Adult Dental Medicaid Benefits, Smile Michigan, October 22, 2009. http://www.smilemichigan.com/NewsArticles/Archives/tabid/429/articleType/ArticleView/articleId/377/Womans-Death-Spotlights–Need-to-RestoreBRAdult-Dental-Medicaid-Benefits.aspx. Accessed 21 June, 2011.

Miller L, Manwell M, Newbold D. The relationship between reduction in periodontal inflammation and diabetes control: a report of 9 cases. J Periodontol. 1992;63:843–8.

Mombelli A, Casagni F, Madianos PN. Can presence or absence of periodontal pathogens distinguish between subjects with chronic and aggressive periodontitis? A systematic review. J Clin Periodontol. 2002;29:10–21.

Montana Business Journal. Employer survey on health insurance in Montana. 2006. From the free library: http://www.thefreelibrary.com/2006+Employer+Survey+on+health+insurance+in+Montana.-a0172012572. Retrieved Mar 21 2011.

Mucci LA, Bjorkman L, Douglass CW, Pedersen NL. Environmental and heritable factors in the etiology of oral diseases – a population-based study of Swedish twins. J Dent Res. 2005;84(9):800–5.

Mullins C, Cohen L, Magder L, Manski R. Medicaid coverage and utilization of adult dental services. J Health Care Poor Underserved. 2004;15(4):672–88.

Nadeau JH. Transgenerational genetic effects on phenotypic variation and disease risk. Hum Mol Genet. 2009;18:R202–10.

Nagelberg RH (2011) The convergence of dental and medical care. Dental Economics.

Narcisi JP. The American dental association's commitment to electronic data interchange. J Dent Educ. 1996;60(1):28–32.

National Institute of Dental and Craniofacial Research. Dentistry's role in responding to bioterrorism and other catastrophic events. 2004. URL: http://www.nidcr.nih.gov/CareersAndTraining/DentistryCatastrophicEvents.htm. Accessed May 2011.

National Institute of Dental and Craniofacial Research. (2011). National Institutes of Health Website: http://www.nidcr.nih.gov/DataStatistics/FindDataByTopic/DentalCaries/. Accessed 18 June 2011.

Nesbitt MJ, Reynolds MA, Shiau H, Choe K, et al. Association of periodontitis and metabolic syndrome in the Baltimore longitudinal study of aging. Aging Clin Exp Res. 2010;22(3):238–42.

Ng SB, Buckingham KJ, Lee C, Bigham AW, et al. Exome sequencing identifies the cause of a mendelian disorder. Nat Genet. 2010;42(1):30–5.

Nikolopoulos GK, Dimou NL, Hamodrakas SJ, Bagos PG. Cytokine gene polymorphisms in periodontal disease: a meta-analysis of 53 studies including 4178 cases and 4590 controls. J Clin Periodontol. 2008;35(9):754–67.

Oral Health America. Keep America smiling: oral health in America. Chicago: Oral Health America; 2003.

Paju S, Scannapeico F. Oral biofilms, periodontitis and pulmonary infections. Oral Dis. 2007;13(6):508–12.

Palmer C. Dental leaders review roles in bioterrorism response. American Dental Association NEWS. 2003. ADA.org URL: http://web.archive.org/web/20060219190632/, http://www.ada.org/prof/resources/pubs/adanews/adanewsarticle.asp?articleid=390. Accessed May 2011.

Partnership for Solutions National Program Office. Chronic conditions: making the case for ongoing care. Baltimore: Johns Hopkins University; 2004.

Patir A, Seymen F, Yildirim M, Deeley K, et al. Enamel formation genes are associated with high caries experience in Turkish children. Caries Res. 2008;42(5):394–400.

Poage GM, Christensen BC, Houseman EA, McClean MD, et al. Genetic and epigenetic somatic alterations in head and neck squamous cell carcinomas are globally coordinated but not locally targeted. PLoS One. 2010;5(3):e9651.

Pokholok DK, Harbison CT, Levine S, Cole M, et al. Genome-wide map of nucleosome acetylation and methylation in yeast. Cell. 2005;122:517–27.

Polverini P. The Ann Arbor dental deans forum: crafting a response to the emerging tiered system of dental education global. Health Nexus, College of Dentistry, New York University Summer 2010 Vol. 12, No. 2. 2010.

Rabinowitz HK, Diamond JJ, Markham FW, Wortman JR. Medical school programs to increase the rural physician supply: a systematic review and projected impact of widespread replication. Acad Med. 2008;83:235–43.

Rao NV, Rao GV, Hoidal JR. Human dipeptidyl-peptidase I. J Biol Chem. 1997;272:10260–5.

Ram S, Teruel A, Kumar SK, Clark G. Clinical characteristics and diagnosis of atypical odontalgia: implications for dentists. J Am Dent Assoc. 2009;140(2):223–8.

Rassoulzadegan M, Grandjean V, Gounon P, Vincent S, et al. RNA-mediated non-mendelian inheritance of an epigenetic change in the mouse. Nature. 2006;441:469–74.

Redman D, Jones M, Rangan B, Reimold R, Mikuls T, Amdur R, et al. Association of periodontitis with rheumatoid arthritis: a pilot study. J Periodontol. 2010;81(2):223–30.

Ren B, Robert F, Wyrick JJ, Aparicio O, et al. Genome-wide location and function of DNA binding proteins. Science. 2000;290:2306–9.

Reshetin VP, Regens JL. Simulation modeling of anthrax spore dispersion in a bioterrorism incident. Risk Anal. 2003;23(6):1135–45.

Rhodes PR. The computer-based oral health record. J Dent Educ. 1996;60(1):14–8.

Rioux JD, Xavier RJ, Taylor KD, Silverberg MS, et al. Genome-wide association study identifies new susceptibility loci for Crohn disease and implicates autophagy in disease pathogenesis. Nat Genet. 2007;39:596–604.

Ripa LW. A half-century of community water fluoridation in the United States: review and commentary. J Public Health Dent. 1993;53(1):17–44.

Risch N, Merikangas K. The future of genetic studies of complex human diseases. Science. 1996;273(5281):1516–7.

Robert Wood Johnson Foundation Pipeline Study. Evaluation of pipeline, profession and practice: community-based dental education. 2007. http://www.rwjf.org/pr/product.jsp?id=15455. Accessed 26 June 2011.

Rodriguez-Lozano FJ, Sanchez-Perez A, Moya-Villaescusa MJ, Rodriguez-Lozano A, Saez-Yuguero MR. Neuropathic orofacial pain after dental implant placement: review of the literature and case report. Oral Surg Oral Med Oral Pathol Oral Radiol Endod. 2010;109(4):e8–12.

Rosenblum Jr R. Oral hygiene can reduce the incidence of and death resulting from pneumonia and respiratory tract infection. J Am Dent Assoc. 2010;141(9):1117–8.

Rothwell PM, Fowkes FG, Belch JF, Ogawa H, et al. Effect of daily asprin on long-term risk of death due to cancer: analysis of individual patient data from randomized trails. Lancet. 2010;377(9759):31–41.

Rubenstein H. Access to oral health care for elders: mere words or action? J Dent Educ. 2005;69(9):1051–8.

Ryan ME. Reconnecting the head to the body. Dental considerations for the optimal medical management of people with diabetes. Seattle: Institute for Oral Health; 2007. p. 15–7.

Safrany E, Melegh B. Functional variants of the interleukin-23 receptor gene in non-gastrointestinal autoimmune diseases. Curr Med Chem. 2009;16(28):3766–74.

Saiki RK, Scharf S, Faloona F, Mullis KB, et al. Enzymatic amplification of b-globin genomic sequences and restriction site analysis for diagnosis of sickle cell anemia. Science. 1985;230:1350–4.

Saikku P, Leinonen M, Mattila K, Ekman MR, et al. Serological evidence of an association of a novel *Chlamydia*, TWAR, with chronic coronary heart disease and acute myocardial infarction. Lancet. 1988;2(8618):983–6.

Saito I, Miyamura T, Ohbayashi A, Harada H, et al. Hepatitis C virus infection is associated with the development of hepatocellular carcinoma. Proc Natl Acad Sci USA. 1990;87(17):6547–9.

Saito T, Shimazaki Y, Kiyohara Y, Kato I, Kubo M, Lida M, et al. The severity of periodontal disease is associated with the element of glucose intolerance in non-diabetics. J Dent Res. 2004;83:485.

Salyer KE, Xu H, Portnof JE, Yamada A, Chong DK, Genecov ER. Skeletal facial balance and harmony in the cleft patient: principles and techniques in orthognathic surgery. Indian J Plast Surg. 2009;42(Suppl):S149–67.

Saremi A, Nelson R, Tulloch-Reid M. Periodontal disease and mortality in type 2 diabetes. Diabetes Care. 2005;28:27–32.

Scannapieco FA. Pneumonia in nonambulatory patients. J Am Dent Assoc. 2006;137(2):21S–5.

Schaefer AS, Richter GM, Groessner-Schreiber B, Noack B, et al. Identification of a shared genetic susceptibility locus for coronary heart disease and periodontitis. PLoS Genet. 2009;5(2):e1000378.

Schaefer AS, Richter GM, Nothnagel M, Manke T, et al. A genome-wide association study identifies *GLT6D1* as a susceptibility locus for periodontitis. Hum Mol Genet. 2010;19(3):553–62.

Schleyer TK. Integrating dental office technology – the next frontier. Dent Abstr. 2003;48(3):112–3.

Schleyer T, Eisner J. The computer-based oral health record: an essential tool for cross-provider quality management. J Calif Dent Assoc. 1997;22(11):57–64.

Schleyer TK, Spallek H, Bartling WC, Corby P. The technologically well-equipped dental office. J Am Dent Assoc. 2003;134(1):30–41.

Schleyer TK, Thyvalikakath TP, Spallek H, Torres-Urquidy MH, Hernandez P, Yuhaniak J. Clinical computing in general dentistry. J Am Med Inform Assoc. 2006a;13(3):344–52.

Schlotterer C. The evolution of molecular markers – just a matter of fashion? Nat Rev Genet. 2004;5:63–70.

Sebat J, Lakshmi B, Malhotra D, Troge J, et al. Strong association of de novo copy number mutations with autism. Science. 2007;316(5823):445–9.

Seddon JM, Reynolds R, Maller J, Fagerness JA, et al. Prediction model for prevalence and incidence of advanced age-related macular degeneration based on genetic, demographic, and environmental variables. Invest Opthalmol Vis Sci. 2008;50(5):2044–53.

Sfikas PM. HIPAA security regulations protecting patients' electronic health information. J Am Dent Assoc. 2003;134:640–3.

Sharrett AR, Hubbard LD, Cooper LS, Sorlie PD, Brothers RJ, Nieto FJ, Pinsky JL, Klein R. Retinal arteriolar diameters and elevated blood pressure: the atherosclerosis risk in communities study. Am J Epidemiol. 1999;150:263–70.

Simpson TC, Needleman I, Wild SH, Moles DR, Mills EJ. Treatment of periodontal disease for glycaemic control in people with diabetes. Cochrane Database Syst Rev. 2010;12(5): CD004714.

Slade G, Ghezzi E, Heiss G, Beck J, Riche E, Offenbacher S. Relationship between periodontal disease and C-reactive protein among adults in the atherosclerosis risk in communities study. Arch Intern Med. 2003;163:1172–9.

Social Security and Medicare Boards of Trustees. Actuarial Publications, Status of the Social Security and Medicare Programs: A Summary of the 2011 Annual Reports. http://www.ssa.gov/oact/trsum/index.html. Accessed 25 Sept. 2011.

Song YL, Wang CN, Fan MW, Su B, Bian Z. Dentin phosphoprotein frameshift mutations in hereditary dentin disorders and their variation patterns in normal human populations. J Med Genet. 2008;45:457–64.

Speliotes EK, Massaro JM, Hoffmann U, Vasan RS, et al. Fatty liver is associated with dyslipidemia and dysglycemia independent of visceral fat: the Framingham heart study. Hepatology. 2010;51(6):1979–87.

Spencer CJ, Neubert JK, Gremillion H, Zakrzewska JM, Ohrbach R. Toothache or trigeminal neuralgia: treatment dilemmas. J Pain. 2008;9(9):767–70.

Stark PC, Kalenderian E, White JM, Walji MF, Stewart DCL, Kimmes N, Meng Jr TR, Willis GP, DeVries T, Chapman RJ. Consortium for oral health-related informatics: improving dental research, education, and treatment. J Dent Educ. 2010a;74:1051–65.

Stefansson H, Rujescu D, Cichon S, Pietilainen OPH, et al. Large recurrent microdeletions associated with schizophrenia. Nature. 2008;455:232–6.

Steinbacher DM, Glick M. The dental patient with asthma: an update and oral health considerations. J Am Dent Assoc. 2001;132:1229–39.

Stewart JE, Wager KA, Friedlander AH, Zadeh HH. The effect of periodontal treatment on glycemic control in patients with type 2 diabetes mellitus. J Clin Periodontol. 2001;28:306–10.

Swartz K. Projected costs of chronic disease. Health care cost monitor. 2011. http://healthcarecostmonitor.thehastingscenter.org/kimberlyswartz/projected-costs-of-chronic-diseases/. loose lind Accessed 25 June 2011.

Szekely DG, Milam S, Khademi JA. Legal issues of the electronic dental record: security and confidentiality. J Dent Educ. 1996;60(1):19–23.

The International HapMap 3 Consortium. Integrating common and rare genetic variation in diverse human populations. Nature. 2010;467:52–8.

The National Electronic Disease Surveillance System Working Group. National Electronic Disease Surveillance System (NEDSS): a standards-based approach to connect public health and clinical medicine. J Public Health Manag Pract. 2001;7(6):42–50.

The Pew Center on the States. Help wanted: a policy maker's guide to new dental providers. National Academy for State Health Policy, WK Kellogg Foundation. 2009. http://www.pewcenteronthestates.org/uploadedFiles/Dental_Report_final_Low%20Res.pdf. Accessed 26 June 2011.

Thorpe K, Ogden L, Galactionova K. Chronic conditions account for rise in Medicare spending from 1987 to 2006. Health Aff. 2010;29(4):718–25.

Thorstensson H, Kuylensteima J, Hugoson A. Medical status and complications in relation to periodontal disease experience in insulin-dependent diabetics. J Clin Periodontol. 1996;23:194–202.

Toomes C, James J, Wood AJ WUCL, et al. Loos-of-function mutations in the cathepsin C gene result in periodontal disease and palmoplantar keratosis. Nat Genet. 1999;23(4):421–4.

Torres-Urquidy MH, Wallstrom G, Schleyer TK. Detection of disease outbreaks by the use of oral manifestations. J Dent Res. 2009;88(1):89–94.

Tsui FC, Espino JU, Dato VM, Gesteland PH, Hutman J, Wagner MM. Technical description of RODS: a real-time public health surveillance system. J Am Med Inform Assoc. 2003;10(5):399–408.

U.S. Department of Health and Human Services. Oral health in American; surgeon general's call to action. Rockville: USDHHS, National Institute of Dental and Craniofacial Research, Nation Institutes of Health; 2003.

Uemura N, Okamoto S, Yamamoto S, Matsumura N, et al. *Helicobacter pylori* infection and the development of gastric cancer. N Engl J Med. 2001;345:784–9.

UnitedHealth Center for Health Reform & Modernization. The United States of diabetes: challenges and opportunities in the decade ahead. Minnetonka: UnitedHealth Group; 2010.

US Census Bureau. Statistical abstract of the US. Washington, D.C.: US Government Printing Office; 2011.

US Department of Health and Human Services. Healthy people 2020. 2010. http://www.healthypeople.gov/2020/topicsobjectives2020/pdfs/HP2020objectives.pdf. Accessed 26 June 2011.

Valachovic R. Opportunities abound for new dental schools. How will we seize them? American dental education association charting progress. 2009. http://www.adea.org/about_adea/Documents/Charting%20Progress/ADEAs_Charting_Progress_August_2009.htm. Accessed 26 June 2011.

Valachovic R. Holding ourselves to the highest standard: doing what's best for patients. American dental education association charting progress. 2010. http://www.adea.org/about_adea/Documents/Charting%20Progress/ADEAs_Charting_Progress_October_2010.htm. Accessed 26 June 2011.

van Houte J. Role of micro-organisms in caries etiology. J Dent Res. 1994;73(3):672–81.

Venter JC, Adams MD, Myers EW, Li PW, et al. The sequence of the human genome. Science. 2001;291(5507):1304–51.

Vieira AR, Marazita ML, Goldstein-McHenry T. Genome-wide scan find suggestive caries loci. J Dent Res. 2008;87:435–9.

Visscher PM, Hill WG, Wray NR. Heritability in the genomics era – concepts and misconceptions. Nat Rev Genet. 2008;9:255–66.

Wagner MM, Moore AW, Aryel RM. Handbook of biosurveillance. Burlington: Elsevier Academic Press; 2006a.

Walboomers JMM, Jacobs MV, Manos MM, Bosch FX, et al. Human papillomavirus is a necessary cause of invasive cervical cancer worldwide. J Pathol. 1999;189:12–9.

Wangsrimongkol T, Jansawang W. The assessment of treatment outcome by evaluation of dental arch relationships in cleft lip/palate. J Med Assoc Thai. 2010;93 Suppl 4:S100–6.

Watson C, Alp NJ. Role of *Chlamydia pneumoniae* in atherosclerosis. Clin Sci. 2008;114: 509–31.

Weber JL, May PE. Abundant class of human DNA polymorphisms which can be typed using the polymerase chain reaction. Am J Hum Genet. 1989;44:388–96.

Weiss R, Dziura J, Burgert TS, Tamborlane WV, et al. Obesity and the metabolic syndrome in children and adolescents. N Engl J Med. 2004;350(23):2362–74.

Wellcome Trust Case Control Consortium. Genome-wide association study of 14,000 cases of seven common diseases and 3,000 shared controls. Nature. 2007;447(7145):661–78.

Werther W, Chu L, Holekamp N, Do D, Rubio R. Myocardial infarction and cerebrovascular accident in patients with retinal vein occlusion. Arch Ophthalmol. 2011;129:326–31.

White House Office of the Press Secretary. Fact sheet project bioshield. 2003. URL: http://web.archive.org/web/20090116121142/, http://www.whitehouse.gov/news/releases/2003/02/print/20030203.html. Accessed: May 2011.

White JM, Kalenderian E, Stark PC, Ramoni RL, Vaderhobli R, Walji MF. Evaluating a dental diagnostic terminology in an electronic health record. J Dent Educ. 2011;75:605–15.

Wiegand A, Buchalla W, Attin T. Review on fluoride-releasing restorative materials – fluoride release and uptake characteristics, antibacterial activity and influence on caries formation. Dent Mater. 2007;23(3):343–62.

Wolff A, Waldman B, Milano M, Perlman S. Dental students' experiences with and attitudes toward people with mental retardation. J Am Dent Assoc. 2004;135:353–7.

Wong TY, McIntosh R. Hypertensive retinopathy signs as risk indicators of cardiovascular morbidity and morality. Br Med Bull. 2005;73/74:57–70.

Wong TY, Klein R, Couper DJ, Cooper LS, Shahar E, Hubbard LD, Wofford MR, Sharrett AR. Retinal microvascular abnormalities and incident stroke: the atherosclerosis risk in communities study. Lancet. 2001;258:1134–40.

Wong TY, Hubbard LD, Klein R, Marino EK, Kronmal R, Sharrett AR, Siscovick DS, Burke G, Tielsch JM. Retinal microvascular abnormalities and blood pressure in older people: the cardiovascular health study. Br J Ophthalmol. 2002a;86:1007–13.

Wong TY, Klein R, Sharrett AR, Schmidt MI, Pankow JS, Couper DJ, Klein BE, Hubbard LD, Duncan BB. Retinal arteriolar narrowing and risk of diabetes in middle-aged persons. JAMA. 2002b;287:2528–33.

Wong TY, Klein R, Nieto FJ, Klein BE, Sharrett AR, Meuer SM, Hubbard LD, Tielsch JM. Retinal microvascular abnormalities and ten-year cardiovascular abnormality: a population-based case-control study. Ophthalmology. 2003a;110:933–40.

Wong WK, Moore A, Cooper G, Wagner M. WSARE: What's strange about recent events? J Urban Health. 2003b;80(2 Suppl 1):i66–75.

Wong TY, Rosamund W, Chang PP, Couper DJ, Sharrett AR, Hubbard LD, Folsom AR, Klein R. Retinopathy and risk of congestive heart failure. JAMA. 2005a;293:63–9.

Wong TY, Shankar A, Klein R, Klein BEK, Hubbard LD. Retinal arteriolar narrowing, hypertension and subsequent risk of diabetes mellitus. Arch Intern Med. 2005b;165:1060–5.

Wu T, Trevisan M, Genco R, Dorn J, Falkner K, Sempos C. Periodontal disease and risk of cerebrovascular disease. Arch Intern Med. 2000;160:2749–56.

Yelin E, Cisternas M, Foreman A, Pasta D, Centers for Disease Control and Prevention (CDC). National and state medical expenditures and lost earnings attributable to arthritis and other rheumatic conditions – United States, 2003. MMWR Morb Mortal Wkly Rep. 2007;56(1):4–7.

Zackrisson AL, Lindblom B, Ahlner J. High frequency of occurrence of CYP2D6 gene duplication/multiduplication indicating ultrarapid metabolism along suicide cases. Clin Pharmacol Ther. 2010;88:354–9.

Zhang J. The digital pioneer. The Wall Street Journal. 2009. http://online.wsj.com/article/SB10001424052970204488304574428750133812262.html. Accessed 26 June 2011.

Zhang Y, Syed R, Uygar C, Pallos D, et al. Evaluation of human leukocyte N-formylpeptide receptor (FPR1) SNPs in aggressive periodontitis patients. Genes Immun. 2003;4:22–9.

Integration of Pediatric Medical and Pediatric Dental Care

Acs G, Shulman R, Ng MW, Chussid S. The effect of dental rehabilitation on the body weight of children with early childhood caries. Pediatr Dent. 1999;21:109–13.

American Academy of Pediatrics Bright Futures Guidelines. 2008. http://brightfutures.aap.org/pdfs/AAP%20Bright%20Futures%20Periodicity%20Sched%20101107.pdf Accessed 7 June 2011.

American Academy of Pediatrics. Recommendations for preventive pediatric health care (periodicity schedule). 2008. http://practice.aap.org/content.aspx?aid=1599 Accessed 28 June 2011.

American Academy of Pediatric Dentistry. Dental care for your baby. 2011. http://www.aapd.org/publications/brochures/babycare.asp. Accessed 28 June 2011.

Broadbent JM, Thomson WM, Williams SM. Does caries in primary teeth predict enamel defects in permanent teeth? A Longitudinal Study. J Dent Res. 2005. doi:10.1177/154405910508400310.

California Dental Association. Oral health during pregnancy and early childhood: evidence-based guidelines for health professionals. Sacramento: California Dental Association; 2010.

Casamassimo PS, Thikkurissy S, Edelstein BL, Maiorini E. Beyond the dmft: the human and economic cost of early childhood caries. J Am Dent Assoc. 2009;140(6):650–7.

Caspary G, Krol DM, Boulter S, Keels MA, Romano-Clarke G. Perceptions of oral health training and attitudes toward performing oral health screenings among graduating pediatric residents. Pediatrics. 2008;122(2):e465–71.

Catalanotto F. Role of the medical team in preventing early childhood caries. 2010. http://allkids.mediasite.com/mediasite/Viewer/?peid=bab7ac16fa624951b3d1a4f604fc92c0. Accessed 5 Feb 2011.

CDC. Centers for disease control and prevention. Vital and health statistics. Series 10, No. 244. 2008. http://www.cdc.gov/nchs/data/series/sr_10/sr10_244.pdf. Accessed 17 Jul 2011.

Census Bureau (2010) Census Bureau quick facts. (2010). http://quickfacts.census.gov/qfd/states/00000.html. Accessed 17 Jul 2011.

Dye B, Thornton-Evans G. Trends in oral health by poverty status as measured by HP 2010 objectives. Public Health Rep. 2010;125(6):817–30.

Edelstein BL, Chinn CH. Update on disparities in oral health and access to dental care for America's children. Acad Pediatr. 2009;9(6):415–9.

Ezer MS, Swoboda NA, Farkouh DR. Early childhood caries: the dental disease of infants. Oral Hlth J. 2010; 1–7.

Ferullo A, Silk H, Savageau JA. Teaching oral health in U.S. Medical Schools: results of a national survey. Acad Med. 2010;86(2):226–30.

Fiks AG, Alessandrini EA, Forrest CB, Khan S, Localio AR, Gerber A. Electronic medical record use in pediatric primary care. J Am Med Inform Assoc. 2011. doi:10.1136/jamia.2010.004135.

Han YW, Fardini Y, Chen C, Iacampo KG, Peraino VA, Shamonki JM, et al. Term stillbirth caused by oral fusobacterium nucleatum. Obstet Gynecol. 2010;115(2):442–5.

Heuer S. Integrated medical and dental health in primary care. J Spec Pediatr Nurs. 2007;12(1):61–5.

IOM (Institute of Medicine). Advancing oral health in America. Washington, D.C.: The National Academies Press; 2011a.

IOM (Institute of Medicine). Improving access to oral health care for vulnerable and underserved populations. Washington, D.C.: The National Academies Press; 2011b.

Lannon CM, Flower K, Duncan P, Moore KS, Stuart J. The bright futures training project: implementing systems to support preventive and developmental services in practice. Pediatrics. 2008. doi:10.1542/peds.2007-2700.

Lewis CW. Dental care and children with special health care needs: a population-based perspective. Acad Pediatr. 2009;9(6):420–6.

Lewis C, Johnston B, Linsenmeyer K, Williams A, Mouradian W. Preventive dental care for children in the US: a national perspective. Pediatrics. 2007;119:E544–53.

Lewis CW, Boulter S, Keels MA, Krol DM, Mouradian WE, O'Connor KG, et al. Oral health and pediatricians: results of a national survey. Acad Pediatr. 2009;9(6):457–61.

Li Y, Wang W. Predicting caries in permanent teeth from caries in primary teeth: an eight-year cohort study. J Dent Res. 2002;81(8):561–6. http://jdr.sagepub.com/content/81/8/561.full.pdf Accessed 17 Jul 2011.

Mabry CC, Mosca NG. Interprofessional educational partnerships in school health for children with special oral health needs. J Dent Educ. 2006;70(8):844–50.

Marrs J, Trumbley S, Malik G. Early childhood caries: determining the risk factors and assessing the prevention strategies for nursing intervention. Pediatr Nurs. 2011;37(1):9–15.

Mertz E, Mouradian W. Addressing children's oral health in the new millennium: trends in the dental workforce. Acad Pediatr. 2009;9(6):443–9.

Mouradian W. Making decisions for children. Angle Orthod. 1999;69(4):300–5.

Mouradian WE, Wehr E, Crall JJ. Disparities in children's oral health and access to dental care. J Am Med Assoc. 2000;284(20):2625–31.

Mouradian W, Slayton R, Maas W, Kleinman DV, Slavkin H, DePaola D, et al. Executive summary: progress in children's oral health since the 2000 surgeon general's report. Acad Pediatr. 2009;9(6):374–9.

Nash DA. Adding dental therapists to the health care team to improve access to oral health care for children. Acad Pediatr. 2009;9(6):446–51.

New York State Department of Health. Oral health care during pregnancy and childhood. 2006. Available at: http://www.health.state.ny.us/publications/0824.pdf.

Otto M. For want of a dentist. 2007. Washington Post, February 28, B01.

Ramos-Gomez FJ, Shepherd DS. Cost-effectiveness model for the prevention of early childhood caries. J Calif Dent Assoc. 1999;1999:1–11.

Ressler-Maerlender J, Krishna R, Robison V. Oral health during pregnancy: current research at the Division of Oral Health, Centers for Disease Control and Prevention. J Womens Health. 2005. doi:10.1089/jwh.2005.14.880.

Savage MF, Lee JY, Kotch JB, Vann Jr WF. Early preventive dental visits: effects on subsequent utilization and costs. Pediatrics. 2004. doi:10.1542/peds.2003-0469-F.

Seale N, McWhorter A, Mouradian W. Dental education's role in improving children's oral health and access to care. Acad Pediatr. 2009;9(6):440–5.

Wolfe JD, Weber-Gasparoni JD, Kane MJ, Qian F. Survey of Iowa general dentists regarding the age 1 dental visit. Pediatr Dent. 2006;28(4):325–31.

Integration of Patient Records and Clinical Research: Lack of Integration as a Barrier to Needed Research; Integration as a Prerequisite to Research

Atkinson JC, Zeller GG, Shah C. Electronic patient records for dental school clinics: more than paperless systems. J Dent Educ. 2002;66(5):634–42.

Barasch A, Cunha-Cruz J, Curro FA, Hujoel P, Sung AH, Vena D, et al. Risk factors for osteonecrosis of the jaws: a case–control study from the CONDOR dental PBRN. J Dent Res. 2011;90(4):439–44.

Blumenthal D, Tavenner M. The "meaningful use" regulation for electronic health records. N Engl J Med. 2010;363(6):501–4.

Brown EG, Wood L, Wood S. The medical dictionary for regulatory activities (MedDRA). Drug Saf. 1999;20(2):109–17.

Buntin MB, Burke MF, Hoaglin MC, Blumenthal D. The benefits of health information technology: a review of the recent literature shows predominantly positive results. Health Aff (Millwood). 2011;30(3):464–71.

Chambers S, Spence J, Taylor D, Walji M, Valenza JA. Assessing user perceptions of an electronic patient record (EPR) before implementation. AMIA Annu Symp Proc. 2007;2007:896.

Chute CG, Cohn SP, Campbell KE, Oliver DE, Campbell JR. The content coverage of clinical classifications. For the computer-based patient record Institute's Work Group on codes & structures. J Am Med Inform Assoc. 1996;3(3):224–33.

Cimino JJ. From data to knowledge through concept-oriented terminologies: experience with the Medical Entities Dictionary. J Am Med Inform Assoc. 2000;7(3):288–97.

Congressional Budget Office. Research on the comparative effectiveness of medical treatments: issues and options for an expanded federal role Pub. No. 2975. 2007. http://www.cbo.gov/ftpdocs/88xx/doc8891/12-18-ComparativeEffectiveness.pdf. Accessed 10 June 2011.

Day S, Fayers P, Harvey D. Double data entry: what value, what price? Control Clin Trials. 1998;19(1):15–24.

Deshmukh VG, Meystre SM, Mitchell JA. Evaluating the informatics for integrating biology and the bedside system for clinical research. BMC Med Res Methodol. 2009;9:70.

El Emam K, Jonker E, Sampson M, Krleza-Jeric K, Neisa A. The use of electronic data capture tools in clinical trials: web-survey of 259 Canadian trials. J Med Internet Res. 2009;11(1):e8.

Fellows JL, Rindal DB, Barasch A, Gullion CM, Rush W, Pihlstrom DJ, et al. ONJ in Two dental practice-based research network regions. J Dent Res. 2011;90(4):433–8.

Goldberg LJ, Ceusters W, Eisner J, Smith B. The significance of SNODENT. Stud Health Technol Inform. 2005;116:737–42.

Grabowski H, Vernon J, DiMasi JA. Returns on research and development for 1990s new drug introductions. Pharmacoeconomics. 2002;20 Suppl 3:11–29.

Harris PA, Taylor R, Thielke R, Payne J, Gonzalez N, Conde JG. Research electronic data capture (REDCap)–a metadata-driven methodology and workflow process for providing translational research informatics support. J Biomed Inform. 2009;42(2):377–81.

Hosking JD, Newhouse MM, Bagniewska A, Hawkins BS. Data collection and transcription. Control Clin Trials. 1995;16(2 Suppl):66S–103S.

Kalenderian E, Ramoni RL, White JM, Schoonheim-Klein ME, Stark PC, Kimmes NS, et al. The development of a dental diagnostic terminology. J Dent Educ. 2010;75(1):68–76.

King DW, Lashley R. A quantifiable alternative to double data entry. Control Clin Trials. 2000;21(2):94–102.

Kleinman K. Adaptive double data entry: a probabilistic tool for choosing which forms to reenter. Control Clin Trials. 2001;22(1):2–12.

Langabeer 2nd JR, Walji MF, Taylor D, Valenza JA. Economic outcomes of a dental electronic patient record. J Dent Educ. 2008;72(10):1189–200.

Manheimer E, Anderson D. Survey of public information about ongoing clinical trials funded by industry: evaluation of completeness and accessibility. BMJ. 2002;325(7363):528–31.

McCray AT. Better access to information about clinical trials. Ann Intern Med. 2000;133(8):609–14.

Rondel RKVS, Webb CF. Clinical data management. 2nd ed. Chichester: Wileys; 2000.

Schleyer TK, Thyvalikakath TP, Spallek H, Torres-Urquidy MH, Hernandez P, Yuhaniak J. Clinical computing in general dentistry. J Am Med Inform Assoc. 2006b;13(3):344–52.

Singer SW, Meinert CL. Format-independent data collection forms. Control Clin Trials. 1995;16(6):363–76.

Spence J, Valenza JA, Taylor D. Documentation of clinical workflow: a key step in a plan to facilitate implementation of an electronic patient record. AMIA Annu Symp Proc. 2007;2007:1119.

Stark PC, Kalenderian E, White JM, Walji MF, Stewart DC, Kimmes N, et al. Consortium for oral health-related informatics: improving dental research, education, and treatment. J Dent Educ. 2010b;74(10):1051–65.

Strang N, Cucherat M, Boissel JP. Which coding system for therapeutic information in evidence-based medicine. Comput Methods Programs Biomed. 2002;68(1):73–85.

Taylor D, Valenza JA, Spence JM, Baber RH. Integrating electronic patient records into a multimedia clinic-based simulation center using a PC blade platform: a foundation for a new pedagogy in dentistry. AMIA Annu Symp Proc. 2007;2007:1129.

Valenza JA, Walji M. Creating a searchable digital dental radiograph repository for patient care, teaching and research using an online photo management and sharing application. AMIA Annu Symp Proc. 2007;2007:1143.

Walji M, Loeffelholz J, Valenza JA. A human-centered design of a dental discharge summary (DDS) for patients. AMIA Annu Symp Proc. 2007;2007:1146.

Walji MF, Taylor D, Langabeer 2nd JR, Valenza JA. Factors influencing implementation and outcomes of a dental electronic patient record system. J Dent Educ. 2009;73(5):589–600.

Zelenski S, Hood H, Holder M. Continuum of Quality Care Series, American Academy of Developmental Medicine and Dentistry. 2008. http://aadmd.org/articles/medicine-i-introduction. Accessed 15 May 2011

Chapter 5
International Perspectives

Miguel Humberto Torres-Urquidy, Jeffrey R. Glaizel, Rodrigo Licéaga-Reyes, André Ricardo Maia Correia, Filipe Miguel Araújo, Tiago Miguel Marques, Filipa Almeida Leite, and Angus W.G. Walls

Learning from different cultures provides an opportunity for discovering solutions which can only become evident if seen from a multicultural perspective. By reviewing the issues faced by other countries, one can learn what the common problems are and most likely identify their key underlying causes. In this chapter we review the experiences and status of medical and dental data integration in two continents including the countries of Canada, Mexico, Portugal and the United Kingdom.

M.H. Torres-Urquidy (✉)
Department of Biomedical Informatics, University of Pittsburgh, Pittsburgh, PA, USA

J.R. Glaizel
myDDSnetwork.com, Toronto, ON, Canada

R. Licéaga-Reyes
Department of Oral and Maxillofacial Surgery, Juarez Hospital in Mexico City, Mexico, DF, Mexico

A.R.M. Correia
Department of the Portuguese Catholic University (DCS-UCP), Dental Medicine, University of Porto (FMDUP), Health Sciences, Porto, Portugal

F.M. Araújo
Health Sciences Department, Universidade Católica Portuguesa - Campus de Viseu, Porto, Portugal

T.M. Marques
Health Sciences Department, Portuguese Catholic University, Porto, Portugal

F.A. Leite
Teotónio Hospital, Viseu, Portugal

A.W.G. Walls
School of Dental Sciences, Newcastle University, Newcastle, UK

5.1 Canada – National Perspective

Jeffrey R. Glaizel

As of 2011 there is very little integration of Dental and Medical records in Canada. However as we move forward into an era of patient-centered care and the increasing adoption of the Electronic Health Record, we can see that foundation is being laid for possible integration.

5.1.1 Barriers for Integration

There are two systemic issues that have traditionally provided barriers to the integration of medical and dental care. The first is the discrepancies in the delivery of medical and dental care in Canada which make integration of records very difficult. The second is the traditional physician-centric health care system which is currently in place. This system leaves all health care practitioners in independent silos both inter- and intra-professionally.

The Canadian Health Care system is controlled by the federal government which mandates reasonable access to health care services and enforces basic principles for all Canadians. Health Canada provides policy, leadership and technical assistance to the provinces and territories. The provincial and territorial governments are tasked with delivering health care to their citizens within the scope of the Canada Health Act through provincial and territorial insurance plans (Baris 1998).

In contrast dentistry in Canada is for the most part a private enterprise. Dental services are paid for by the patient and supplemented by private insurance if applicable. There are a patchwork of provincial social programs which provide emergency and/or basic dental services to children, the elderly and those on social assistance. Some hospitals provide emergency care and certain services which are covered through provincial health care insurance plans. For example, according to the Ontario Association for Public Health Dentistry (OAPHD 2011a).

> In Ontario, access to oral and dental care is limited to those who can pay (either out of pocket or from 'dental insurance' plans received as a benefit of employment). There are limited programs that address the needs of children with acute problems. For those children eligible for Ontario Works, CINOT (Children in Need of Treatment) or the new Healthy Smiles Ontario program, they have access to a provincial dental treatment program. Others may be eligible for dental care on an emergency basis only (OAPHD 2011b).

5.1.2 Governance Model

There is a provincial governance model over the profession of dentistry within its jurisdiction. In the province of Ontario this is the Regulated Health Professions Act. This act lays out the framework and professional governance model of dentists within Ontario. It also provides guidance to the regulatory bodies on how to govern its membership.

This fundamental difference in the provision and delivery of systemic health care services and oral health care services has led to a divide in the Canadian dental-medical world specifically in private practice. There is no significant infrastructure in place to allow for the integration of medical and dental care in Canada.

For the most part private dentists are successful in providing dental services to the population with support of organized dentistry organizations such as the Canadian Dental Association (CDA) and their provincial counterparts. The success of the business of dentistry has fostered an environment which supports the status quo of providing dental services outside of the medical health care system. Historically, there appeared to be a political concern, whether well-founded or not, that dentistry needs to remain as a silo and entirely walled off from the medical health care system to remain autonomous. Currently, in private practice there is no integration of health care records. That being said, the expanded list of services provided by private practitioner dentists including for sleep apnea, pain management and temporomandibular disorder (TMD) treatment, are forcing dentists to become more collaborative in approaching patient care. Specifically this is seen in the Royal College of Dental Surgeons of Ontario (RCDSO); guidelines for the "Diagnosis and Management of Temporomandibular Disorders and Related Musculoskeletal Disorders" published in July 2009 (Royal College of Dental Surgeons of Ontario 2009). There are numerous references in the document for the need of collaboration with other health care practitioners for the proper diagnosis and treatment of TMDs.

5.1.3 Steps Toward Integration

Furthermore, the increased use of information technology in society and in the profession is helping organized in dentistry to recognize the importance of integration to improve patient care. This recognition is demonstrated through the actions of dental associations and regulatory bodies in Canada. At the time of the drafting of this perspective, the RCDSO has produced for review by stakeholders an electronic records management systems guideline. It is the first dental regulatory body in Canada to produce such a document and the guidelines themselves will begin to provide the regulatory foundation that will allow dentistry to standardize and connect to a provincial EHR.

In January 2011, the Ontario Dental Association formed an eHealth Records Taskforce to review and evaluate the impact and implications for the dental profession of eHealth initiatives, and the related interoperability issues for the dental profession.

With respect to hospital-based care there are areas of integration of dental and medical care that attempt to improve patient care. One example of this can be found at the Wasser pain clinic at Mount Sinai Hospital in Toronto, Ontario, Canada. This clinic is a multidisciplinary and multiprofessional clinical research, assessment and treatment centre for adults with chronic, non-cancer, disabling pain disorders (Mount Sinai 2011).

Looking forward as there is a very large push both politically and financially to deliver on an electronic health record (EHR) in Canada to improve patient care and decrease ever growing delivery costs. On a federal level the initiative is being spearheaded by Canada Health Infoway (Canada Health 2011) which has been funded by the federal government as of January 28, 2009 to the total of 2.1 billion Canadian Dollars. This funding is not directed to develop the Canadian EHR per se but it is meant to be invested "in partnership with the country's federal, provincial, and territorial governments to create and implement electronic health record (EHR) systems that will build a legacy of health care distinguished by improved access, quality, privacy and productivity."

The Canadian Dental Association has representation at Canada Health Infoway however there has been no focus, strategy or programs to this date that on any dental specific issues or dental-medical integration issues.

There are numerous pan-Canadian organizations that address Canadian health information and integration. Two of the more prominent groups are the Canadian Institute for Health Information (CIHI) (CIHI 2011) and the Canadian Council on Integrated Health Care (CCIH) (CCIH 2011). According to CCIH, "The original intent of the CCIH was to bring together key opinion leaders from across the Canadian private healthcare sector to exchange views and propose solutions for the evolving management of healthcare in Canada. More recently, the Council has broadened its membership to include expertise from consumer, health professional and political perspectives." Both of these organizations (CIHI and CCIH) have not addressed and are not looking to address dental data and integration at this time. Apparently the focus of CCIH is on public-private payer issues, rather than on multidisciplinary integration of care delivery (CCIH 2009).

On a provincial level there have been no significant government efforts to integrate medical and dental information. The provinces of Alberta and Ontario are leading the EHR charge, however medical-dental integration is not at the forefront of discussion.

Ontario recently procured a C$46.2 million (CAD) diabetes registry. Unfortunately there was no involvement of organized dentistry in the development of the specifications or requirements.

Ontario has recently created the Ontario Health Study (OHS) (OHS 2011) which is tasked to "be the biggest community-based health study ever done in Ontario, and one of the biggest in the world." "The Ontario Health Study is a long-term study that will help us understand the causes, prevention and treatment of diseases such as cancer, heart disease, asthma, and diabetes." Although the Ontario Health Study would be an opportunity to address integration of medical and dental care, the study presents only one dental question to its participants as shown here.

When was the last time you saw a dental professional, including a dentist or a hygienist?

- Less than 6 months ago
- 6 months to less than 1 year ago
- 1 year to less than 2 years ago

- 2 years to less than 3 years ago
- 3 or more years ago
- Never
- Don't know
- Prefer not to answer

The one sign of integration of medical and dental care is that both medical and dental health plans are announced on a single web site, Insurance Direct Canada (IDC 2011).

5.2 Integration of Medical and Dental Data: Mexico

Rodrigo Licéaga-Reyes and Miguel Humberto Torres-Urquidy

Mexico, a country whose population is around one third of that of the US, is constituted by a mix of cultures resulting from its long history. The last five decades have witnessed a surge in the economic development of Mexico and in population numbers. Therefore, the healthcare delivery system had to adapt in order to maximize the use of resources and improve the effectiveness of caregivers. In this chapter we provide insights into the issues that will influence the adoption of new technologies and the conundrums faced by those interested in the integration of medical and dental data.

5.2.1 Healthcare as a Legal Right

The Mexican Constitution establishes in its fourth article that all Mexicans have the right to health. This was defined in the General Health Law of 1984 (Secretaria de Salud 1984). In this law, article 27 details the types of services and benefits that should be available for the Mexican population. Prevention and control of oral diseases are considered a part of the basic services to be provided by the State.

In Chap. 2 of the General Health Law "Benefits of Social Health Protection" (article 77b), it is possible to identify the minimum requirements for care. These include an integrated clinical record, whose implementation characteristics are, however, not specified.

Additionally, 15 years ago the government issued a norm for the prevention and control of oral diseases. In chapter IX, "Beneficiary Obligations", it is stated that patients have the right to a clinical record. This norm mentions the existence of records where the patient's clinical data is collected and that need to be signed by the treating dentist. The norm further specifies that the clinical document should contain a clinical history with minimum elements including a general medical history and a dental chart for capturing oral conditions.

Mexican laws do not specify the format in which the clinical document should be captured or how it can be exchanged with other authorities or medical institutions (Secretaria de Salud 1984). Consequently, it appears that the clinical record becomes property of the provider (i.e. dentist) and not the patient.

One of the main aims of the National Health Program for 2007–2012 is to promote investment in Information Technology and Communications, therefore increasing efficiency and integration in the healthcare system (Villareal Levy 2007). This plan specifically aims "… to establish base infrastructure for adopting an electronic clinical record and management of services." As of this writing, this program has attained an advanced development stage, and is expected to be launched in pilot states in 2012.

The electronic health record (EHR) aims to include demographic data, the medical history, and all bio-psycho-social information related to the patient (Gómez and Triana 2001). Specific benefits that are expected from an EHR include the immediate availability of data, independent geographic of the location of data, standardized communication between health professionals, and decision support for diagnosing and treating diseases (Vivanco-Cedeño 2009). In addition to improving care, widespread adoption of the EHR is expected to improve clinical research. Researchers will now have access to a reservoir of clinical information that can be used for basic, translational, and population level research and aid in the development of evidence based medicine (Tapia Vazquez 2010).

Arredondo Velazquez et al. (2005) found that among 300 dentists only 63% met the required norms when preserving the clinical history of their patients. Specifically, according to state norms, the record should not only follow the appropriate format, but also be filled out correctly (González et al. 2004). They showed that there is misinformation about the regulations and laws among oral care practitioners and that dentists and their staff sometimes do not completely fill electronic records, even if they are the copy of paper files. In other words, the simple translation of paper files into electronic records does not guarantee that the appropriate information is collected (Fig. 5.1).

As described by the Division of Innovation and Quality in Health of the Mexican Ministry of Health, the public sector covers about 80% of the healthcare demand in hospitals and 65% of ambulatory services. The total budget of the health sector is equivalent to 3.1% of Gross Domestic Product. In comparison, the private sector covers about 20% of hospitalizations and almost one third of the ambulatory visits (Figs. 5.1 and 5.2 respectively). The expenses of the private sector can reach up to 3% of the GDP.

Currently, the Mexican Health Ministry and the Federal Institute for Access to Public Information are developing a project named "Electronic Clinical Record". The goal of this Project is to develop a repository to maintain clinical information online and to constitute a unified source for all patient information. This will likely bring several benefits, including avoiding having duplicate prescriptions, laboratory and test results. In addition, the repository will also guarantee full complete treatments. Finally, the project will make the clinical record property of the patient and not the institution. In terms of information ownership, a legal restriction exists since

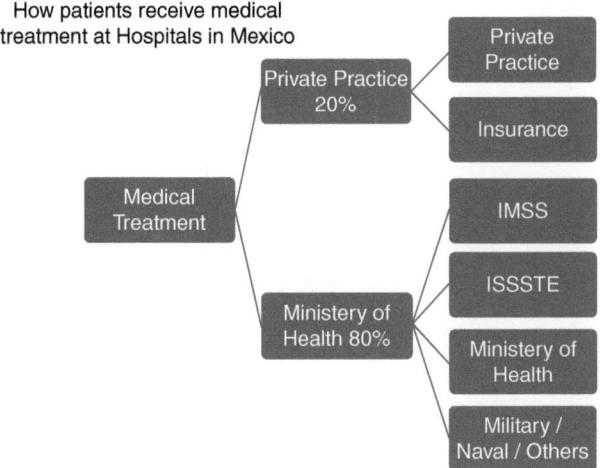

Fig. 5.1 Breakdown of hospital treatments provided in Mexico by type of institution/source of funding

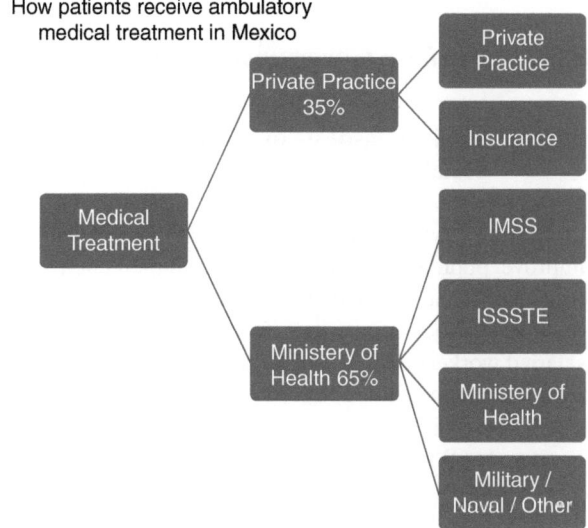

Fig. 5.2 Breakdown of ambulatory treatments provided in Mexico by type of institution/source of funding

regulation considers institutions as owners of the records. In addition, these organizations are required to keep these records for a period of up to 5 years, after which the records can be destroyed or transferred for archiving. As a result, if a patient did not receive care in the previous 5 years, it is possible that his/her records were destroyed. New records would then have to be developed again. There is therefore a risk of clinical records providing incomplete data, since some information may no longer available or may be too difficult to obtain.

Fig. 5.3 Distribution of governmental medical treatment services by institution

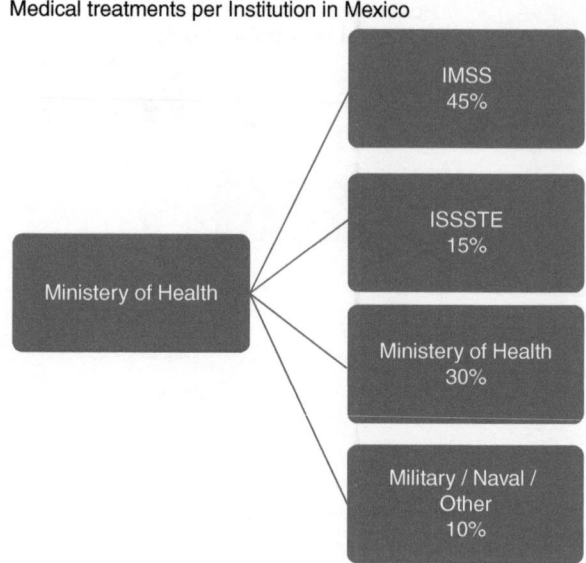

5.2.2 Mexican Government: Advances

5.2.2.1 Mexican Institute for Social Security (Instituto Mexicano del Seguro Social – IMSS)

In Mexico, two governmental institutions are leading these efforts to not only improve population health but also implement modern information technology (Fig. 5.3). One of them is the *Instituto Mexicano del Seguro Social* (Mexican Institute of Social Security). The institute was founded in 1943 as an answer for salaried workers demanding for quality medical services. The Institute aims to have an electronic medical record for each one of their affiliates as a unique patient record available in all of their facilities. According to official estimates, the Mexican Institute for Social Security, in 2010, covered 43 million people. This is for example, four times the population of countries like Portugal or Sweden.

IMSS has embarked in an ambitious enterprise by adapting the US' Veterans Health Information Systems and Technology Architecture (VistA) medical record and making it available to all its affiliates (Webster 2011). Despite the benefits of having a unique collection of patient records, there are still challenges to be faced when trying to take advantage of the full electronic application within the institution, as of the time of this writing. One example is that not all patients have their electronic record enabled. Another is that the interdependence between medical and dental elements is the less developed aspect of the application. Also, the system only provides a limited amount of options for capturing information regarding the treatments the patient received, even at simple levels. For instance, recording of data focuses on simple procedures such as extractions and fillings. Patients who have

Fig. 5.4 The Mexican Institute of Social Security (Instituto Mexicano del Seguro Social – IMSS) is one of the major health care providers in Mexico

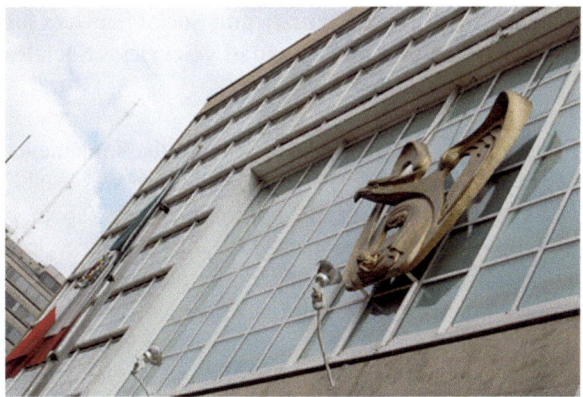

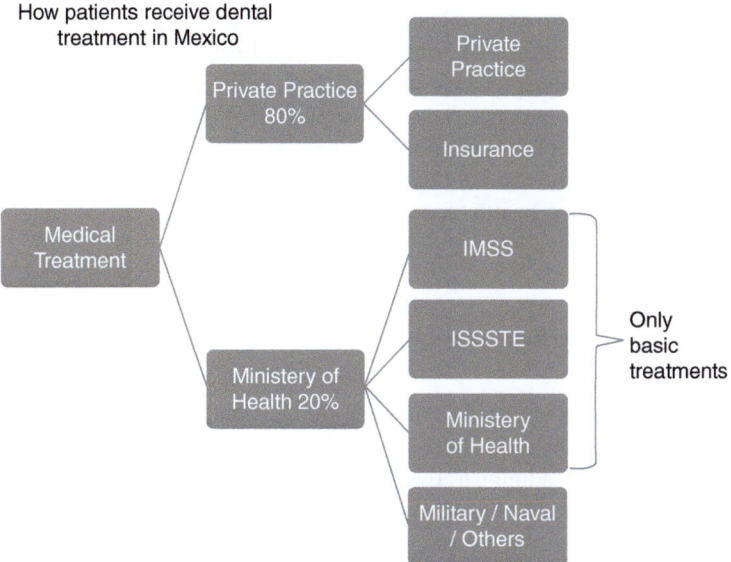

Fig. 5.5 Distribution of dental treatment services by sector

more elaborate treatments such as prosthesis or other full oral rehabilitations not performed at the institute do not have their information registered in the record. In addition, when these patients see a provider outside of IMSS, they do not have access to their own record (Fig. 5.4).

Nowadays, the institute provides dental services to its affiliates. These services are limited to some treatment options including extractions, amalgams, and initial prophylactic phases plus the application of fluoride. The services provided by the institute do not include root canal treatments or prosthetics. This means that all patients that require visits to private providers cause data to be distributed among different entities and this can be one of the reasons why a significant portion of dental services occur in the private sector (Fig. 5.5).

5.2.2.2 Institute of Security and Social Services for State Workers (Instituto de Seguridad y Servicios Sociales de los Trabajadores del Estado – ISSSTE)

ISSSTE is the other institution leading the implementation of electronic records in Mexico (ISSSTE 2009). This organization was established 51 years ago and provides care for about the 10 million members (about 10% of the Mexican population). ISSSTE has also planned creating a unique electronic record for its patients. The electronic record should incorporate medical and dental information. The institution has planned that the development and implementation of this electronic record should be phased, starting at the general practice level, followed by the regional hospitals, and, in the final stage, implementing it at the national centers. As of this writing, the precise dates of this process are unknown.

However, for some patients in ISSSTE, a reduced form of this system is already functioning. Through software called SIMEF 2.0, physicians can now review patient information including surgeries, consultations, and discharges. The system currently does not allow the exchange of this information with other institutions and most data still remains in paper form, requiring double data entry (paper and electronic). Yet, currently, it is not possible to access a dental chart or any other type of patient dental data. However, the organization plans to include more areas and procedures when expanding health records for all patients.

5.2.3 Private Medical and Dental Care

Currently, information exchange between the private and public sector is not required, even for the benefit of the patient. Even though there are many software products that assist in administrative tasks, capturing clinical information, these programs are meant for internal use only. They are not designed to share or exchange information via a universal format. Each software captures patient information according to its particular architecture.

For the private sector, one of the available Electronic Medical Records is SineMed, a multiuser system that allows accessing an online clinical chart from different computers. SineMed uses several standards including HXP and HL7 that have been adapted to meet official Mexican Regulations (Norma Oficial Mexicana 1995) that establishes the use of electronic records as mandatory and requires the exchange of information among different institutions in the country.

This software is able to store most patient information and history, and also allows for different analyses according to specialties. Regarding dental information, the software does not include a dental chart and does not record specific dental conditions. However, SineMed allows for customization, so it would be possible to integrate dental information.

Another application that allows accessing clinical information is available through the web portal www.consultorioweb.com. This website proposes to store patient information, schedule, images, and files for a monthly fee. The website also generates prescriptions, reports, vaccination registry among other features.

5.2.4 Transitioning into Electronic Health Records: Lessons from the Field

Dr. Antonio Manrique, Director of the Juarez Hospital of Mexico (part of the Federal system of Hospitals, which is a part of the Ministry of Health) says he is concerned about the perceived importance of transforming the clinical health record in an electronic clinical file, something that is planned to be working in the next 2 years.

One of the most important parts of the project, which will involve several areas of the hospital, is decision support and structuring of content. Although the clinical file must fulfill Official Mexican Norm No.24, it should include major hospital work areas including Pharmacy, Social Work and Billing. This project contemplated the integration of an odontogram that allows registering buccal diagnoses and treatments. At the moment an image network permits the visualization in different areas from the hospital as the different doctor's offices of external consultation the studies of simple x-rays and tomographies that or are taken with digital format [Dr. Antonio Manrique, personal interview].

Dr. Manrique considers that one of the advantages of the electronic clinical file will be its use for academic research. Currently, healthcare data from the hospital is not easy to document and paper files being difficult to store and handle. Indeed, the necessity of physical space causes paper files to be stored solely for 5 years as requested by the Official Norm. This makes retrospective analyses difficult or impossible in the long run. Thus, the interest of moving into the digital realm.

5.2.5 Conclusions

According to the 2009–2010 World Economic Forum Technology report, Mexico occupied the 78th place in terms of technological implementation (a decrement of 11 places from the previous year). Mexico had been 44th in the 2001–2002 report. The ranking included assessment of individual, private and governmental advancement. Demographically, Mexico grew from approximately 15 million people in 1910 to 112 million in 2010, making it the 11th most populous country in the planet (Fig. 5.6).

In the short term, one of the biggest challenges for the implementation of widespread electronic health records is access to technology. In 2010, only 29.8% of homes in Mexico owned a computer, while 22.2% had internet connectivity. In

Fig. 5.6 Access to communication technologies in Mexico

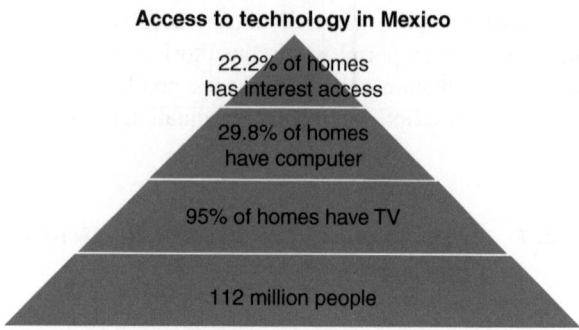

Mexico only 2.8% of the population has access to high speed internet; 40% of citizens above 6 years old are considered to be a computer user, but only 33% of the population older than 6 years are considered an internet user. (Fig. 5.5) (National Institute for Geography Statistics and Informatics – INEGI) (National Institute for Geography Statistics and Informatics 2011).

In order to implement the Electronic Health Record and required computer hardware, the Mexican government expects to invest 5 billion pesos among all public healthcare institutions. One of the most challenging aspects will be the integration of medical and dental records. Other is the portability of information between public health providers and the private sector. This process will require governmental efforts and widespread collaborations between medical and dental organizations and the private sector.

5.3 Portugal: A Case for Medical and Dental Data Integration

André Ricardo Maia Correia, Filipe Miguel Araújo, Tiago Miguel Marques, Filipa Almeida Leite, and Miguel Humberto Torres-Urquidy

5.3.1 Portugal: Perspectives and Comparisons

Portugal is a coastal nation in southwestern Europe, located at the western end of the Iberian Peninsula and bordering Spain on its northern and eastern frontiers. The country territory also includes a series of archipelagoes in the Atlantic Ocean: Azores and Madeira. In total, the country occupies an area of 92,090 sq km of which 91,470 sq km is land and 620 sq km is water (Central Intelligence Agency 2011).

According to the 2001 Census of the Portuguese National Institute of Statistic (*Instituto Nacional de Estadistica – INE*) the population was about 10,356,117, being 51.7% female and 48.3% male. The Portuguese population is relatively homogeneous for most of its history: a predominant single religion (Catholicism) and a single language have contributed to this ethnic and national unity (Instituto Nacional de Estadistica 2002).

Currently, Portugal is a member of the European Union and the United Nations, as well as a founding member of the Latin Union, the Organization of Ibero-American States, OECD, NATO, Community of Portuguese Language Countries, Eurozone and Schengen state. It is considered to be a developed country (United Nations 2010) and it has the world's 19th highest quality-of-life, according to *The Economist Intelligence Unit* (Franklin 2004). It is the 13th most peaceful (Institute for Economics and Peace 2010) and the 8th-most globalized country in the world (Dreher et al. 2008).

Portugal has enjoyed substantial improvements in the health status of its population over the last 25 years and life expectancy has converged to the European Union (EU) average. In the 2006–2008 period, average life expectancy at birth was 78.9 years while the average for the EU 15 group in 2007 was 80.4 years. Despite remarkable improvements, there are still important inequalities in health between gender, regions and socioeconomic groups, and most health system performance indicators have not yet reached the level of the EU or OECD averages (Barros and Simões 2007). The GDP spent on Health in Portugal was 10.2% in 2006, being 70.6% of this spent by the government (Kravitz and Treasure 2008). The GDP spent on Oral Health was 0.36% in 2004, being 40% of oral health expenditure private (Kravitz and Treasure 2008).

5.3.2 Health Subsystems

Healthcare in Portugal is controlled by a Minister of Health who delegates powers to each one of the 18 continental districts, plus Madeira and Azores archipelagos, headed by a politically appointed President (usually a Public Health Doctor) (Kravitz and Treasure 2008). At the district level, there are no health boards. However there is a Regional Administration that is responsible for large Hospitals and Health Centers that provide primary and secondary care, and Clinics which only have primary care facilities (Kravitz and Treasure 2008).

The National Health Service (NHS) employs doctors, nurses, other health professionals, and supporting staff. Concerning dental care providers, there are only a small number of stomatologists (MD) and a very few dentists (DMD) working in the Portuguese NHS (Kravitz and Treasure 2008).

5.3.2.1 Private Health Insurance

The Private Healthcare insurance market in Portugal is growing and some companies already have dental medicine care plans. These plans are more expensive and can have two options: reimbursement and co-pay. In the first system, the patient pays the total cost of treatment to the clinician and then seeks reimbursement, as

Table 5.1 Medical schools in Portugal

University	Medical school	City	URL
University of Porto	Faculty of Medicine	Porto	http://www.med.up.pt
University of Porto	Institute of Biomedical Sciences Abel Salazar	Porto	http://www.icbas.up.pt
University of Coimbra	Faculty of Medicine	Coimbra	http://www.uc.pt/fmuc/
Universidade de Lisboa	Faculty of Medicine	Lisboa	http://www.fm.ul.pt/
New University of Lisbon	Faculty of Medical Sciences	Lisboa	http://www.fcm.unl.pt/
University of Minho	School of Health Sciences	Braga	http://www.ecsaude.uminho.pt
University of Covilhã	School of Health Sciences	Covilhã	http://www.fcsaude.ubi.pt/

appropriate, from the insurance company. Prior approval is used through reports from the clinician. In the second system, which is cheaper and the most common, the clinician earns a certain amount for each treatment defined by the insurance company. The insurance company pays a part of this amount and the patient has to make a co-payment directly to the clinician that varies in function of the treatments and the contract established between the company and the patient (Kravitz and Treasure 2008).

5.3.3 Medical Education and Practice

There are seven medical schools in Portugal (Table 5.1).

The Medical training programs at the first five medical schools (Lisbon, Oporto and Coimbra) follow the same curriculum adjusted to the Bologna Process, which is probably the most important educational change in Europe in the last 50 years. The aim of the Bologna Process is to make the education and training provided in the higher education more intelligible and comparable, allowing and promoting mobility of the students and academic staff through a system of credits in the different countries that signed the Declaration (ECTS – European Credit Transfer and Accumulation System) (Plasschaert et al. 2005, 2006; Cowpe et al. 2010).

In this system there are usually two cycles leading to a Master's degree (1st cycle of 3 years and a 2nd cycle of 2 years). Due to its particularities, the Medical Degree has a 6 year program leading to an Integrated Master Degree in Medicine. The first 3 years have a core program covering the basic sciences and the last 3 years have a clinical program based on practice and specialized procedures, with the 6th year being a professional year with programmed and oriented training (Barros and Simões 2007; Medical Education Center FMUP 2010).

The Ministry of Health and the Portuguese Medical Association (*OM – Ordem dos Médicos*) have a role in determining the content of training program and educational standards in the intern period, at postgraduate specialist training level and in continuing medical education (Rowe and García-Barbero 2005).

After university, all graduates must undertake an exam to access a medical specialization, after which they will perform a common year internship (general) for 12 months, with 3 months of training in general practice, and public health, and 9 months in hospital training. After this internship, they will begin a training for the specialty that they have been accepted (hospital specialties: 4–6 years; general practice/family medicine: 4 years; and public health medicine: 4 years (Barros and Machado 2010; Portuguese Medical Association 2011).

According to the Portuguese Medical Association there are 44,390 medical doctors in Portugal (Portuguese Medical Association 2009). Data from the General Directorate of Health showed that 23,389 of these were employed by the NHS in 2004 (hospitals and PCCs), the majority in secondary and tertiary care. GPs/family doctors, those specialized in family medicine, accounted for 29.5% of the total number of doctors in the NHS; 42.5% were hospital doctors and 2% were public health doctors (Barros and Simões 2007).

5.3.3.1 Regulation of Medical Practice

The Minister of Health is responsible for the licensing of Physicians and, in accordance with the legislation, delegates this task to the Portuguese Medical Association (Rowe and García-Barbero 2005).

The Portuguese Medical Association is responsible for regulation of the profession including medical ethics. The full License for independent practice is awarded after the basic degree and Internship. There is also a license to practice as a specialist (including general practice). An additional license concerning professional qualifications is required in relation to the standards of the medical premises in which medical practice will take place (Rowe and García-Barbero 2005).

5.3.3.2 Providing Medical Care to the Population

A mix of public and private health service providers delivers primary health care in Portugal. In the public sector it is mostly delivered through publicly funded and managed health centers. Each of them covers an average of 28,000 people although some of them cover more than 100,000 people and others fewer than 5,000 people. They employ in total 30,000 professionals (including regional health administration personnel). Of these, 25% are doctors (mostly general practitioners) and 20% are nurses. There are on average 80 health professionals per center, although some have as many as 200 and others as few as one medical doctor (Bentes et al. 2004).

General Practitioners/family doctors and nurses deliver most primary health care in the health center setting. However, some health centers also provide a limited range of specialized care. The specialists who work in HCs belong to the so-called ambulatory specialties, such as mental health, psychiatry, dermatology, pediatrics, gynecology and obstetrics and surgery (Bentes et al. 2004).

The range of services provided by GPs in HCs is as follows: general medical care for the adult population, prenatal care, children's care, women's health, family planning and perinatal care, first aid, certification of incapacity to work, home visits and preventive services, including immunization and screening for breast, cervical and other preventable diseases (Bentes et al. 2004).

Patients must register with a GP, and can choose among the available clinicians within a geographical area. Many patients prefer to go directly to emergency care services in hospitals or the private sector where the full range of diagnostic tests can be obtained in a few hours. This leads to excessive demand on emergency departments and considerable misuse of resources as expensive emergency services are used for relatively minor complaints (Bentes et al. 2004).

5.3.4 Dental Education and Practice

5.3.4.1 Higher Education in Dental Medicine

There are five Universities and two Institutes teaching Dental Medicine in Portugal:

As listed in Table 5.2, the first three Universities are Public, and are ruled by the Portuguese Government (Ministry of Science, Technology, and Higher Education). The Catholic University enjoys a special status (agreement) – "*Concordata*" – between Portugal and the Vatican, which is recognize by the Portuguese State. The last three schools are private educational corporations, also recognized by the Portuguese State. Due to this number of dental schools, Portugal has one of the highest rates in Europe of graduating dentists (Bentes et al. 2004).

Dental Education in the referred training programs has two distinct parts: biomedical sciences and dental sciences. The former is related to education and training in some areas like health and biology sciences (e.g. anatomy, physiology, pathology, pharmacology among others). The later is an advanced education in specific areas of Dentistry (e.g. endodontics, oral pathology, periodontics, prosthodontics, oral surgery, restorative dentistry, among others).

This Dental Education has undergone some changes in the recent years due to the Bologna Process. Now, all Portuguese Universities and Institutes undertook this curricular change and adopted the profile and competences principles. Bologna Process recommends the "3–5–8" model (Bachelor – Master – Doctor) (Cowpe et al. 2010). This establishes that Dental Education and training should compromise a total of at least 5 years of full-time theoretical and clinical study (300 ECTS credits), given in a University or other recognized higher education institution, and leading to a Dental Master's Degree.

Table 5.2 Higher education in dental medicine in Portugal

University	Dental school	Course	City	URL
University of Porto	Faculty of Dental Medicine	Master's Degree in Dental Medicine	Porto	http://www.fmd.up.pt
University of Lisbon	Faculty of Dental Medicine	Master's Degree in Dental Medicine	Lisbon	http://www.fmd.ul.pt
University of Coimbra	Faculty of Medicine	Integrated Master's in Dentistry	Coimbra	http://www.uc.pt/fmuc/
Advanced Institute of Health Sciences – North	Master's Degree in Dental Medicine		Paredes (Gandra)	http://www.cespu.pt
Advanced Institute of Health Sciences Egas Moniz	Master's Degree in Dental Medicine		Almada (Caparica)	http://www.egasmoniz.com.pt/
University Fernando Pessoa	Master's Degree in Dental Medicine		Porto	http://www.ufp.pt/
Portuguese Catholic University	Health Sciences Department	Master's Degree in Dental Medicine	Viseu	http://www.crb.ucp.pt

Achieving European Convergence in Higher Education also raised the question about what should be the profile and minimum set of generic and specific professional competences of the European Dentist (Plasschaert et al. 2005, 2006, 2007; Oliver et al. 2008; Cowpe et al. 2010), which is similar to the standardization of training between states in the United States of America.

From the European dentist it is expected to co-operate in achieving the total health of patients through oral health management (Cowpe et al. 2010). Thus, a set of competences and abilities are essential to begin independent, unsupervised dental practice (Cowpe et al. 2010).

Seven domains have been identified, and each one has a major competence, and several supporting competences (Cowpe et al. 2010, Table 5.3):

These domains are the basic levels of professional behavior, knowledge and skills necessary for a graduating student to meet the future challenges of Dental Practice.

5.3.4.2 Dental Medicine Practice

In Portugal, Dental Medicine is mainly practiced under private practice and it requires an advanced degree (Bachelor's Degree, before Bologna Process, or Master

Table 5.3 Outline of domains and competences, Europe

I. Professionalism
  (a) Major competence
    (i) Professional attitude and behavior
    (ii) Ethics and Jurisprudence

II. Interpersonal, communication and social skills
  (a) Major competence
    (i) Communication

III. Knowledge base, information and information literacy
  (a) Major competence
    (i) Application of basic and biological, medical, technical and clinical sciences
    (ii) Acquiring and using information

IV. Clinical information gathering
  (a) Major competence
    (i) Obtaining and recording a complete history of the patient's medical, oral and dental state

V. Diagnosis and treatment planning
  (a) Major competence
    (i) Decision-making, clinical reasoning and judgment

VI. Therapy: establishing and maintaining oral health
  (a) Major competence
    (i) Establishing and maintaining oral health

VII. Prevention and health promotion
  (a) Major competence
    (i) Improving oral health of individuals, families and groups in the community

Degree, after Bologna Process implementation) in order to obtain a professional license from the Portuguese Dental Association (*OMD – Ordem dos Médicos Dentistas*). This allows every Dental Medicine Graduate to practice and perform any type of dental treatment, within the limits of their skills and knowledge (Barros and Simões 2007; Kravitz and Treasure 2008; OMD 2011a).

However there are a few exceptions in this practice. Some professionals are linked and develop their work in public institutions, as part of the National Health Service, especially in Hospitals or Oncology Services as the Portuguese Institute of Oncology (*IPO – Instituto Português de Oncologia*) (Kravitz and Treasure 2008, Table 5.4).

According to the Manual of Dental Practice: Council of European Dentists (Kravitz and Treasure 2008) approximately 50% of the population is not provided with dental care, due mainly to financial reasons.

Regulation of the Dental Practice: Portuguese Dental Association (*OMD*)

The OMD is a public entity, autonomous, independent from the Portuguese State, which regulates dental practice in Portugal. It has a General Assembly, a Board of

Table 5.4 Dental medicine practice in Portugal

Dental medicine practice	N
General Private Practice	6,974
Public Dental Service	43
University	200
Hospital	90
Armed Forces	31
General Practice as a proportion	95%

Adapted from the Manual of Dental Practice (Kravitz and Treasure 2008)

Table 5.5 Number of dentists graduated in Portuguese Dental Schools

Dental school	Dentists graduated since foundation (N)
Faculty of Dental Medicine of the University of Porto (FMDUP)	1,227
Faculty of Dental Medicine of the University of Lisbon (FMDUL)	761
Dental Medicine Course of the Faculty of Medicine of the University of Coimbra (FMUC)	501
Advanced Institute of Health Sciences of the North (ISCS-N)	1,228
Advanced Institute of Health Sciences Egas Moniz (ISCS-Egas Moniz)	1,400
Dental Medicine Course of University Fernando Pessoa (UFP)	382
Dental Medicine Course of the Portuguese Catholic University (UCP)	83

Directors, a Fiscal Board and also a Disciplinary Board. The President (*Bastonário*) of the OMD, as well as the Board of Directors and the Fiscal Board, are directly elected by all members. The Disciplinary Board is also directly elected but within an autonomous election. The OMD provides relevant professional information to its members, including international and national legislation and also transnational recommendations such as CED information (Kravitz and Treasure 2008; OMD 2011a).

According to the latest data provided by the OMD (OMD 2010), there were 6,595 Dentist, from 29 different nationalities, practicing Dental Medicine in Portugal, generating a population ratio of one dentist per 1,611 residents. The average age of the practitioner is 36.9 years old (Table 5.5).

In 2015, the OMD estimates that the number of Dentists affiliated are expected to exceed the 10,000.

However, the practice of Dentistry in Portugal has some particularities, since it is not limited to Dentists. Other professional classes such as Stomatologists (MD) and Odontologists (without academic training, legalized administratively for restricted activities in oral care) are allowed to practice Dentistry (Kravitz and Treasure 2008; OMD 2010). According to the Manual of Dental Practice of the Council of European

Table 5.6 Article 64th (Health) of the Constitution of the Portuguese Republic, 7th review

Constitution of the Portuguese Republic

Article 64 – (Health)
1. Everyone has the right to the protection of health and the duty to defend and promote health.
2. The right to the protection of health shall be fulfilled:
   (a) By means of a universal and general national health service which, in regards to the economic and social conditions of the citizens who use it, shall tend to be free of charge;
   (b) By creating economic, social, cultural and environmental conditions that particularly guarantee the protection of childhood, youth and old age; by systematically improving living and working conditions, and promoting physical fitness and sports in school and among the people; and also by developing the people's health and hygiene education and living practices.
3. In order to ensure the right to the protection of health, the state is charged, as a priority, with:
   (a) Guaranteeing access by every citizen, regardless of his economic situation, to preventive, curative and rehabilitative medical care;
   (b) Guaranteeing a rational and efficient nationwide coverage in terms of human resources and healthcare units;
   (c) Working towards the socialization of the costs of medical care and medicines;
   (d) Disciplining and inspecting entrepreneurial and private forms of medicine and articulating them with the national health service, in such a way as to ensure adequate standards of efficiency and quality in both public and private healthcare institutions;
   (e) Disciplining and controlling the production, distribution, marketing, sale and use of chemical, biological and pharmaceutical products and other means of treatment and diagnosis;
   (f) Establishing policies for the prevention and treatment of drug abuse.
4. Management of the national health service shall be decentralised and participatory.

Dentists there are, in total, 7,514 professionals practicing Dentistry in Portugal (Kravitz and Treasure 2008).

Currently, the Portuguese Dental Association only recognizes two specialties: Oral Surgery and Orthodontics; with a small number of specialists in the country: 40 orthodontists and 4 oral surgeons (OMD 2010). Recently, efforts are being developed to create and recognize Periodontology, Odontopediatrics and Prosthodontics specialties.

This Association also supervises and regulates continuing education for dentists, mandatory from January 2009 (Kravitz and Treasure 2008).

5.3.4.3 Providing Dental Care to the Population

Portugal has a Public National Health Service which should be free for all the Portuguese population, according to Article 64th of the Constitution of the Portuguese Republic (Assembly of the Republic 2005, Table 5.6).

However, the publicly funded oral health care system in Portugal is not comprehensive (Barros and Simões 2007). There are very few NHS dental care professionals in this sector, so people normally use the private sector (Barros and Simões 2007). Due to this discrepancy, the Portuguese Government creates National

Table 5.7 Groups currently included in the PNPSO

PNPSO: population groups included
• Children and teenagers (<16 yo).
• Pregnant women.
• Low income elderly people.
• HIV infected people.

Programs to provide dental care through the private sector. It is the competence of the General Directorate of Health to guarantee health promotion, prevention of oral illnesses and afford assistance of oral health capable of being performed in the National Health Service (SNS). This intervention is assured by the professionals of the Local Medical Centers (*Centros de Saúde*), through actions directed to the individual, the family and the school community (Kravitz and Treasure 2008).

In 2005 it was introduced the National Program for Oral Health Promotion (PNPSO). Its aim was to improve oral health thought an intervention based on oral health promotion and on oral illness prevention on children and teenagers (3 yo–16 yo). It contemplated also a curative perspective to a small part of school population reached by the program. For admission to the PNPSO regarding dental intervention, only dentists (DMD) and stomatologists (MD) enrolled in the respective professional associations could apply (Kravitz and Treasure 2008).

In 2008, the PNPSO was widened to include pregnant women enrolled in the National Health Service and aged people, beneficiaries of the Solidarity Complement for Seniors (SCI). For its first time, a part of the public budget was consigned to oral health through the "National Oral Health Promotion Program – *Cheque-dentista*" (€21.000.000 budget). This referred groups benefit from some public expenditure on oral treatments, with the possibility to choose freely from a list of private adherent dentists (Kravitz and Treasure 2008). The low income elderly people may benefit also from a contribution up to €250 in a 3 year period regarding prosthetic procedures (Kravitz and Treasure 2008). In 2009, HIV infected people were also included in this program (Government of Portugal 2010; Ministry of Health, 24 de Março de 2009, Table 5.7).

The rest of the publicly funded oral health care system in Portugal is quite complex. Dentists may apply for a contract to one or more fund schemes.

There are a large number of other funds which provide additional cover for individual professions, for example for, lawyers, banks, industry, the military and civil servants. Each fund has its own administrative structure and each one pays a different level of benefit as a contribution towards the cost of care. Payments to each fund vary and the system is progressive with higher paid personnel contributing more than those with lower salaries. Payments are collected by employers from salaried personnel and the self-employed pay a quarterly amount based on the previous year's income. The level of contributions is calculated annually according to expenditure and deficits are not allowed (Kravitz and Treasure 2008).

Each fund is self-regulated, with its own rules, and has its own list of eligible treatments and scale of fees, which tends to be low (Barros and Simões 2007; Kravitz and Treasure 2008). Few provide cover for advanced prosthodontics and those that do, usually require prior approval (ex. *SAMS quadros*, for bankers) (Kravitz and Treasure 2008).

Most oral healthcare is provided in private (liberal) practices although a few hospitals and Health Centers from the National Health Service have dentists (Kravitz and Treasure 2008).

5.3.4.4 Health Information Systems

According to the Benchmarking ICT use among General Practitioners (European Commission 2008), Portugal has a classification of 1.7 (0–5) on e-health solutions, which means that there is still much to do in this field.

All health institutions of the NHS are connected through a Health Information Network (RIS – *Rede de Informação em Saúde*), which is run by an Health System Central Administration (ACSS – *administração central do sistema de saúde*) (Ministry of Health 2008).

Portuguese NHS has a Patient National Record (RNU – *Registo Nacional do Utente*) available since March 2007. This is an informatics platform of the Health Minister created to contain NHS patient's unique and consolidated information, and it was created with the migration of 400 local databases of a National Information System of Health Users (SINUS – *Sistema de Informação Nacional de Utentes de Saúde*) (Ministry of Health 2010).

The RNU is updated daily, in a synchronic process with SINUS, and with the Citizen Card and the Justice Information Technology Institute Database (in order to obtain information contained in the death certificates) (Ministry of Health 2010). As of this writing, SINUS remains active, until RNU system is fully implemented. Today, every newborn is registered in the same day in the RNU, which assures a better access to health care.

Besides the RNU, the Portuguese NHS has four information systems developed to monitor the access to health care: (Ministry of Health 2010)

- Information System to Manage Surgery Inscriptions (SIGIC – *Sistema de informação de gestão de inscritos para cirurgia*)
- This system was created in 2004 with the aim of decreasing the time elapsing between the indication for a surgical intervention and the day of surgery. Between 2005 and 2009 it has reduced the number of patients registered in SIGIC by 34%.
- Appointment in time and hours (CTH: *Consulta a Tempo e Horas*)
- This electronic system was developed to improve the management of access to medical specialties including first visits in the NHS Hospitals, through local medical centers and hospitals.
- Information system for oral health (SISO: *Sistema de informação para a saúde oral*) (see below)
- Information system of the program for medically assisted procreation. (FERTIS: *sistema de informação do programa de apoio à procriação medicamente assistida*).
- System developed to allow a better access to information related to the epidemiology of cases, access to MAP techniques, control of information regarding

Table 5.8 Description of services

Service name	URL	Description
e-SIGIC	https://servicos.min-saude.pt/acesso/faces/Login.jsp	Allows patient on-line access to SIGIC and monitoring of its processes.
e-Agenda		Allows citizen to schedule an appointment in its Local Medical Center.
e-Prescription		Allows cronic patient to request, through Internet, new medications.

couples, reducing waiting times and assuring a correct referral between the public and the private health sector.

The NHS has also developed on-line services for the citizen, which promote autonomy and direct access to health services and information (Ministry of Health 2010, Table 5.8).

e-Health Record

In the majority of the hospitals, the application SONHO is the backbone of the electronic health records. In the Health Centers, this function is completed with SINUS. Both of these applications were developed in the late '80s. These operate in UNIX platforms; they use Oracle database and a client–server architecture (telnet) that allows communications between different institutions (Araújo 2007; Espanha and Fonseca 2010; Health System Central Administration 2010).

SONHO is mainly an administrative application developed by the IGIF (former Institute of Informatics and Financial Management of Health, extinguished and included in the ACSS) that is used in some Hospital departments, such as the emergency room, outpatient, inpatient, clinical records and complementary diagnosis means. Its major aim is to control the flow of patients inside the institution. Sinus, also developed by IGIF, aims to support the daily activities of the Health Centers, implementing some features like patients registry, schedule appointments, immunization record and patients card (Araújo 2007; Espanha and Fonseca 2010; Health System Central Administration 2010).

However, both of these computer applications needed to have a complete and exhaustive electronic health record that allowed the doctor to easily access and records patients' information. To fulfill this need, a module was developed designed to support physician activities (SAM), based and integrated on the clinical and administrative information systems SINUS and SONHO. Opposite to these late systems, SAM uses web technology, has a user-friendly interface, includes JAVA technology, Oracle Developer tools and is typically installed in Windows 2000 servers. SAM allows the physician to record the clinical information of the consultation, inpatient and emergency room; prescribe additional means of diagnosis and therapy; prescribe drugs; schedule appointments; check and record personal and family history; consult reports and access patients clinical history, among others functionalities (Araújo 2007; Espanha and Fonseca 2010; Health System Central Administration 2010).

Fig. 5.7 Health Information Network in Portugal (RIS)

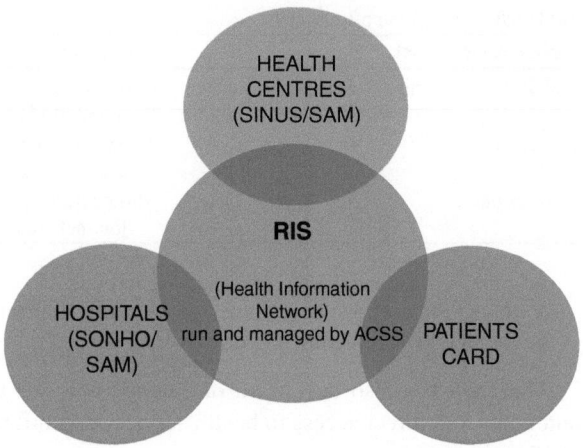

To facilitate access to health care the "Patient Card" was created. It allows each patient to be identified in any National Health System Institution. The Health Information Network (Fig. 5.6), one of the largest networks in the country, supports inter-institutional communications among Hospitals, Health Centers and other institutions related to the Portuguese NHS (Araújo 2007; Espanha and Fonseca 2010; Health System Central Administration 2010, Fig. 5.7).

In the case of regulation, currently, Portuguese law is seen as a key determinant of use of records electronic. The applicable laws are the following (Health System Central Administration 2009):

- Law on the 'Protection of Personal Data' (№ 67/98, 26th October), according to the directive 95/46/CE of the European Parliament and Council.
- Law on 'Health and Genetic Personal Information' (№ 12/2005, 26th of January)
- Law on the 'Access to official documents and reuse' (№ 46/2007, 24th August).

Institutions are legally required to keep records on paper, regardless of whether the records are made electronically (Health System Central Administration 2009). Even if the paper record is scanned, it cannot be destroyed, in which at least its microfilm is required. During the creation of the electronic health records opinions from the national commission on data protection were required *(CNPD – comissão nacional de protecção de dados)* in order to maintain harmony with the legal system (Health System Central Administration 2009). Concerning the introduction of data in the EHR of the patient, the European Commission recommends semantic interoperability to ensure an accurate interpretation of exchanged information that is understandable by any system or application not initially developed for this purpose (European Commission 2009; Health System Central Administration 2009). However, there are no orientations or general rules / models in Portugal on this matter, allowing the ACSS, or the Professionals Associations (ex. Nursing) to control

Table 5.9 Examples of PMS developed and commercialized in Portugal

PMS name	Company	URL
Newsoft DS	Imaginasoft Healthcare Solutions	http://www.imaginasoft.eu/
Novigest	Tactis	http://www.tactis.pt
Gestrato	Gestrato	http://www.gestrato.pt/
Dentoral	Duas Ribeiras	http://www.duasribeiras.com/dentoral.htm

the use of certain terminologies, reducing its interoperability (European Commission 2009; Health System Central Administration 2009).

Actually efforts are being developed to define an EHR model, and by the end of 2012, the Portuguese Government seeks to ensure that all patients have an Electronic Health Record, according to the XVIII Constitutional Government Program (Portuguese Government 2009–2013; Ministry of Health 2010). No information is available about the inclusion of oral health in this EHR, since most of the dental procedures are performed on a private basis.

e-Oral Health Record

The Information System for Oral Health (SISO) has been developed under the rules of the National Program for Oral Health Promotion (PNPSO). This is a web-based application created to allow access to professional participation in the program, by any connection of any information system, from public or private services.

This system allows access to dental appointments, payment of medical services, handling of information related to dental prosthesis expenses and management of the program (Ministry of Health 2008, 2010). This system is not intended to be handled by the patient directly, but directed for use by Health Professionals, including dentists, family doctors and other health management entities (ex. Health System Central Administration). The main limitation of this information system is that it is consigned only to the Health Professionals and Patients adherent to the PNPSO program.

Besides this national public program, most of the clinical procedures in the dental practice are performed through a private basis. Patient's information is then registered in an electronic oral-health record (e-OHR) included in a practice management system (PMS) (Table 5.9 and 5.10).

The two systems, public (SISO / PNPSO) and private, do not integrate with each other, which means that a dentist that works in private practice and has also a contract with the PNSPSO has to introduce clinical records in two different systems (Figs. 5.8–5.11).

In this e-OHR, all treatment names have a specific designation included in a "Nomenclature Table" created by the Portuguese Dental Association (OMD 2011b). This is the basis for the nomenclature tables in every PMS. However, this table may be modified by the dentist or by the PMS company, if required.

Table 5.10 Examples of PMS developed and commercialized in Portugal and related data

PMS	Year[a]	Versions[a]	Scientific Data (Dias 2009)	Companies data[a]	
			Users %	Users	Other information
Newsoft DS	1997	Light, Professional, Dentistery College	31.9%	3200 users 910 clinics	Installed in 4 Portuguese Dental Schools (FMDUP, FMDUL, ISCS-EM, UCP) Internationalization perspective to: Spain, England, Brazil and Angola.
Novigest	2003		4.3	225 clinics	No internationalization perspetive.
Gestrato	NDR	NDR	2.1%	NDR	NDR
Dentoral	NDR	NDR	12.8%	NDR	NDR

[a]Information given by the companies representative
NDR no data received

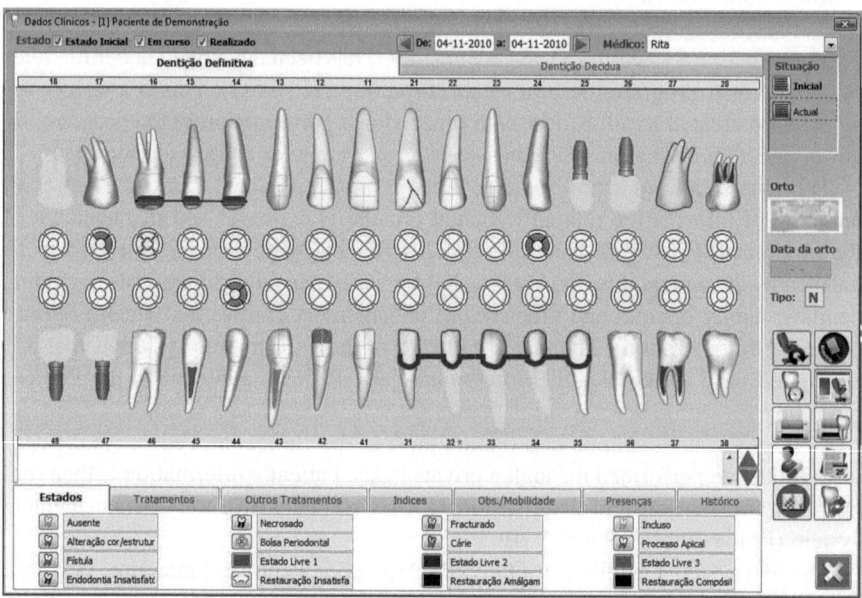

Fig. 5.8 Newsoft Dente® odontogram (with permission)

Concerning "Diagnostic Names", currently there is no Nomenclature followed by Portuguese Dentists. Usually, the dentist inserts in the Clinical Record the treatment performed according to the previously described "Nomenclature Table", but no information about the diagnosis of the situation, since there is not a "Classification of Diseases" as such ICD-9, for use by dentists.

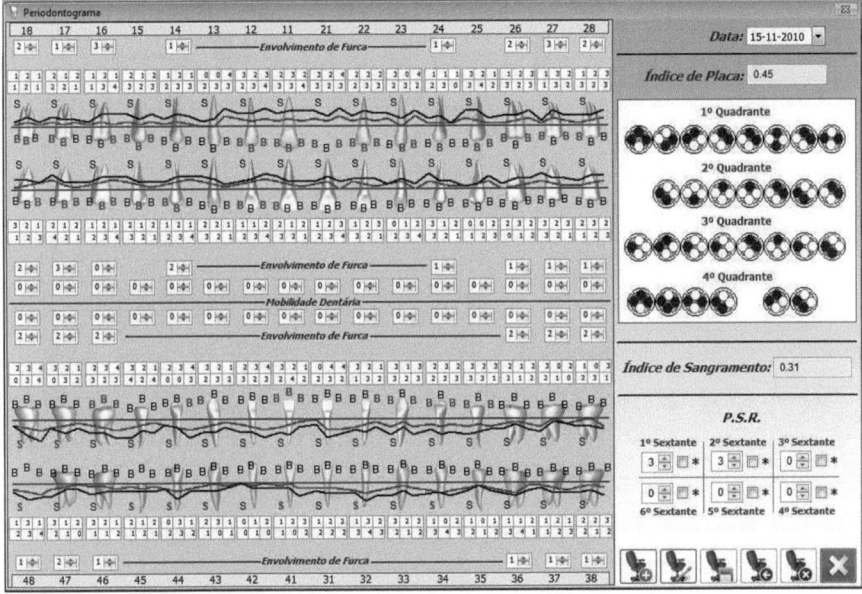

Fig. 5.9 Newsoft Dente® periogram (with permission)

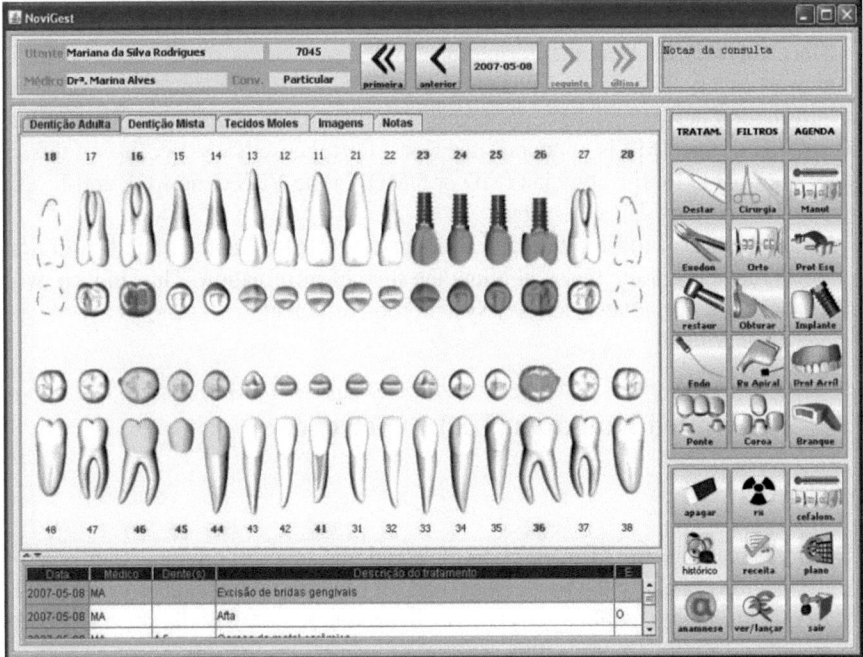

Fig. 5.10 Novigest® odontogram (with permission)

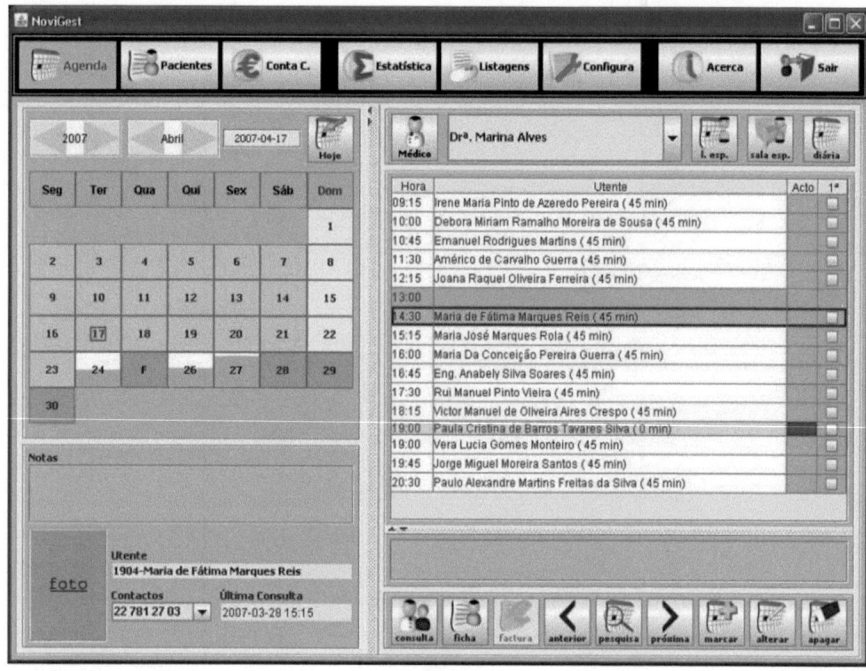

Fig. 5.11 Novigest® e-agenda (with permission)

Since there is no Dental Information Model defined by the Portuguese legal framework, every PMS company develops its own software, preventing the exchange of information between distinct packages. In addition, the information contained in the e-OHR of this PMS is not connected to the Portuguese NHS. Because of this, it is not impossible for the clinician (MD or DMD) in the NHS to now the oral-health status of his patient, and vice-versa.

It will be task of those interested in integrating medical and dental data to first establish the appropriate that will allow the flow of information. This, in turn, will likely make the Portuguese delivery system more efficient.

5.4 The United Kingdom (UK) Experience

Angus W.G. Walls

The theoretical benefits of integration of dental and medical clinical records were clearly demonstrated by the pioneering work of Mason and colleagues in the 1990s (Mason et al. 1994; Haughney et al. 1998; Jones et al. 1999). Sadly there has been no significant development in this area subsequently despite the increased awareness of bidirectional relationships between oral and systemic health.

The reasons for this are unclear but are probably based in two distinct challenges:

Firstly, there is no single electronic record of patient medical care in the UK. Each care provider hosts their own electronic system and while there is a requirement for the capacity to share data in primary medical care (this allows patients to change their practitioner with minimal disruption), there is currently no similar requirement either in the secondary care sector or in dental practices. There isn't even a reliable method for one dentist's records, either paper or electronic to be transferred between dentists if a patient decides to change their practitioner. Most patient-retained information is in the form of paper records which are also likely to be out of date. Further patients do not have "ownership" of their personal health information; it is maintained for them by their medical and dental practitioners. There are some notable exceptions but these all revolve around hypersensitivity reactions and bleeding disorders rather than aspects of routine care.

Secondly, medical practitioners are employed by the NHS to provide the services they provide for patients, which are largely free at the point of delivery. Dental practitioners are largely self-employed undertaking a mixture of NHS and private care for patients. Even where practitioners share premises there is no linkage between practice lists and whilst the vast majority of people are registered with a general medical practitioner 30% of dentate adults in the UK only seek care when they are in pain rather for routine care and maintenance (Steele and O' Sullivan 2009). There is no incentive for either dental or medical practitioners to share data about patients, indeed under the UK's data protection legislation explicit consent would need to be sought from every patient to allow this to happen.

There are obvious benefits to such data sharing but differences in software, hardware and legislation make the obvious impractical.

References

Araújo S Segurança na Circulação de Informação Clínica. Department of Electrical and Computer Engineering. Porto, Master in Communication Networks and Services. Faculty of Engineering of the University of Porto. Master: 2007. p. 1–180.

Arredondo Velásquez EL; Gómez Cazares Luatani; Hernández Rodríguez JA, et al. Evaluación de los cirujanos dentistas que cumplen con los criterios del Expediente clinico según la Norma Oficial Mexicana NOM-168-SSA1-1998 "Expediente clínico" y la NOM-013-SSA2-1994. 2005. http://www.odontologia.iztacala.unam.mx/contenido/indice_oral_archivos/trab%coloq%20oral/html Accessed 25 Apr 2011.

Assembly of the Republic. Constitution of the Portuguese Republic – Seventh Revision. 2005. http://app.parlamento.pt/site_antigo/ingles/cons_leg/Constitution_VII_revisao_definitive.pdf Accessed 10 Nov 2011.

Baris E Reforming health care in Canada. Salud Publica Mex 1998; 40: 276–80. http://www.scielosp.org/pdf/spm/v40n3/Y0400309.pdf. Accessed 18 May 2011.

Barros PP, Machado SR. Money for nothing? The net costs of medical training. Health Care Manag Sci. 2010;13(3):234–55.

Barros PP, Simões JA. Portugal health system review. Health Syst Transit. 2007;9(5):1–140.

Bentes M, Dias C, Sakellarides C, Bankauskaite V. Health care systems in transition: Portugal. Copenhagen: The European Observatory on Health Care Systems; 2004.
Canada Health. Canada Health Infoway. 2011. https://www.infoway-inforoute.ca/. Accessed 24 May 2011.
Canadian Institute for Health Information. CIHI Home page. 2011. http://www.cihi.ca/. Accessed 24 May 2011.
Canadian Council on Integrated Health Care. Bridging the divide between public and private payer communities in Canada's Health Care System. 2009. http://www.ccih.ca/docs/CCIH_Paper_From_Isolation_to_Integration_February2009.pdf. Accessed 24 May 2011.
Canadian Council on Integrated Health Care. 2011 http://www.ccih.ca/. Accessed 24 May 2011.
Central Intelligence Agency. CIA world factbook. 2011. https://www.cia.gov/library/publications/the-world-factbook/geos/po.html. Accessed 26 May 2011.
Cowpe J, Plasschaert A, Harzer W, Vinkka-Puhakka H, Walmsley AD. Profile and competences for the graduating European dentist – update 2009. Eur J Dent Educ. 2010;14(4):193–202.
Dias R Computers use in the Dental Clinic (Utilização de computadores na clínica de Medicina Dentária). Dental Informatics (Informática Médico-Dentária). Viseu, Portuguese Catholic University (Universidade Católica Portuguesa). Master Degree in Dental Medicine: 2009. p. 107.
Dreher A, Gaston N, Martens P. Measuring globalisation gauging its consequences. New York: Springer; 2008.
Espanha R, Fonseca R (2010) Plano Nacional de Saúde 2011–2016. Tecnologias de Informação e Comunicação. Alto Comissariado da Saúde. 2010. p. 1–43.
European Commission. Benchmarking ICT use among General Practitioners in Europe – Final Report. Information Society and Media Directorate General; 2008.
European Commission. Semantic Interoperability for Better Health and Safer Healthcare, Research and Deployment Roadmap for Europe. Semantic Health Report; 2009.
Franklin D. The world in 2005. London: The Economist Intelligence Unit; 2004.
Gómez GR, Triana EJ. Guía de autoevaluación del expediente clínico Odontológico. Rev ADM. 2001;58(6):233–6.
González Barrón S, Rivera Cisneros AE, Tena Tamayo C, Sánchez González JM, Manuell Lee GR, Triana Estrada J, et al. Recomendaciones para mejorar la práctica odontológica. Comisión de Arbitraje médico. Rev ADM. 2004;61(3):109–16.
Government of Portugal. Office of the Assistant Secretary of State and Health – Order n. 16159/2010 (in Portuguese); 2010.
Haughney MG, Devennie JC, Macpherson LM, Mason DK. Integration of primary care dental and medical services: a three-year study. Br Dent J. 1998;184(7):343–7.
Health System Central Administration. RSE – Registo de Saúde Electrónico. R1: Documento de Estado da Arte (in Portuguese); 2009. p. 1–130.
Health System Central Administration. Health Information Directory. 2010. http://www.acs.min-saude.pt/dis/bases-de-dados/. Accessed 9 Apr 2011.
Jones R, McConville J, Mason D, Macpherson L, Naven L, McEwen J. Attitudes towards, and utility of, an integrated medical-dental patient-held record in primary care. Br J Gen Pract. 1999;49(442):368–73.
Institute for Economics and Peace. Global peace index GPI map 2010. Sydney, Australia: Institute for Economics and Peace; 2010.
Instituto Nacional de Estadistica. Censos 2001. Resultados definitivos. Lisboa, Portugal, Instituto Nacional de Estatística; 2002.
ISSSTE. "Proceso de despliege del expediente clínico electrónico", Issstemed, Dirección Médica, Internal Communication; 2009.
Insurance Direct Canada. 2011. http://www.medicalhealthplans.com/. Accessed 24 May 2011.
Kravitz A, Treasure E. Portugal. Manual of Dental Practice. Council of European Dentist; 2008. p. 287–96.
Mason DK, Gibson J, Devennie JC, Haughney MG, Macpherson LM. Integration of primary care dental and medical services: a pilot investigation. Br Dent J. 1994;177(8):283–6.

Medical Education Center (FMUP) Relatório – Acerca da concretização dos objectivos do Processo de Bolonha. Faculty of Medicine of the University of Porto; 2010. p. 1–58.

Ministry of Health. Order n. 301/2009 (in Portuguese). Diário da República 1ª Série(58); 2009. p. 1858–60.

Ministry of Health. Sistema de Informação – Novo Programa Nacional de Promoção da Saúde Oral (in Portuguese); 2008. p. 1–97.

Ministry of Health. Relatório anual sobre o acesso a cuidados de saúde no SNS (in Portuguese); 2010. p. 13–23.

Mount Sinai Hospital Joseph and Wolf Lebovic Health Complex. Wasser Pain Management Center. 2011. http://www.mountsinai.on.ca/care/pain_management. Accessed 24 May 2011.

National Institute for Geography Statistics and Informatics. http://www.inegi.org.mx/. Accessed 25 Apr 2011.

Norma Oficial Mexicana. NOM 013-SSA-1994, Diario Oficial de la Federación. 1995. Published: Jan 21, 1995.

Oliver R, Kersten H, Oliver R, Kersten H, Vinkka-Puhakka H, Alpasan G, et al. Curriculum structure: principles and strategy. Eur J Dent Educ. 2008;12 Suppl 1:74–84.

OMD. Os Números da Ordem – Estatísticas (in Portuguese); 2010.

OMD. Ordem dos Médicos Dentistas / Portuguese Dental Association (in Portuguese); 2011a. http://www.omd.pt/. Accessed May 2011.

OMD. Tabela de Nomenclatura – Ordem dos Médicos Dentistas (in Portuguese). 2011b. http://doc.omd.pt/docs/nomenclatura/tabela.swf. Accessed May 2011.

Ontario Association for Dental Public Health. 2011. http://www.oaphd.on.ca/. Accessed 24 May 2011.

Ontario Association for Dental Public Health. 2011b http://www.oaphd.on.ca/index.php?option=com_content&view=article&id=54&Itemid=60. Accessed 24 May 2011.

Ontario Health Study. 2011 www.ontariohealthstudy.ca. Accessed 15 Apr 2011.

Plasschaert AJ, Holbrook WP, Delap E, Martinez C, Walmsley AD, Association for Dental Education in Europe, Profile and competences for the European dentist. Eur J Dent Educ. 2005;9(3):98–107.

Plasschaert AJ, Lindh C, McLoughlin J, Manogue M, Murtomaa H, Nattestad A, et al. Curriculum structure and the European Credit Transfer System for European dental schools: part I. Eur J Dent Educ. 2006;10(3):123–30.

Plasschaert AJ, Manogue M, Lindh C, McLoughlin J, Murtomaa H, Nattestad A, et al. Curriculum content, structure and ECTS for European dental schools. Part II: methods of learning and teaching, assessment procedures and performance criteria. Eur J Dent Educ. 2007;11(3):125–36.

Portuguese Government. Programa do XVII Governo Constitucional (in Portuguese); 2009–2013. p. 78.

Portuguese Medical Association. Estatísticas Nacionais – Distribuição por Especialidade, Idade e Sexo – 2009. Portal Oficial da Ordem dos Médicos (in Portuguese). 2009. https://www.ordemdosmedicos.pt/. Accessed May 2011.

Portuguese Medical Association. Colégios – Especialidades (in Portuguese). 2011. https://www.ordemdosmedicos.pt/. Accessed May 2011.

Royal College of Dental Surgeons of Ontario. Diagnosis and Management Temporomandibular Disorders and related Musculoskeletal Disorders. 2009. http://rcdso.org/pdf/guidelines/Guidelines_TMD_Jul09.pdf. Accessed 24 May 2011.

Rowe A, García-Barbero M. Regulation and licensing of physicians in the WHO European Region, World Health Organization Europe; 2005.

Secretaria de Salud. Ley General de Salud. Reglamento de la Ley General de Salud en materia de Prestación de Servicios de Atención Medica. Secretaria de Salud. Diario Oficial de la Federación. 1984. Published: Feb 7, 1984.

Steele J., O' Sullivan I. Executive summary. Adult Dental Health Survey 2009. London: The Health and Social Care Information Centre; 2009. p. 21.

Tapia Vázquez JL. El expediente clínico electrónico. Rev Odontol Mex. 2010;14(2):76–7.

United Nations. Human development report 2010: overcoming barriers: human mobility and development. Basingstoke: Palgrave Macmillan; 2010.

Villarreal-Levy G (2007) Expediente Clínico Electrónico, Comunicación de la Subsecretaría de Innovación y Calidad Dirección General de Información en Salud. Programa Nacional de Salud. 2007–2012; 2007.

Vivanco-Cedeño B. La realidad de la historia clínica odontológica. Rev ADM. 2009;65(1):10–4.

Webster PC. The rise of open-source electronic health records. Lancet. 2011;377(9778):1641–2.

Chapter 6
An Integrated Medical-Dental Electronic Health Record Environment: A Marshfield Experience

Amit Acharya, Natalie Yoder, and Greg Nycz

6.1 Rationale and Need to Articulate Medical and Dental Data

National investments in biomedical science and other scientific studies are helping us to better understand the interrelationships between oral and systemic disease. The large number of interrelationships being studied suggests that medicine's historic neglect of the oral cavity and dentistry's limited understanding of systemic nature should be addressed. While the emerging science base has implications for medical and dental training programs, it is important to consider approaches to facilitate translation and adoption of scientific advances by those currently practicing in dentistry and medicine.

Techniques that support better integration, not only hold the promise of improved care for patients, but the application of emerging knowledge on oral systemic interactions that improve patient care simultaneously elevates the value of national investments in scientific discovery.

Strategies to support care for oral and systemic disease in a more coordinated fashion, and to enable more rapid translation of future scientific discoveries in this area are needed. A promising approach would be to facilitate better collaboration through seamless communication between dental and medical providers. The use of integrated medical-dental electronic health record technology by clinicians from both disciplines would allow bidirectional access to relevant patient information enabling a more comprehensive approach to their overall health care treatment and prevention needs. The potential to deploy decision support tools and to modify those tools as new discoveries are made has great potential to both shorten the time between discovery and adoption, and improve population health outcomes.
– *Greg Nycz, National Institutes of Health Director's Council of Public Representatives*

A. Acharya (✉)
Biomedical Informatics Research Center, Marshfield Clinic Research Foundation, Marshfield, WI, USA

N. Yoder
Biomedical Informatics Research Center, Marshfield Clinic Research Foundation, Marshfield, WI, USA

G. Nycz
Family Health Center of Marshfield, Inc, Marshfield, WI, USA

6.2 Marshfield Clinic – A Pioneer in the Development of an Integrated Medical-Dental Electronic Health Record Environment

6.2.1 Introduction

Established in 1916, Marshfield Clinic in Wisconsin (WI) is one of the largest multi-specialty group practices in the Unite States. Marshfield Clinic currently employs approximately 780 physicians representing 84 different specialties and 6,500 additional staff working on the main campus in Marshfield, WI or one of 54 regional clinics serving the population of Northern, Central, and Western Wisconsin, and the Upper Peninsula of Michigan. The Marshfield Clinic records over 3.4 million patient encounters annually. The Marshfield Clinic, a not-for-profit 501(c) (3) tax-exempt organization, has developed this regional system of care structure to address the health needs of the rural population. Marshfield Clinic works closely with St. Joseph's Hospital (a 524-bed acute care facility), providing primary, secondary, and tertiary care for individuals regardless of financial status. Marshfield Clinic maintains a joint electronic medical record system with St. Joseph's Hospital, including computerized diagnostic files dating back to 1963 (Fig. 6.1).

6.2.2 Electronic Health Record at Marshfield Clinic

The Marshfield Clinic also has an impressive track record in applied Clinical Informatics. The internally-developed Electronic Health Record (EHR) is one of the oldest and most comprehensive in the country, containing coded diagnoses data back to 1960, with other coded data and digital documents back to the mid-1980s. Through the development of the Medical Event Coding by Clinicians Application (MECCA) system, Marshfield Clinic has several decades of experience in the use of coded terminology in an EHR. In addition, the EHR contains roughly 70 million text documents. Marshfield Clinic provides an unique environment for informatics research and has been the perfect laboratory to develop new tools for clinicians and their staff. Marshfield Clinic physicians have been routinely using computers as a part of every patient encounter for over a decade. Marshfield Clinic develops much of its own clinical software, allowing new ideas to be implemented quickly. With the introduction of hand-held wireless tablet PCs, Marshfield Clinic was among the first health care providers in the country to put electronic medical record truly at the source of health care decisions – in physicians' hands (Fig. 6.2).

6.2.3 Integrated Medical-Dental Electronic Health Record Environment

As an early adopter, Marshfield Clinic, with financial support from Delta Dental of Wisconsin and Family Health Center, integrated dental clinical and practice management functions into its comprehensive, proprietary electronic health record

6 An Integrated Medical-Dental Electronic Health Record Environment

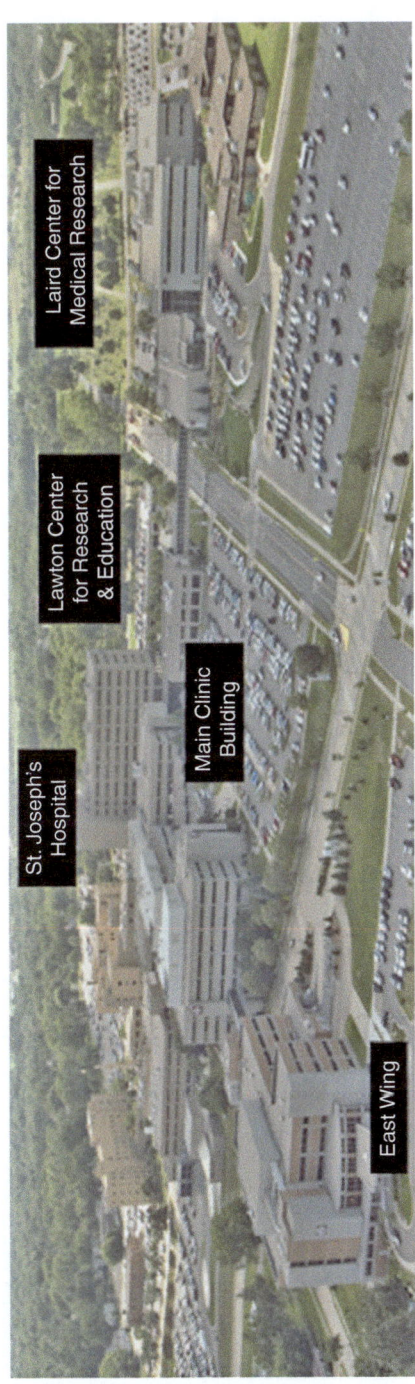

Fig. 6.1 Marshfield Clinic Health Center Complex

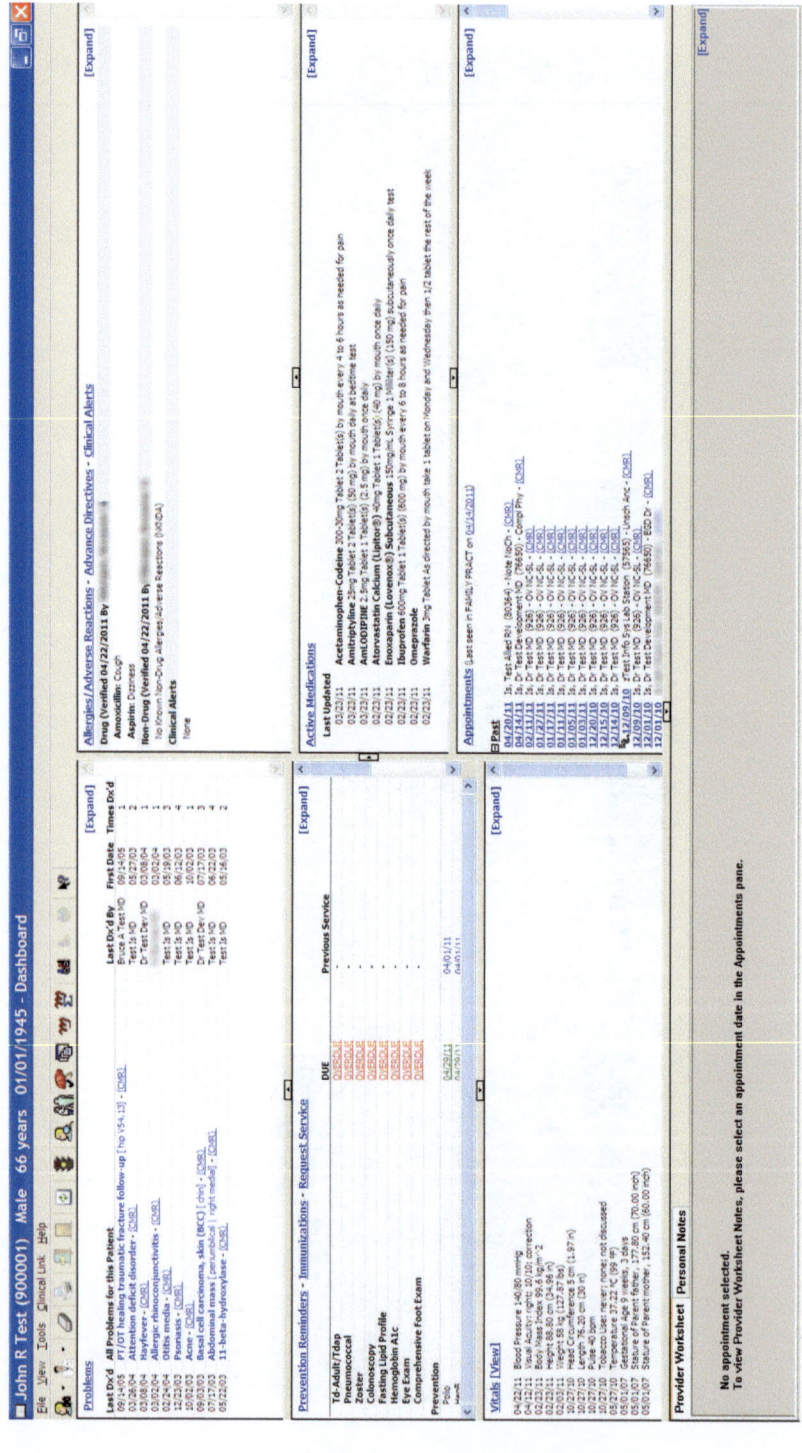

Fig. 6.2 Physicians' Dashboard application

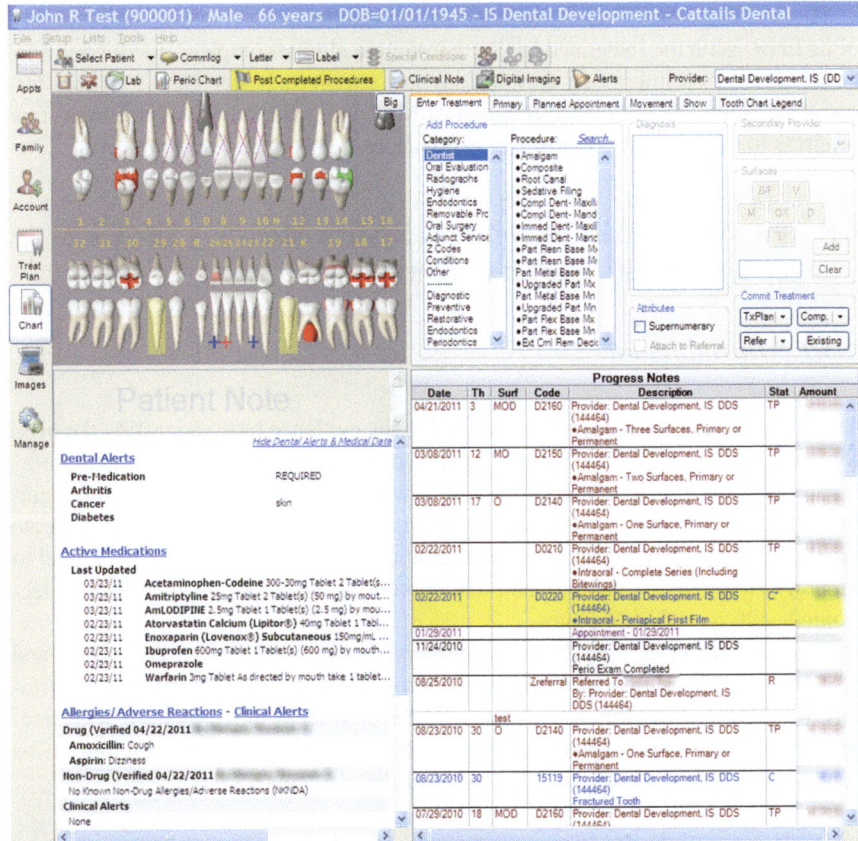

Fig. 6.3 Dentists' Dashboard application

known as CattailsMD™. With medical/dental diagnoses, hospital information, imaging studies such as X-rays, prescription information, as well as potential drug interactions all available at the touch of a button, Marshfield Clinic clinicians have in their hands the information needed to make the best clinical decisions. The dental module, CattailsDental, has been successfully implemented in all seven Marshfield Clinic dental centers. CattailsDental is based on an open-source dental software platform, Open Dental of Salem, Oregon.

The integrated medical-dental EHR system was designed primarily for Marshfield Clinic physicians and dentists to access and share patient health information. CattailsDental includes a dental dashboard (Fig. 6.3); workflow management tools including tooth charting, periodontal charting and treatment planning; access to centralized medications, allergies, special conditions, problems list, demographics and HIPAA forms; access to medical appointments to support better coordination of care; and highly secure remote access supporting devices such as laptops and computer tablets.

Historically, Marshfield Clinic has focused efforts on maximizing the capability of its EHR. With the Integrated EHR environment almost complete, attention is now being focused on improving decision support at point-of-care. This is an area targeted for improvement by the Institute of Medicine, who has recognized that true progress in this arena is possible due to advances in informatics technology.

6.3 Fit Within Existing Delivery System Models – The Case of Community Health Centers

6.3.1 Introduction

The research community continues to add to the evidence base suggesting the need for better integration between medicine and dentistry. Emerging advances in information technologies hold the promise of new tools that can facilitate such integration. Given that dentistry and medicine in the United State largely remain separate entities, an important question is whether a market demand is present at a level to properly stimulate the creation and deployment of integrated medical-dental electronic health record technology.

Who, for instance, might be early adopters? Within the United States a large and growing federally supported primary care program may represent the best opportunity for creating the demand for software developers to move forward with integrated products. These potential early adopters are generically referred to as *"community health centers" or "federally qualified health centers."*

6.3.2 History of the Community Health Center Model

The community health center model with its' emphasis on community control, equitable access to comprehensive primary care services, and an interest in improving the health of communities is present in many countries. Within the United States the community health center program was born out of the 'War on Poverty', which had its roots in the Kennedy and Johnson Administrations (Lefkowitz 2007).

The first two community health centers were launched in an urban public housing project called Columbia Point in Boston and in rural Mound Bayou, Mississippi. Key architects of the program were Dr. Jack Geiger and Dr. Count Gibson of Tufts University. The inspiration for the comprehensive primary care center model came from a Rockefeller Foundation Fellowship that brought Dr. Jack Geiger to South Africa in 1957 during his senior year at Western Reserve Medical School. In South Africa, Dr. Geiger worked with Sidney and Emily Kark at a health center that they had established in a 500 square mile Zulu Tribal Reserve. The Kark's had established 40 such community health centers throughout South Africa to attend to the health of the African workers. It was this experience that was the inspiration for the first two health centers in the United States in 1965.

After some experimentation, the 94th Congress amended Public Law 94-63 on July 29, 1975 creating Section 330 of the Public Health Service Act, establishing a statutory template for community health centers. When implementing regulations were passed in 1976 mandatory services were defined to be diagnostic, treatment, consultative, referral and other services rendered by physicians, diagnostic laboratory services and diagnostic radiologic services, preventive health services, emergency medical services, transportation services and preventive dental services. Although not mandated, health centers could apply to provide supplemental health services, which included dental services other than those provided as primary health services (i.e., preventive dental services). It is significant that this early legislation recognized that at least preventive dental services should be incorporated within the primary health care service set.

Twenty-four years later in the year 2000, the Surgeon General of the U.S. Public Health Service published the first-ever comprehensive report on Oral Health in America. The preface boldly announced: "we know that the mouth reflects general health and well-being." The report also noted that "those who suffer the worst oral health are found among the poor of all ages with poor children and poor older Americans particularly vulnerable" (US Department of Health and Human Services 2000). The very same populations are served by community health centers. At the time of the report, there were 730 community health centers providing services to approximately 9,600,158 people. 8,606,022 people received medical services and 1,329,655 people received dental services. Given that the principle target population for health centers was underserved minorities and low-income individuals and families, the health center program was seen as a potential resource to address the disparities highlighted in the Surgeon General's report.

In 2003, the National Call to Action to promote oral health was issued under the leadership of the Office of Surgeon General. The Call to Action was described as "...an invitation to expand plans, activities, and programs designed to promote oral health and prevent disease, especially to reduce the health disparities that affect members of racial and ethnic groups, poor people, many who are geographically isolated, and others who are vulnerable because of special oral health care needs" (US Department of Health and Human Services 2003). The partners in this effort included the National Association of Community Health Centers. For the year in which the Call to Action was made, the Nation's community health centers had grown to serve 11,014,677 medical patients and 1,885,359 dental patients.

Between 2001 and 2006 the community health center program underwent a major expansion under a special initiative of President George W. Bush. At the start of the President's initiative a shift in federal policy was implemented to assure that all new community health center sites would have a comprehensive oral health component (BPHC PIN 2001-18). This policy shift helped to assure that the Nation's community health centers would be more actively engaged in oral health service delivery. To further accelerate the development of oral health programs among existing community health centers without them, the Health Resources and Services Administration offered numerous oral health service expansion grant opportunities over the course of the expansion period.

Both Healthy People 2010 and Healthy People 2020 initiatives prioritized improvements in the number of community health centers having a dental component. Baseline data for the 2010 plan indicated "by the late 1990's nearly 60% of community-based health centers had a dental component." The target for these centers and local health departments was 75%. The 2020 plan listed as its' baseline for 2007, 75% of federally qualified health centers having had an oral health component and listed as its' target for 2020, 83% of such health centers having an oral health component.

By 2009 there were 1,131 community health centers providing services at 7,900 locations. Total medical patients served reached 16,166,416. Total dental patients served reached 3,438,340. The percent of dental to medical patients stood at 15.5% in 2000 when the Surgeon General's report was released. It rose to 17.1% in the year of the Call to Action. Following the Presidential Initiative it reached 21.3% in 2009.

The Patient Protection and Affordable Care Act of 2010 provided $11 billion in mandatory spending to further expand the Nation's community health center network. The National Association of Community Health Centers set a goal of 40 million people served by community health centers following the 5 years of mandatory federal spending. With a growing proportion of community health centers offering comprehensive primary care services including oral health and with a rapidly expanding number of community health centers assured as part of America's health reform plan, the Nation's community health centers represent a growing market for Electronic Health Records (EHR) that fully integrate medical and dental, clinical and administrative systems.

The most recent survey data on EHR adoption in community health centers is from 2009. The results indicate for the 362 health centers surveyed, that 49% of respondents were using an EHR and were either "all electronic" (23%) or "part paper and part electronic" (26%) (Lardiere 2009). While not all community health centers have adopted EHRs in 2010, the pace of EHR adoption is accelerating and special provisions providing incentives for meaningful use of EHR will help to accelerate that pace.

6.4 Family Health Center of Marshfield, Inc. – A Pioneer in the Adoption of Integrated Medical-Dental Electronic Health Record

Family Health Center of Marshfield, Inc. began providing services to underserved populations in the northern section of the State of Wisconsin, United States as a federally funded health center in March of 1974. Dental services for children and preventive dental services for adult patients of Family Health Center were managed through a contract network with local dentists. Beginning the 1980s and throughout the 1990s the contract network began to fail with a growing number of dentists refusing to renew their contracts. During this same period the State of Wisconsin's Medicaid agency experienced a decline in dentist participation in the Medicaid program.

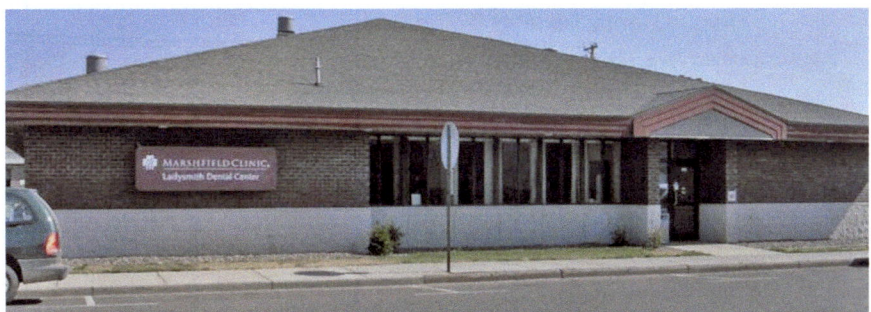

Fig. 6.4 Ladysmith Dental Center – Family Health Center of Marshfield, Inc. and Marshfield Clinic's first Dental Center

Following publication of the Surgeon General's Oral Health Report and a 2001 strategic planning meeting by the Family Health Center Board, improving oral health access for low-income residents of the service area was prioritized. Family Health Center opened its' first dental center in November 2002 (Fig. 6.4).

The new center was immediately inundated with patients, many with very significant dental disease. Many patients with dental emergencies drove in excess of 100 miles to obtain care. In the first full year of operation the center served over 5,500 patients from 45 of Wisconsin's 72 counties (Fig. 6.5).

After gaining experience with oral health service delivery a second larger dental center was opened in 2007, along with a small center in Owen, Wisconsin. Together these three centers housed 17 dentists and 19 hygienists. Early in 2007, at the request of the Secretary of the Department of Health Services, a comprehensive 10 year plan was drafted to outline how our State's oral health access problems could be positively addressed by its' federally funded community health centers. The plan called for the rapid expansion of the State's community health centers' dental capacity, and the creation of a second dental school as a partnership between Marshfield Clinic and Family Health Center of Marshfield, Inc. Family Health Center opened a third large (5 dentist/6 hygienist) dental center in March of 2008. As progress on the dental school continued, Family Health Center committed to both increase the pace of the dental center expansion and to install dedicated clinical training and classroom space in all of its new dental centers (Fig. 6.6).

By the end of 2010 the smaller center in Owen, Wisconsin was closed following the opening of a larger center nearby. With 7 centers operational, 34,293 patients were seen in 2010 (Fig. 6.7).

As the pace of expansion grew, Family Health Center's leadership recognized that its' goals of: (1) reversing oral health access disparities; (2) eliminating oral health disease disparities; and (3) integrating medicine and dentistry could not be reached without the continued growth of dental capacity, coupled with an approach that would facilitate virtual teaming across medicine and dentistry. As additional dental centers were built, Family Health Center sought and received help from Delta Dental of Wisconsin in the form of $500,000 donation that would be matched with

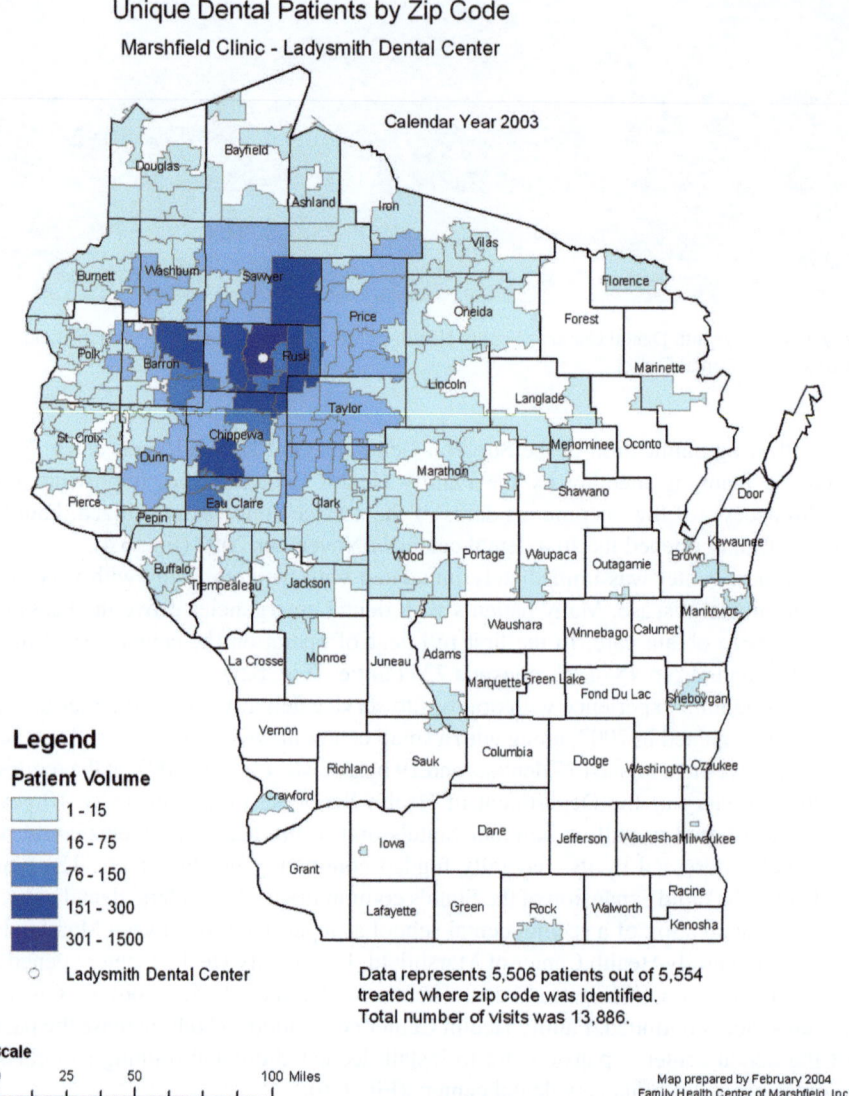

Fig. 6.5 Unique dental patients at Ladysmith Dental Center after first full year of operation (calendar year 2003)

$400,000 from Family Health Center to support Family Health Center's partner, Marshfield Clinic, in adapting their advanced electronic health record system to fully incorporate, on both clinical and administrative levels, our dental operations. The fully integrated electronic record was implemented at all of Family Health Center's dental centers in March 2010.

As new dental centers were built patients who had been traveling significant distances for care at an older clinic were transferred to the new center closer to their residence. This

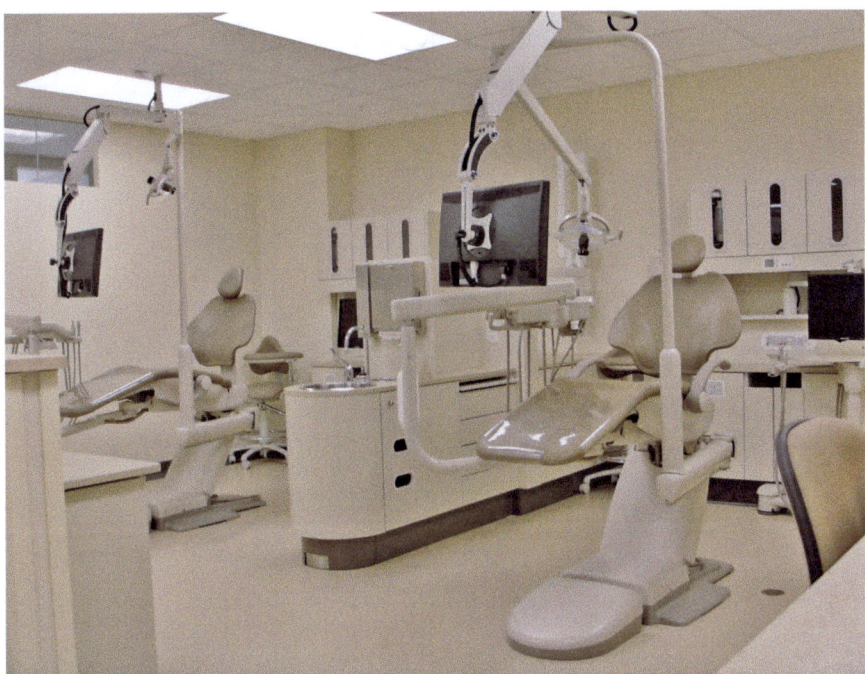

Fig. 6.6 Dedicated clinical training space at Marshfield Dental Center

created opportunities to serve more patients from the immediate area of the older center, increasing the penetration of the target population (Fig. 6.8).

The Health Resources and Services Administration has helped to define the community health center model as providing comprehensive primary care where primary care spans medical, behavioral and oral health disciplines. Fueled by national investments in science, the growing evidence base on oral systemic disease and treatment relationships strongly suggest the need to refine our education and delivery systems to accommodate this new evidence by developing better integration and closer working relationships between dentists and physicians. The investment Family Health Center made with support from Delta Dental of Wisconsin in fully integrating its electronic medical and dental records was done to achieve a number of important objectives. On the practice management side integration would promote efficiency and patient centeredness by allowing appointments to be linked across medicine and dentistry, saving transportation time and improving convenience for the patients while helping to boost compliance with preventive visits and reduce no-shows. From a quality of care perspective, safety could be enhanced by sharing information on the prescription drugs patients were using and their drug allergies. For frail patients or patients with multiple medical conditions, access to the medical record assists FHC's dentists in developing comprehensive treatment plans.

For Family Health Center to be successful in addressing its goals related to access and oral health disparities as it expands its' dental capacity, it must more heavily

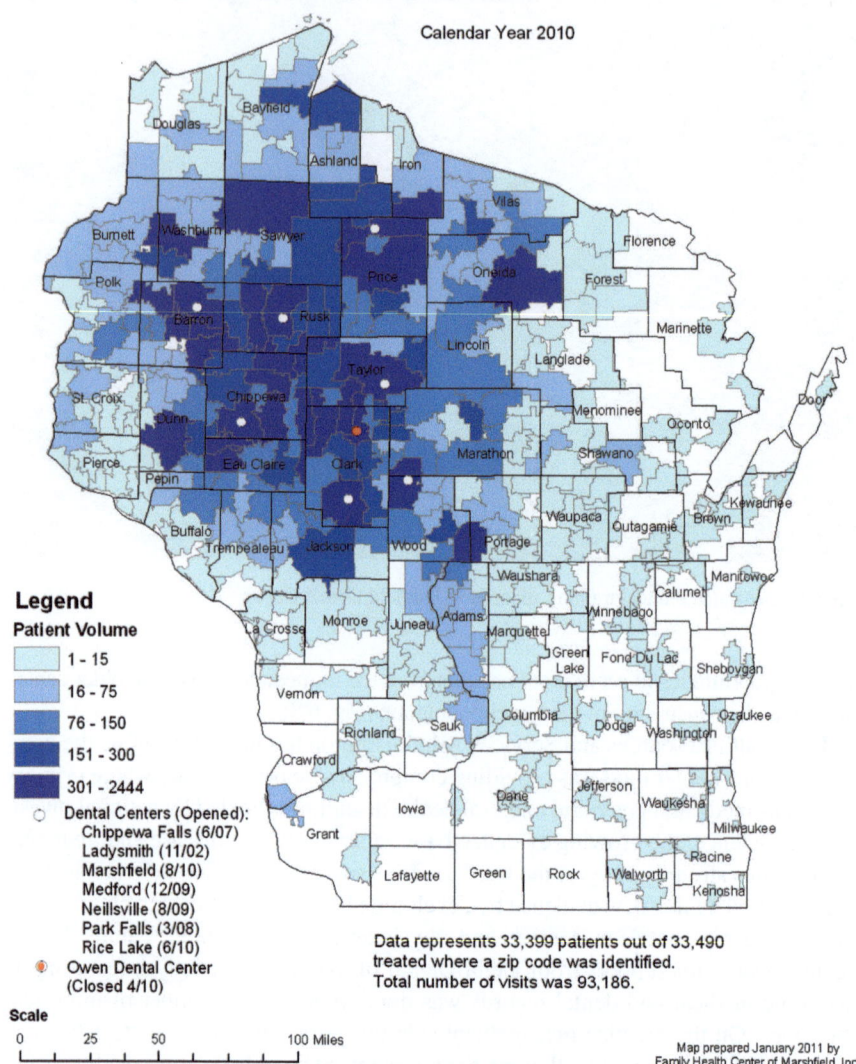

Fig. 6.7 Unique dental patients at all of Marshfield Clinic Dental Centers in the 2010 calendar year

rely on the integrative record platform. The development of decision tools physicians can use to identify patients lacking dental care enables them to address patient oral health literacy issues and facilitate referral into dental care. This in turn will allow earlier less costly dental intervention and orient our target population to preventive services and good daily oral hygiene habits.

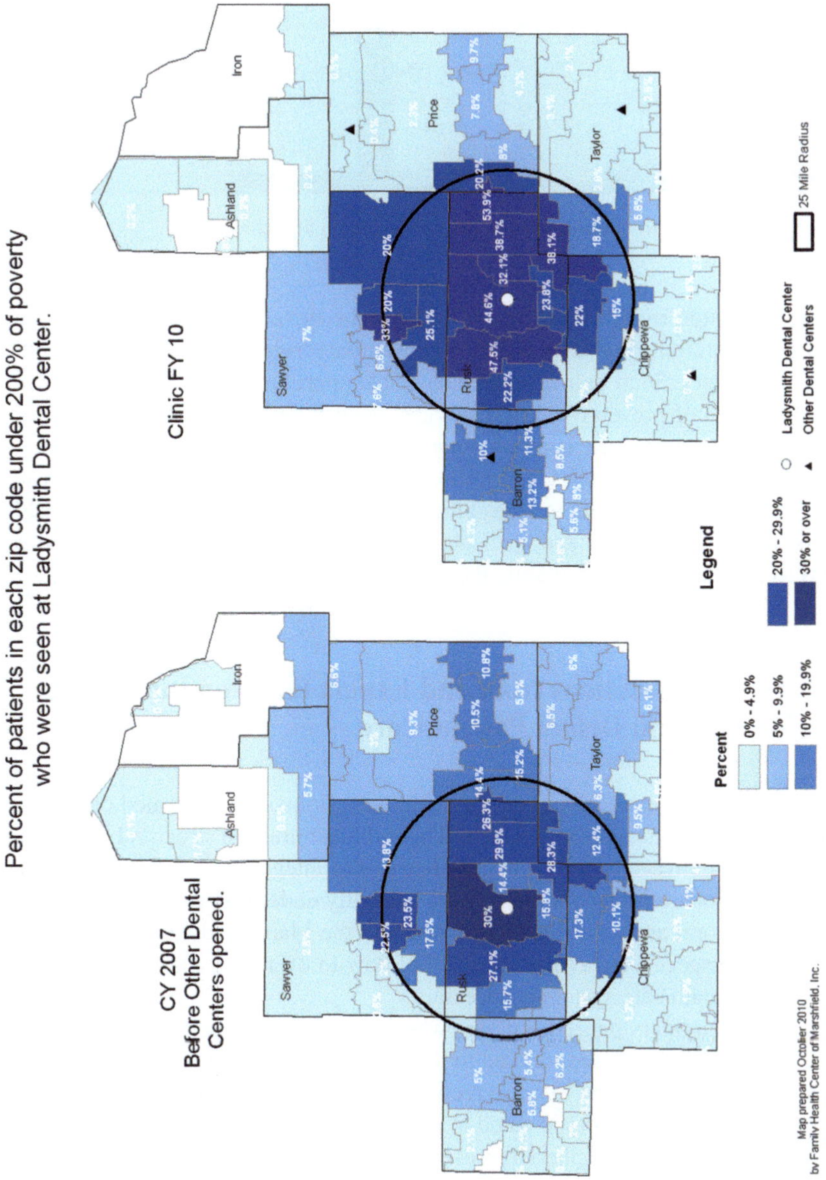

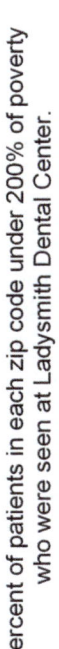

Fig. 6.8 Percent of patients in each zip code under 200% poverty who were seen at Ladysmith Dental Center

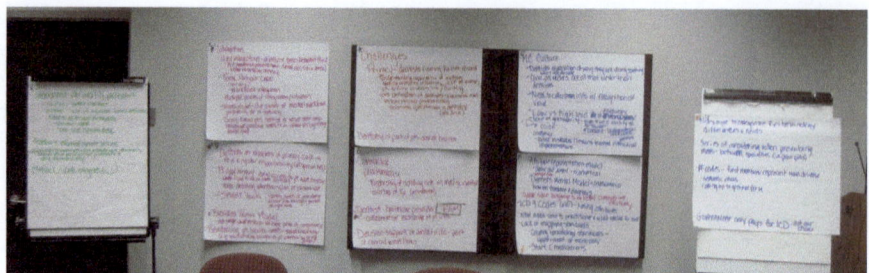

Fig. 6.9 Key concepts from the discussion panel recorded on flips charts

The integrated record platform will allow the development of bidirectional decision support tools to improve clinical preventive service provision in both medicine and dentistry. Such bidirectional decision support would enable physicians to remind patients of preventive dental services needed while dentists could support physician efforts in the provision of clinical preventive services, such as mammography, immunization, pap tests, and well-child exams. Once such improvements are achieved it will be important to spread these capabilities to other community health centers, increasing the demand, as health centers themselves grow, for integrative record technologies and stimulating the market to produce them.

6.5 Recommendations from and Expert Panel on Integrating Medical and Dental Patient Care

The division of the medical and dental health care domains has created deep roots in the United States health care systems. This solid cultural and structural separation of health care delivery poses significant barriers to integrating medical and dental patient care. However, many initiatives are currently under way to achieve cohesive integration of oral and systemic health care and the Marshfield Clinic is clearly a leader in this aspect. Further investigation of how to overcome these hurdles at all levels of the health care system is necessary.

An interdisciplinary panel discussion was held at the Marshfield Clinic on March 7, 2011 to identify key issues related to the integration of medical and dental care, education, and research and to make recommendations to address these challenges. Fourteen expert panelists participated in the panel discussion, including the co-editors of this book. The members represented a variety of research, education and health care subspecialties including dentistry, genomics, epidemiology, and biomedical, clinical, imaging and dental informatics.

A dental informatics scientist, also an editor of the book, chaired the panel. An usability analyst wrote key concepts on flips charts during the discussion for the panel to reference and review. The panel lasted approximately 1 h and 45 min (Fig. 6.9).

The session was audio recorded and transcribed for further analysis. A modified grounded theory approach was used to analyze the content of the discussion.

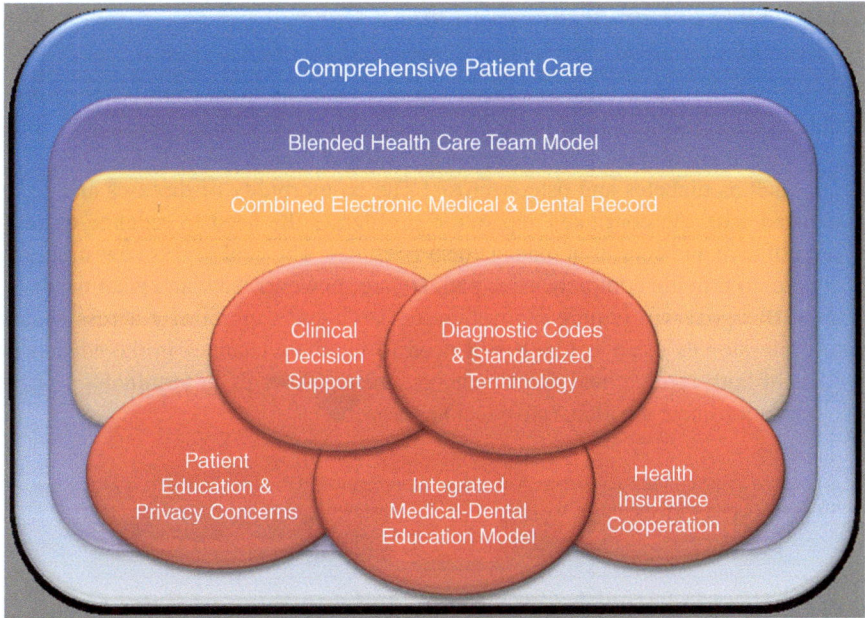

Fig. 6.10 Overarching themes identified as part of the panel discussion analysis

Grounded theory is a thematic analysis method used to identify, analyze and report patterns in qualitative data. The method was used to deconstruct the transcript into key words and phrases and then used to visualize and identify important concepts. These concepts and phrases built overarching themes identifying issues and recommendations for integrating medical and dental patient care. An iterative analysis of the transcript was utilized to allow flexible refinement and reinterpretation of the themes. These themes are described in the sections to follow (Fig. 6.10).

6.5.1 Acceptance of a Combined Electronic Medical and Dental Record

Panel members recognized that combining medical and dental electronic records is an essential component to successfully integrating the two streams of patient care. They discussed how the division of patient data leads to patient safety risks, such as adverse reactions to medication, and communication gaps between dental and medical providers. On the other hand, the group also acknowledged that this huge step comes with a set of challenges to address prior to fully integrating electronic patient health records.

Quote#1
… the informatics piece could actually make that happen pretty seamlessly if you're all on the same record system.

6.5.2 Shift to Comprehensive Patient Care

Members of the panel fully embraced the bidirectional connection between oral health care and medical health care for the rest of the body. More specifically, they discussed the significant relationship of periodontal conditions with systemic diseases, such as diabetes and osteonecrosis. The co-morbidity of diseases and risks associated with the continued separation proliferate the need to redefine current system of care and condition management practices. The goal of this new structure is simple, to provide comprehensive patient care; however, how and what needs to achieve this goal will require innovation, research and commitment across health care professionals in all fields. It will need to facilitate changes in the education models of both medical and dental schools, create standards in terminology mapping and coordinate a collaborative team approach.

Quote#2
There are some conditions such as, you know, you mentioned diabetes where it is truly easy to connect one with the other, we don't want the treatment effect one has on the other.

6.5.3 Blended Health Care Team Model to Support Total Care of Patient

The panel collectively emphasized cultivating a blended team model to unify the concept of comprehensive patient care. A collaborative framework that combines the strengths of each provider has great potential to overcome some of the challenges of integrating dentistry and medicine, as well as, delivering high quality health care more effectively and efficiently. They discussed a shared responsibility in the overall care of a patient across all medical and dental specialties. This would entail a role in creating patient awareness of necessary preventive health care services and mutual reinforcement of health concerns and interventions. One member gave an example of a dentist taking the opportunity to intervene in the reduction of the consumption of soft drinks for a patient with osteoporosis and presenting extensive caries and lower bone levels.

Several members noted that this workforce integration will require a structured approach with defined roles as to who intervenes and when. On the other hand, they also expressed concerns about the lack of time for providers to coordinate efforts and the risk of increasing providers' mental workload. The group further described potential solutions through an integrated electronic medical and dental patient record. For example, it could help facilitate quick and easy communication between dental and medical providers, provide a simple display of patient's combined medical and dental appointment history and present a merged list of preventive care reminders. One panelist described this as "virtual teaming."

Quote#3
Think of how working together we can achieve much greater penetration in providing clinical preventive services across both of those disciplines if they both reinforced each other.

Quote#4
But I think it's too much to ask physicians or dentists to really do a good job on that unless there's some sort of structured way of helping them know when they should engage and when they don't have to engage.

6.5.4 Clinical Decision Support

The concept of clinical decision support was reflected in discussions on integrating patient records, attaining a collaborative blended team, standardizing terminology and establishing evidence based dentistry. For example, a combined systemic and oral electronic preventive care reminder list empowers medical and dental providers to take part in making a patient aware of relevant services. Another member proposed the development of a "smart tool" with a comprehensive ontology that could interpret almost any free text entry and transform the data for optimal exchange and interoperability.

Panel members noted that clinical decision support in dentistry has limitations. They explained that there is a lack of oral health data to establish evidence based practice; a panelist noted part of the issue is due to the failure to collect the reason for treatment. Panelists sharing this perspective identified collecting a diagnostic code will help facilitate more research to establish thresholds and enable the use of the data to reduce treatment variability.

The panel described several characteristics of an effective clinical decision support system to support the integration of oral and systemic care. They emphasized the importance of seamless integration with providers' workflow and good usability. With substantial differences in the cognitive workflow between dental and medical providers, a system needs to accommodate the diversity and manage the information accordingly, including content, data granularity and task flow. Careful consideration of users' mental model and avoiding information overload on screens are keys to success. The next section further discusses the issues associated with diagnostic codes and data management.

Quote#5
Software could also be helpful in terms of looking at when was the last time a dental exam was done, are there any diagnosable oral health issues, and this may also impact upon the use of chemotherapy as well in terms of making it part of the routine of the workflow, to make sure that the dental health is attended to before these drugs are prescribed.

6.5.5 Diagnostic Codes and Standardized Terminology

The panel revealed that currently dentists are not comfortable working with diagnostic codes because documenting a patient diagnosis is not a normal part of their workflow. Moreover, there is no drive for dentistry to add an extra step to providers' busy workflow since it is not required for the reimbursement of dental services. Besides, there is no standard set of diagnostic codes for dentistry to utilize. Consequently, the failure to collect diagnostic codes for treatment creates barriers to obtaining oral health data needed for good research and quality improvement, as well as communication gaps preventing collaboration that would be beneficial for the total care of a patient.

There was common agreement that implementing the documentation of diagnostic codes in dentistry would be met with resistance. To help facilitate acceptance, the group discussed a variety of recommendations in the development and adoption of dental diagnostic codes. Most predominant was the concept of matching the mental model of dentists for both terminology and workflow integration. A panelist stated that dentists perceive the documentation of a dental treatment as equivalent to a diagnosis. Further, another panelist stated that dentists must recognize the value to entering a diagnosis since adding this task would not be balanced out by the removal of another.

On the other hand, there is not a universal vocabulary used throughout health care for patient documentation and order entry (e.g. medication). The lack of consistent data management and terminology mapping standards presents an enormous challenge when implementing clinical decision support and establishing interoperability of electronic records. A panel member discussed current limitations experienced with some of the ICD-9 codes, including lack of separation for certain diagnosis, loss of specificity and absence of plurality.

Panel members highlighted several considerations for standardized terminology. First, a panelist stated that government involvement is needed to intercede and enforce a controlled vocabulary. Second, the loss of specificity and failure to distinguish between certain diseases in diagnostic coding needs to be addressed. Furthermore, providing different levels of data granularity will be important in preventing information overload pushed on providers. This would involve managing the level of abstraction for patient data, such as appointment history and diagnoses, depending on the specialty or profile of the provider. However, this would not limit a provider's capability to seek out further detail if desired.

Quote#6
ICD is extremely limited, and very bizarre. It's a very bizarre, you know, nomenclature. For example, the two most common cancers in the human race both have the same code, basal cell skin cancer and squamous cell skin cancer.

6.5.6 Integrated Dental-Medical Education Model

The panel concluded that the culture of the current education models in dental and medical schools inhibit integration of the oral health and medical domains. The medical and dental education system plays a very important role in developing health care professionals' perception on how they see their own discipline, as well as other health care fields. These perceptions foster the artificial division of these streams of health care and contribute to the lack of inertia in establishing a blended health care team.

A panel member asserted that it is imperative to change the current curricula in dental and medical school to help facilitate an individual and cultural attitude shift. Such a transformation would have the potential to make the connection between dentistry and medicine more transparent. It would involve cross training of medical into dental schools and vice versa. Thus direct interaction between dental and medical students could flourish within the same environment, yielding a cohesive relationship of the disciplines. Furthermore, a coordinated education model would enable a controlled vocabulary to be instituted at the learning stage. This structure would help bridge the communication gap between medicine and dentistry.

Quote#7
If we are speaking the same language then our communications are effective, and then care is more effective, hence more cost effective and efficient.

6.5.7 Patient Education and Privacy Concerns

Panel members discussed patients' privacy concerns about their medical records being shared and viewed by dental providers and staff. This preempted notion is correlated to some patients' perception of dentistry as a business rather than a health care establishment. This cultural disconnect regarding dentistry would likely minimize dentists' access to medical information pertinent to the "total care" of patient and patient safety. The group recognized the need to be proactive at an earlier stage to overcome the culture barriers. They recommended that patients become more aware and educated on the integral role dentistry plays on their overall health and the connection between their dental and medical health care. This would include information on the benefits of granting dentists access to their medical record. One member suggested another component of this educational process is to include an informed consent that acknowledges that the patient understands the consequences that could be incurred by restricting dentists' access. Furthermore, this would remove liability from the dentists making patient care decisions for patients who still refuse.

Quote#8
I think one of the interesting challenges that will come out and that we will need to address is as the push for privacy occurs, I think that we have to be very up front and proactive in making sure that we are not restricted in being able to do what we know needs to be done, namely the integration of dentistry into medicine.

6.5.8 Health Insurance Cooperation

The segregation of medical and dental health insurance reinforces the artificial disconnect of systemic and oral health care. One member asserted that medical insurance companies are resistant to recognizing the cross-disease model. Another reflected on the disparities in dental coverage for patients. Panel members expressed concerns about patients not receiving proper dental care when they need it, resulting in the possibility of future harm and development of diseases that could have been prevented. Some of the panelists ascertained that cooperation of insurance companies to merge medical and dental health coverage is necessary to allow access to both types of care, promote patient safety and improve quality of care.

> **Quote#9**
> And I second what you just said because unfortunately I have had situations where I am treating a patient with diabetes and blood sugar is not controlled because he had infection in his mouth and literally you have to wait till he gets an abscess because then I can refer him to a dental surgeon who is in the clinic, but he does not have insurance or ways to go to a dentist, who treat the earlier stages of infection.

6.5.9 Conclusion

The interdisciplinary panel recognized the fundamental value and benefits of achieving cohesive integration of medical and dental patient care. The expertise and experiences of the group facilitated discussions on a wide variety of potential barriers and provided recommendations to coordinate and merge these domains to deliver the best care.

Integrating dental and medical electronic patient records is necessary, but not sufficient, to unifying systemic and oral health care. All levels of the health care system must recognize the cross-disease framework and cultivate a shift towards a more holistic treatment of patients. Patient education and cross training of providers in dentistry and medicine could help foster these changes. Furthermore, a blended team model would enhance the comprehensive care of the patient and may be more effective by defining a framework for workforce integration. Clinical decision support could assist providers to share responsibility and manage mental workloads. Development of dental diagnostic codes and standardized terminology will improve the effectiveness of the latter. Lastly, dental and medical insurance companies need to acknowledge the co-morbidity of oral and systemic health and merge coverage to increase patients' access to both care domains.

There are many possible areas to initiate the integration of oral and systemic patient care. However, further investigation is needed to determine how to successfully implement these strategies and to identify the most effective place to start harmonizing dentistry and medicine.

References

Lardiere MR (2009) A national Survey of Health Information Technology (HIT) Adoption in Federally Qualified Health Centers. National Association of Community Health Centers. http://www.nachc.com/client/NACHC%202008%20HIT%20Survey%20Analysis_FINAL_6_9_091.pdf Accessed 10 Oct 2011.

Lefkowitz B. Community health centers: a movement and the people who made it happen. New Brunswick: Rutgers University Press; 2007.

US Department of Health and Human Services. Oral health in America: a report of the surgeon general. Rockville: US Department of Health and Human Services, National Institute of Dental and Craniofacial Research, National Institutes of Health; 2000.

US Department of Health and Human Services. A national call to action to promote oral health. Rockville: US Department of Health and Human Services, Public Health Service, National Institutes of Health, National Institute of Dental and Craniofacial Research; 2003.

Chapter 7
Conclusion and Recommendations

Franklin M. Din and Valerie J.H. Powell

The editors of this volume have observed the progress of healthcare informatics and health information technology (HIT) over the years and concluded that while the coalescence of informatics and IT is advancing in general, the progress is uneven. In many ways, the progress reflects the siloization of healthcare itself. Some domains are favored and are well-advanced and others are left isolated and with uncertain direction. If uncorrected, this will lead to a stratification of healthcare in which some domains experience the benefits of an interoperable healthcare information environment and others exist in an information vacuum; a ghettoization of information and care. The editors have determined that we must try to assure that patients can benefit from access to integrated care supported by integrated HIT.

The editors and the contributing authors, to whom the editors are greatly indebted, have introduced the reader to many of the challenges facing dentistry's engagement with healthcare informatics and HIT. We chose to make specific recommendations that will address a range of challenges. We break these recommendations into the following categories:

1. Current activities
2. Path to the future

F.M. Din
HP Enterprise Services, Global Healthcare, Camp Hill, PA, USA

V.J.H. Powell (✉)
Department of Computer and Information Systems, Clinical Data Integration Project,
Robert Morris University, Moon Township, PA, USA
e-mail: powell@rmu.edu

Finally, we cite a couple of de-identified real-life stories about the *true cost of inaction*.

7.1 Current Activities

These are the tasks that need to be addressed immediately. These set the foundation upon which true healthcare information interoperability can be achieved between oral and systemic healthcare.

7.1.1 Electronic Dental Record Certification

While many Electronic Dental Record (EDR) developers and vendors view certification as an unnecessary burden and cost, we tend to disagree. The complexity of healthcare applications dictates that certain minimal standards must be met and that potential purchaser must be confident that the EDR will meet the standards. The alternative is reliance upon a vendor's marketing material with its self assertion of capabilities. This runs the risk of definition creep in which a standard is interpreted in way designed to meet the application's capability rather than force the application to meet the same functionality and capability as all other vendors. Without a trusted certification process, incompatibilities are inevitable.

We call on all EDR developers and vendors to work closely with certification bodies to produce a workable approach to meet the existing certification process with modifications for dentistry. In most cases, if the standard is applicable to both medical and dental data, the dental must be modified to conform to the medical. In cases in which the dental data is unique, distinct, or of greater importance to the dental domain than the medical domain, the standard will be determined by the dental participants. As examples:

- Medical trumps dental: The medical domain is used to recording a coded diagnosis as a routine part of a medical record. The certification process includes the need to capture structured diagnosis as a data element. Dentistry is unaccustomed to recording a diagnosis, instead preferring to record treatment and inferring a diagnosis from the treatment. In this case, the EDR must conform to the requirement to record structured diagnosis as a data element.
- Dental dictates the standard: Dentistry has developed a tooth numbering system and a tooth surface identification system to meet the needs to record the details of dental conditions and treatments. These systems help to identify problems with the specific teeth and to identify a location relative to an easily identifiable tooth ("on the *buccal mucosa* adjacent to the *crown* of *tooth 29*"). Each of the italicized terms may be unused or little used within the medical domain but are not only important to dental care, but provide a way to communicate location

with medical providers. In this case, the needs of dentistry dictate a certification standard in which dental trumps medical.

7.1.2 Data Standards Development, Use, and Training

The use of data standards (concept based, structured, and coded) is well developed for systemic care. Examples include ICD for diagnosis, SNOMED CT as an overall healthcare terminology, LOINC for labs and observations, etc. Dental concepts within these are limited and incomplete. In the field of medicine, a detailed standard for the format and content of patient records known as the Practice for Content and Structure of the Electronic Health Record standard is available. On the contrary, there is no standard for the content and structure of the EDR in general dentistry. Several generic standards for the electronic health records have been developed such as the American National Standards Institute (ANSI)/American Dental Association (ADA) [Dental] ANSI/ADA Specification 1,000: Standard Clinical Data Architecture for the Structure and Content of an Electronic Health Record and Specification 1,039: Standard Clinical Conceptual Data Model, but there is clearly a lack of standard specific for the content and structure of EDR. To achieve semantic interoperability it is important to have standard information models along with the terminology and inference models for the dental practice. In order to achieve the requisite completeness, dentistry must also become involved in the process of developing the appropriate data standards.

The efforts of formal dental organizations to fully engage with Standards Development Organizations (SDOs), such as HL7, is vital. An example of this is ADA/SCDI working with HL7 on developing standards around a functional model for EDR. Organized dentistry must not only support the in-depth and constant participation by knowledgeable individuals (a well meaning but untrained participant may well hinder rather than promote progress) to these organizations, but also commit to the use, dissemination, and training of the end user dental professionals (see also Sect. 2.1.3).

It is the training of the end user dental professional that is the most difficult to accomplish. Without unqualified support in this endeavor, success is unlikely. Typical avenues to support this effort include:

Training workshops tied to dental conferences
Focused presentations at conferences
Unqualified statement of support for the effort
Printed, DVD-based, and web-based training and support material availability
Research support
Establishment of Department of Informatics as a criterion for The Joint Commission (TJC), formerly the Joint Commission on Accreditation of Healthcare Organizations (JCRE-AHO), re-certification of dental schools. This must include the development of a curriculum that includes informatics training.

7.1.3 Provider Designations: Clinical Versus Medical and Clinician Versus Physician; Explicit Inclusion

Do we need to substitute *clinical* for *medical* or *clinician* for *physician* in certain contexts?

In a care delivery environment that is *evidence-focused, patient-centered*, and *outcomes-based*, the answer is likely *no*. Research and care environments can achieve integration of medical and dental care and data without being concerned with such terminology choices. This applies in any culture.

In a context where wording can have an *exclusive* impact, the answer is likely *yes*. Examples are regulations, laws and policies. Failure to include oral health providers on committees, forums, and commissions dealing with healthcare planning has had an unfortunate effect, since no one present at deliberations on setting goals, framing laws and policies, or specifying health information technology is likely to speak up if the oral health dimension is neglected. Making an explicit commitment to inclusive terms (*clinical* or *clinician*) alerts stakeholders to the significance of oral health for the initiative. Where healthcare specialties are designated for the composition of a commission, for example, it is vital that oral health providers be explicitly included.

7.1.4 Recording of Dental Diagnoses: Issues at Hand

Several calls have been made to institute explicit recording of dental diagnoses. Writing down dental diagnosis would be a way to improve research and quality of care. At the same time, there is the possibility (real or perceived) that recording diagnoses in dental care may lead to a loss of autonomy as a profession. However, identifying the reasons why dentists can routinely deliver care without writing down diagnoses is largely overlooked. In comparison, their medical counterparts routinely record diagnoses and have a long tradition of using recorded diagnostic concepts in their clinical functions.

The doctoral work of one of the editors (Torres-Urquidy, in preparation) contributes to the understanding of why dentists do not record diagnosis. Surely, a simple answer could be that dentists do not get reimbursed per diagnosis. However, this is, at best, a partial solution. It leaves unanswered how the practice of dentistry evolved so differently from the medical practice as to make reimbursement mechanisms differ so dramatically between the two areas. Early results of Torres-Urquidy's research suggest that there are differences in the way diagnostic information is used in dentistry and medicine. In particular, it seems that gains in cognitive efficiency allow dentists to focus their attention rapidly into treatment decisions. This suggests that forcing dentists to record diagnosis could have unforeseen consequences. Consequently, additional research is needed to identify the circumstances in which it is appropriate to modify the way dentists conduct clinical activities. Ultimately,

7 Conclusion and Recommendations 357

we need solutions that maximize the ability of clinicians to provide care, and improve the health of our patients.

7.2 Path to the Future

Envisioning a path for the future is a challenging task. However, the occurrence of some elements can be predicted, even though the time of their arrival may be uncertain. Outlines for the future can then be planned, and modified as roadblocks are encountered. With this proviso, we suggest attention to continuing education.

7.2.1 Consistent and Ongoing Training

This is a paradigm shift for most dentists. Most of the opposition to this effort in dentistry stems from fear of the unknown. As with all major changes to the status quo, the antidote to fear is education and training. By leveraging existing dental informaticians as teaching resources, establishment of formal dental school education in Informatics, and constant availability of training, slowly but inevitably, the fear will dissipate and be replaced with a understanding of the benefits. Dentists will become ambassadors of change instead of opponents.

7.2.2 Sharing Experience with Successful Implementations

Look to an existing working EDR implementation for inspiration and as a guide to success. Learn from their experience so that you can avoid the same mistakes. In this book, we have provided a detailed example of the Marshfield clinic implementation, but this is not the only one. Seek out others. Even if the working implementation is limited in scope, you may be able to find useful information. If your implementation experiences a success that others have not had, be generous and share your success with others. Establish and use a working group to periodically share and discuss issues.

7.2.3 Using HIT Adoption Best Practices

The implementation of an EDR and associated software capabilities is a precise activity. While dentists and dental informaticians are knowledgeable, they are largely untrained in software implementation. Clinical and informatics leaders should recognize the advantage of having trained implementation personnel do what they do best and avoid the temptation to oversimplify the complexity and attempt to implement an EDR themselves. Look back to the ideas presented in Sect. 4.3 on how to prepare to acquire an appropriate EHR technology.

7.2.4 Cooperation and Collaboration with HIT and Informatics Consultants and Vendors

This is related to the preceding comment. The typical relationship between software vendors, consultants, and the customer can be somewhat adversarial. Each has a different primary motivation. Dental leaders should engage with the vendors and consultants as a trusted resource with the collective mission to improve healthcare through HIT and informatics. Similarly the vendors and consultants must also engage these implementations as a trusted partner and sublimate the tendency to view implementations as a project with an end point followed by a departure. Ongoing communications and support must include an open discussion of problems and solutions.

7.2.5 Rating and Ranking EHRs

In the future EHR technologies which do not include integration of medical and dental patient records will be regarded as obsolescent and should not be rated as adequate or ranked high in quality. Current rankings of EHR products may neglect medical-dental patient record integration when developing rating criteria, in spite of the widespread presence of such integration in the EHR technologies used in U.S. Federally-sponsored healthcare systems, such as those of the U.S. Department of Veterans Affairs, the Indian Health Service, and the U.S. military and in the product lines of some EHR vendors.

7.2.6 Including the Oral Health Dimension in Quality Measures

In future quality initiatives, performance measures should verify integration of care, initially by including "dental referral" or "dental visit" in "all-in-one" composite measures for diseases such as diabetes. An oral health measure should be expected in assessing the quality of ICU care, for example, considering the American Association of Critical Care Nurses' (AACCN) practice alert on "Oral Care for Patients at Risk for Ventilator-Associated pneumonia" (AACN 2010). Performance measures relevant for care of patients whose diagnoses include several of the diseases and conditions covered in Appendix C should be reviewed to determine whether the oral health dimension for such care has been accounted for in performance measure design.

7.2.7 Including the Oral Health Dimension in Clinical Research Design

Research projects investigating diabetes, cardiovascular, or cerebrovascular care should account for the oral health dimension in the research design. Research projects consulting forensic evidence, as might occur with diabetes, will benefit from access to populations whose EHRs integrate medical and dental records.

7.2.8 Formalize Informatics Training of Dental Students as a Core Requirement and Review Continuing Education Requirements

Training of the next generation is important to cementing the gains of the current generation. That training will also allow new graduates lead the improvement of healthcare IT. There should be review, and where necessary revision, of continuing education (CE) requirements so that dental providers and dental hygienists can receive credit for CE topics dealing with patient records management and health informatics.

7.2.9 Educate Dental and Medical Students in a Cross-Disciplinary Environment

It is important for the next generation of dentists to be trained as oral physicians. The dental students should be comfortable to treat dental patients with systemic conditions. At the same time, the next generation physicians should be trained to be adept in knowledge about oral and craniofacial diseases and its implication and manifestation as a result of systemic diseases. It is also important to train the next generation of healthcare providers within an integrated medical-dental electronic health record environment.

7.3 Patient Experiences: The True Cost of Inaction

We have tried to assure that a range of providers could contribute their ideas to this volume. We must also include the experience of patients. Originally as this project was planned we did not anticipate interviewing patients. As the work progressed, some individuals who noticed what we were doing requested to be able to have input as patients. We set up a research design to accommodate these requests, which also gave us the opportunity to design and evaluate a procedure for collecting patient input (IRB, 2011). In the process of seeking IRB approval this design was shared with the International Centre for Oral-Systemic Health at the University of Manitoba in Winnipeg to gain input.

What we learned from this project was that:

- Patients perceive (on their own) that medical and dental care are not adequately articulated,
- Patients' stress and concern are heightened during a health crisis through lack of adequate articulation of medical and dental care,
- Patients have to make extra effort and spend extra time to deal with the lack of articulation of medical and dental care,
- Delivery of care can be delayed by the lack of adequate articulation of medical and dental care,
- Patients find themselves required to access resources beyond their care settings to solve the problems they face, and
- Patients may find their health and life threatened by the lack of articulation of medical and dental care. Under such circumstances, patients' confidence in the health care system is diminished.

In one example the diagnosis was squamous cell carcinoma of a lymph node; the providers to be articulated included: primary care physician, otolaryngologist, general dentist, chemo oncologist, radiation oncologist. The patient encountered difficulties facilitating communication between the one of the medical providers and the general dentist at the point of care delivery where oral health had to be assured before radiation treatment.

In another example, the diagnoses applying to the patient included:

Diabetes type 1,
Von Leiden Factor V (with anticoagulant medication),
Coronary atherosclerosis-native coronary vessel with stents,
Hypothyroidism,
Need for removal of multiple teeth.

The providers to be articulated included primary care physician, general dentist, oral surgeon at the point in time described. In this case, failure to adequately articulate care contributed to two life-threatening experiences for this patient.

7 Conclusion and Recommendations

We observe that the problems encountered by patients were not necessarily due solely to the medical-dental integration issues, but more likely also to a more general failure to assign priority to articulation of care into the process of delivering healthcare. We express our appreciation to patients who took the initiative to approach us and wished to inform us about their experiences.

7.4 Final Thoughts

We hope that the details provided in this volume will allow the reader to address the integration of medical and dental data with confidence. We hope these efforts will contribute to improvements in delivery of care and ultimately help improve the health of the population.

Appendix A

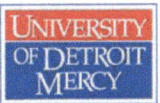

University of Detroit Mercy
School of Dentistry
8200 W. Outer Drive
Detroit, MI 48219-0900
(313) 494-6700

University of Detroit Mercy
Dental Service DRH/UHC
4201 St. Antoine
Detroit, MI 48201

Medical Consultation

Consultant: _____

Address: _____

_____   Date: _____

Patient: _____   UDM Chart Number: _____

Clinic requesting medical consultation:
Emergency/Screening 313-494-6718
Surgical Services 313-494-6739

REASON FOR CONSULTATION:

Dear Dr. _____

Our patient as identified above presented to the University of Detroit Mercy School of Dentistry on ___/___/___. During the medical history review, the patient stated that he/she has Type ____ diabetes mellitus. Please provide the following information requested below so that his/her dental treatment can be initiated.

Your assistance is appreciated. Thank you.

Faculty Signature: _____

RELEASE
I hereby consent to the release of my medical records to the University of Detroit Mercy School of Dentistry including any information regarding HIV status and infectious disease. I understand that this information will remain confidential.

Patient Signature: _____

PHYSICIAN'S RESPONSE

1. The current HbA1c is _____ % as measured on the date of _____.

2. The glycemic control goal for this patient is HbA1c _____ %

Physician Signature: _____
Date: _____

Disposition

Faculty Signature _____
Date _____

Appendix A

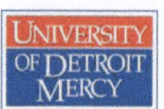

University of Detroit Mercy
School of Dentistry
8200 W. Outer Drive
Detroit, MI 48219-0900

University of Detroit Mercy
Dental Service DRH/UHC
4201 St. Antoine
Detroit, MI 48201

(313) 494-6700

Medical Consultation

Consultant: _____

Address: _____

_____ Date: _____

Patient: _____ UDM Chart Number: _____

Clinic requesting medical consultation:
Emergency/Screening 313-494-6718
Surgical Services 313-494-6739

REASON FOR CONSULTATION:

Dear Dr. _____

Faculty Signature: _____

RELEASE
I hereby consent to the release of my medical records to the University of Detroit Mercy School of Dentistry including any information regarding HIV status and infectious disease. I understand that this information will remain confidential.

Patient Signature: _____

PHYSICIAN'S RESPONSE

Physician Signature: _____
Date: _____

Disposition

Faculty Signature _____
Date _____

Appendix A

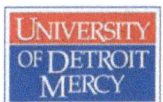

University of Detroit Mercy
School of Dentistry
8200 W. Outer Drive
Detroit, MI 48219-0900

University of Detroit Mercy
Dental Service DRH/UHC
4201 St. Antoine
Detroit, MI 48201

(313) 494-6700

Medical Consultation

Consultant: _____

Address: _____

_____   Date: _____

Patient: _____   UDM Chart Number: _____

Clinic requesting medical consultation:
Emergency/Screening   313-494-6718
Surgical Services   313-494-6739

REASON FOR CONSULTATION:

Dear Dr. _____

In compliance with the American Heart Association 2007 guidelines for infective endocarditis (IE) prevention, and to help us determine the need for antibiotic prophylaxis, please indicate which of the following condition(s) apply to this patient:

Faculty Signature: _____

RELEASE
I hereby consent to the release of my medical records to the University of Detroit Mercy School of Dentistry including any information regarding HIV status and infectious disease. I understand that this information will remain confidential

Patient Signature: _____

PHYSICIAN'S RESPONSE

_____ Prosthetic cardiac valve or prosthetic material used for heart valve repair
_____ Previous infective endocarditis (IE)
_____ Congenital heart disease (CHD) with findings as below
 _____ Unrepaired cyanotic CHD, including palliative shunts and conduits
 _____ Completely repaired CHD defect with prosthetic material or device
  for the first 6 months after procedure
 _____ Repaired CHD with residual defects at the site or adjacent to site of
  prosthetic patch/device which inhibit endothelialization
_____ Cardiac transplantation recipients who develop cardiac valvulopathy

Physician Signature: _____
Date: _____

Disposition _____

Faculty Signature _____

Appendix A

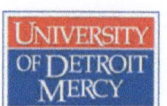

University of Detroit Mercy
School of Dentistry
2700 Martin Luther King Jr Blvs
Detroit, MI 48208

(313) 494-6700

University of Detroit Mercy
Dental Service DRH/UHC
4201 St. Antoine
Detroit, MI 48201

Medical Consultation

Consultant: _____
Address: _____
_____
_____ Date: _____

Patient: _____ UDM Chart Number: _____

Clinic requesting medical consultation:
Emergency/Screening 313-494-6718
Surgical Services 313-494-6739

REASON FOR CONSULTATION:
Dear Dr. _____

Ms./Mrs./Mr._____ needs dental treatment in our dental clinic. She/He informed us that a total prosthetic joint was implanted _____ years ago.
We are aware that dental procedures cause transient bacteremia that might be a risk factor for the prosthetic joint infection. We are also aware of AAOS's recommendation of antibiotic prophylaxis (AP) for dental procedures. However, we do not have complete information about her/him to assess the risk and benefit ratio for AP. Please evaluate her/him accordingly.
If you believe the benefit of AP would outweigh the risk, please provide her/him with prescriptions for antibiotics of your choice and the regimen.

Thank you for your assistance in optimizing hers/his oral health.

Faculty Signature: _____

RELEASE
I hereby consent to the release of my medical records to the University of Detroit Mercy School of Dentistry including any information regarding HIV status and infectious disease. I understand that this information will remain confidential.

Patient Signature: _____

PHYSICIAN'S RESPONSE
Please check one box below

☐ Ms./Mrs./Mr._____'s benefit of AP outweighs the risk and I will provide the prescription.

☐ Ms./Mrs./Mr._____ will not benefit from taking AP for dental procedure.

Physician Signature: _____
Date: _____

Disposition

Faculty Signature_____
Date_____

Appendix B – Wisconsin Diabetes Mellitus Essential Care Guidelines, 2011

The referral and screening tools in Appendices B.1 and B.2 are reproduced by permission of Leah Ludlum, Director of the Wiscon-sin Diabetes Prevention and Control Program, with the explicit support of Warren LeMay, DDS, MPH, Chief Dental Officer, Wisconsin Division of Public Health. This material is available online at http://www.dhs.wisconsin.gov/health/diabetes/PDFs/T-MedDentalTeam.pdf and http://www.dhs.wisconsin.gov/health/diabetes/PDFs/T-ScreenGumsTeeth.pdf both accessed 15 May 2011, respectively.

For the Wisconsin Diabetes Mellitus Essential Care Guidelines section on oral care, see: http://www.dhs.wisconsin.gov/health/diabetes/PDFs/GL09.pdf. According to that section, "people with diabetes are more susceptible to oral infections such as periodontal disease. Susceptibility is further increased during periods of poor glycemic control or prolonged periods of hyperglycemia. The presence of active periodontitis can, in turn, impair glycemic control and increase risk of developing sys-temic complications of diabetes, particularly cardiovascular disease and stroke. Pregnant women with diabetes maybe at increased risk of periodontitis and as a result could be at increased risk of preterm delivery with a low birth weight infant. Individuals can avoid the negative outcomes of periodontitis through early screening, referral, and treatment."

The "Frequency of Essential Tests for People with Diabetes" quick reference guide specifies a "dental exam by general dentist or periodontal specialist at diagnosis" and periodically thereafter; see: http://www.dhs.wisconsin.gov/health/diabetes/PDFs/GLQuickRef.pdf accessed 15 May 2011. The Wisconsin Essential Diabetes Mellitus Guidelines are exemplary for integrating diabetes-related oral health care at the same level of attention as diagnosis and treatment for diabetes-related eye care and foot care.

- B.1 Medical-Dental Team Referral Form, Wisconsin Diabetes Mellitus Essential Care Guidelines

MEDICAL-DENTAL: TEAM REFERRAL FORM

Client Name: _____ Date of Birth: _____

Medical Provider: Complete this section

1. Type of diabetes: ❑ Type 1 diabetes ❑ Type 2 diabetes ❑ Other Year diagnosed: _____
2. List medication(s)/insulin: _____
   _____
   _____
3. Result and date of most recent: A1C: _____ % Date: _____
4. Result and date of most recent blood pressure _____ History of cardiovascular disease: ❑ Yes ❑ No
5. Antibiotic pre-medication required? ❑ Yes ❑ No Drug allergies: _____
6. Inspection of gums and teeth: ❑ Loose, sensitive teeth, and/or separated teeth ❑ Accumulation of food debris and/or plaque around teeth
   ❑ History of abscess ❑ Red, sore, swollen, receding or bleeding gums ❑ Halitosis ❑ Missing teeth ❑ Other _____
7. Medical provider: _____
   Address: _____
   City/State: _____
   Telephone: _____ FAX: _____

Dental Provider: Complete this section

1. Date of dental visit: _____ Next dental appointment or F/U _____
2. Periodontal status (check): ❑ Gingivitis ❑ Early Periodontitis ❑ Moderate Periodontitis ❑ Advanced Periodontitis
3. Dental oral exam findings: _____
   _____
4. Treatment provided: _____
   _____
   _____
5. Dental office recommendations: ❑ F/U with healthcare provider ❑ Other _____
6. Dental provider: _____
   Address: _____
   City/State: _____
   Telephone: _____ FAX: _____

I, _____, consent to the release and exchange of medical/dental information pertinent to
                  Client name
my diabetes management and overall healthcare.

PLEASE FAX THIS FORM TO THE REFERRING DENTAL OR MEDICAL PROVIDER.

Appendix B

- B.2 Wisconsin Diabetes Mellitus Essential Care Guidelines, Diabetes Screening Tool for Inspection of Teeth and Gums

Diabetes: Screening tool for inspection of gums and teeth

Visual inspection of a person's gums and teeth for early signs of periodontal disease at diagnosis, and then at each focused visit can assist with early detection and treatment. The accompanying diagrams may be helpful for understanding the evaluation criteria and the presence of periodontal disease.

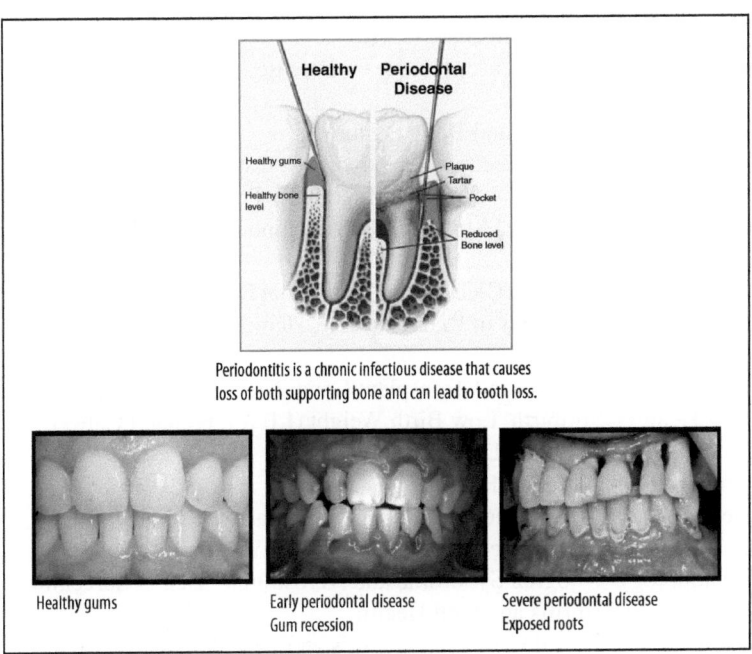

Periodontitis is a chronic infectious disease that causes loss of both supporting bone and can lead to tooth loss.

Healthy gums

Early periodontal disease
Gum recession

Severe periodontal disease
Exposed roots

Assign a score based on current findings. Refer to a dentist for further evaluation if score is 4 or more.

More than 6 months since last dental visit	4
Red, sore, swollen, or bleeding gums	4
Loose, sensitive teeth, and/or separated teeth	4
Visible debris or accumulation of hardened material around teeth	3
Exposed roots in the mouth	2
Strong odor in the mouth	1
Smoking or smokeless tobacco use	1
Total score	

Appendix C

Contact Points Between Medical and Dental Care and Research, C-1–C-37

C-1 Diabetes, Metabolic Syndrome – Periodontal Diseases
C-2 Hypertension
C-3 Manifestations of Thyroid Disease, HPT
C-4 [C] Cardiovascular Disease, [H] Heart Disease, [S] Stroke – Gingivitis and Periodontal Diseases
C-5 Stomatognathic System and Body Posture
C-6 Oral Health and Bone Diseases (Osteoporosis, Osteopenia)
C-7 Obstructive Sleep Apnea – Anterior Mandibular Positioning (AMP) Devices
C-8 [R] Respiratory diseases ([A] Asthma, [P] Pneumonia, [C] COPD) – Periodontal Diseases
C-9 Chronic Kidney Disease (CKD); End Stage Renal Disease (ESRD) – Periodontal Diseases; Oral Manifestations of Renal Disease, Hemodialysis (HD) and Peritoneal Dialysis (PD)
C-10 Organ Failure Patients and Transplant Candidates – Oral Health Care
C-11 Oral Health – Stillbirth, Low Birth Weight (LBW), Prenatal Care [Disputed]
C-12 Mental Health – Eating Disorder Screening
C-13 Oral Health and Mental Health
C-14 Neurologic Topics: Dementia, Alzheimer Disease, Bell Palsy
C-15 HIV/AIDS – Dental Screening
C-16 Immunology – Sjögren Syndrome and Xerostomia – Dental Screening
C-17 Rheumatoid Arthritis and Oral Health
C-18 Rheumatology – Ankylosing spondylitis and Periodontal Disease
C-19 Tobacco/Betel Use Screening and Cessation (Risk Factor for Oral Cancer)
C-20 Oncology – [C] Cancer; [O] Oral Cancer Screening, Oral Premalignant Lesions, Oral Cancer Care;
C-21 Bisphosphonate Osteonecrosis ([B] BON) and Osteoradionecrosis ([R] ORN, Postradiation osteonecrosis)
C-22 Blood Disorders, Iatrogenic or Otherwise: von Willebrand disease, Neutropenia, Polycythemia, Aplastic Anemia, Sickle Cell Anemia, Hemophilia
C-23 Bacterial Diseases
C-24 Archaeal Role in Disease
C-25 Fungal Diseases
C-26 Viral Diseases
C-27 Dermatological Disease Including Nummular Eczema as a Dental Focal Infection
C-28 Special Populations: Children (Pediatric)
C-29 Special Populations, Geriatric Care

C-30 Special Populations, ND/ID
C-31 Congenital Conditions, CL/CP, Hutchinson Teeth, Macroglossia
C-32 Ectodermal Dysplasia and Severe Hypodontia
C-33 Breath Odor: Halitosis
C-34 Cognitive Parameters of Reducing Disparities in Healthcare (Including Dental Care)
C-35 Periodontal Diseases – Systemic Inflammation [Research]
C-36 Biofilms: Cystic Fibrosis, Endocarditis, Cystitis, Dental Plaque, Indwelling Devices and Implants. [Research]
C-37 Anesthesia, Sedation, Pain or Odontalgia Management

Contact Points Between Medical and Dental Care/Research: Categories 1–37 and References

Contributions to this page from Valerie J.H. Powell, Ph.D., M.S., RT(R), Clinical Data Integration Project, Robert Morris University; Franklin Din, DMD, M.A. HP Enterprise Services, Global Healthcare, Amit Acharya B.D.S., M.S., Ph.D., (Marshfield Clinic Research Foundation/Biomedical Informatics Research Center), Edward P. Heinrichs, DMD, Department of Periodontics and Preventive Dentistry, University of Pittsburgh; Titus K. Schleyer, DMD, Ph.D., Director, Center for Dental Informatics, University of Pittsburgh, Shin Mei Rose Yin Geist, DDS, M.S., Diplomate ABOM, University of Detroit Mercy School of Dentistry, Miguel Humberto Torres-Urquidy, DDS, M.S., Ph.D. Candidate, Center for Dental Informatics, University of Pittsburgh. Categories devoted to research (rather than care) are marked [Rsch]. Research results disputed or controversial marked [Dsptd].

Summary of areas of cross-domain (medical/dental) communication	Dental specialties	Medical subspecialties	References (adding references in progress)
1. Diabetes, metabolic syndrome – periodontal diseases; reciprocal screening opportunities	General dentist, periodontist	Primary care, endocrinologist, diabetologist	D'Aiuto F, Sabbah W, Netuveli G, Donos N, Hingorani AD, Deanfield J, Tsakos G. Association of the metabolic syndrome with severe periodontitis in a large U.S. population-based survey. J Clin Endocrinol Metab. 2008;93(10):3989–94.
			Darré L, Vergnes J-N, Gourdy P, Sixou M. Efficacy of periodontal treatment on glycaemic control in diabetic patients: a meta-analysis of interventional studies. Diabetes Metab. 2008;34:497–506.
			Iacopino AM. Periodontitis and diabetes interrelationships: role of inflammation. Ann Periodontol. 2001;6:125–37.
			Kuo LC, Polson AM, Kang T. Associations between periodontal diseases and systemic diseases: a review of the inter-relationships and interactions with diabetes, respiratory diseases and osteoporosis. Public Health. 2008;122:417–33.
			Mealey BL. Periodontal disease and diabetes: a two-way street. JADA. 2006;137:26S–31S.
			Mealey BL, Rose LF. Diabetes mellitus and inflammatory periodontal diseases. Curr Opin Endocrinol Diabetes Obes. 2008;15:135–41.
2. Hypertension	General dentist	Primary care	Desvarieux M, Demmer RT, Jacobs DR Jr, Rundek T, Boden-Albala B, Sacco RL, Papapanou PN. Periodontal bacteria and hypertension: the oral infections and vascular disease epidemiology study (INVEST). J Hypertension. 2010;28(7):1413–21.
			Tumanyan S, Zevallos JC, Joshipura KJ. Relationship between periodontitis and hypertension among older adults, IADR. 2008. http://iadr.confex.com/iadr/2008Toronto/techprogram/abstract_109052.htm. Accessed 17 June 2011.
3. Manifestations of thyroid disease, HPT	General dentist	Primary care, endocrinologist	Padbury AD Jr, Tözüm TF, Taba M Jr, Ealba EL, West BT, Burney RE, Gauger PG, Giannobile WV, McCauley LK. The impact of primary hyperparathyroidism on the oral cavity. J Clin Endocrinol Metab. 2006;91(9):3439–45. doi:10.1210/jc.2005-2282.
			Pinto LA, Glick M. Management of patients with thyroid disease: oral health considerations. J Am Dent Assoc. 2002;133:849–58.

4. [C] Cardiovascular disease, [H] Heart disease, [S] Stroke – gingivitis and periodontal diseases	General dentist, periodontist	Primary care, cardiologist, neurologist

[C] Demmer RT, Desvariaux M. Periodontal infections and cardiovascular disease: the heart of the matter. JADA. 2006;137:14S–20S.

[C] Mochari H, Grbic JT, Msco L. Usefulness of self-reported periodontal disease to identify individuals with elevated inflammatory markers at risk of cardiovascular disease. Am J Cardiol. 2008;102(11):1509–13.

[H] Angeli F, Verdecchia P, Pellogrino C, Pellegrino RG, Pellegrino G, Prosciutti L, Giannoni C, Cianetti S, Bentivoglio M. Association between periodontal disease and left ventricle mass in essential hypertension. Hypertension. 2003;41:488.

[H] Bahekar AA, Singh S, Saha S, Molnar J, Arora R. The prevalence and incidence of coronary heart disease is significantly increased in periodontitis: a meta-analysis. Am Heart J. 2007;154(5):830–7.

[H] Grines CL, Bonow RO, et al. Prevention of premature discontinuation of dual antiplatelet therapy in patients with coronary artery stents: a science advisory from the American Heart Association, American College of Cardiology, Society for Cardiovascular Angiography and Interventions, American College of Surgeons, and American Dental Association, with representation from the American College of Physicians. Circulation. 2007;115(6):813–8. Epub 2007 Jan 15.

[H] Humphrey LL, Fu R, Buckley DI, Freeman M, Helfand M. Periodontal disease and coronary heart disease incidence: a systematic review and meta-analysis. J Gen Intern Med. 2008;23(12):2079–86.

[H] Friedewald VE, Kornman KS, Beck JD, Genco R, Goldfine A, Libby P, Offenbacher S, Ridker PM, Van Dyke PE, Roberts WC. The American journal of cardiology and journal of periodontology editors' consensus: periodontitis and atherosclerotic cardiovascular disease. J Periodontol 2009;80(7):1021–32.

[H] Friedlander AH, Yoshikawa TT, Chang DS, Feliciano Z, Scully C. Atrial fibrillation: pathogenesis, medical-surgical management and dental implications. J Am Dent Assoc. 2009;140(2):167–77;quiz 248.

(continued)

Summary of areas of cross-domain (medical/dental) communication	Dental specialties	Medical subspecialties	References (adding references in progress)
			[S] Dörfer CE, Becher H, Ziegler CM, Kaiser C, Lutz R, Jörß D, Lichy C, Buggle F, Bültmann S, Preusch M, Grau AJ. The association of gingivitis and periodontitis with ischemic stroke. J Clin Periodontol. 2004;31:396–401.
			[C] Saremi A, Nelson RG Tulloch-Reid M, Hanson RL, Sievers ML, Taylor GW, Shlossman M, Bennett PH, Genco R, Knowler WC. Periodontal disease and mortality in type 2 diabetes. Diabetes Care. 2005;28:27–32, http://care.diabetesjournals.org/cgi/content/full/28/1/27. Accessed 17 June 2011.
			[S] Piconi S, Trabattoni D, Luraghi C, Perilli E, Borelli M, Pacei M, Rizzardini G, Lattuada A, Bray DH, Catalano M, Sparaco A, Clerici M. Treatment of periodontal disease results in improvements in endothelial dysfunction and reduction of the carotid intima-media thickness. Fed Am Soc Exp Biol J. 2009;23:1196–204.
5. Stomatognathic system and body posture	General dentist, orthodontist, prosthodontist	Primary care, pediatrician, orthopedist	Cuccia A, Carradonna C. The relationship between the stomatognathic system and body posture. Clinics. 2009;64(1):1–9, http://www.scielo.br/scielo.php?script=sci_arttext&pid=S1807-59322009000100011.
			Fujimoto M, Hayakawa I, Hirano S, Watanabe I. Changes in gait stability induced by alteration of mandibular position. J Med Dent Sci. 2001;48:131–6.
			Gangloff P, Louis JP, Perrin PP. Dental occlusion modifies gaze and posture stabilization in human subjects. Neurosci Lett. 2000;293:203–6.
			Huggare JA, Raustia AM. Head posture and cervicovertebral and craniofacial morphology in patients with craniomandibular dysfunction. Cranio. 1992;10:173–8.
			Milani RS, De Periere DD, Lapeyre L, Pourreyron L. Relationship between dental occlusion and posture. Cranio. 2000;8:127–34.
			See also category: special populations, children (pediatric)

Topic	Dental role	Medical role	References
6. Oral health and bone diseases (osteoporosis, osteopenia)	General dentist	Primary care, orthopedist	Wactawski-Wende J. Periodontal diseases and osteoporosis: association and mechanisms. Ann Periodontol. 2001;6(1):197–208. doi 10.1902/annals.2001.6.1.197. Wactawski-Wende J, Grossi SG, Trevisan M, Genco RJ, Tezal M, Dunford RG, Ho AW, Hausmann E, Hreshchyshyn MM. The role of osteopenia in oral bone loss and periodontal disease. J Periodontol. 1996;67(10 Suppl):1076–84. See category 22, Bisphosphonate Osteonecrosis ([B] BON) and Osteoradionecrosis ([R] ORN, Postradiation osteonecrosis)
7. Obstructive sleep apnea – anterior mandibular positioning (AMP) devices	General dentist, prosthodontist, oral and maxillofacial surgeon	Primary care, sleep specialist	Clark GT, Sohn J-W, Hong CN. Treating obstructive sleep apnea and snoring: assessment of an anterior mandibular positioning device. J Am Dent Assoc. 2000;131(6):765–71.
8. [R] Respiratory diseases ([A] Asthma, [P] Pneumonia, [C] COPD) – periodontal diseases	General dentist, periodontist	Primary care, pulmonologist	[A] Anjomshoaa I, Cooper ME, Vieira AR. Caries is associated with asthma and epilepsy. Eur J Dent. 2009;3:297–303. [A] Stensson M, Wendt L-K, Koch G, Oldeaeus G, Birkhed D. Oral health in preschool children with asthma. Int J Paediatr Dent. 2008;18:243–50. [R] Scannapieco FA. Role of oral bacteria in respiratory infection. J Periodontol. 1999;70:793–802. [P] Scannapieco FA. Pneumonia in nonambulatory patients: the role of oral bacteria and oral hygiene. JADA. 2006;137: 21S-5. [C] Scully C, Ettinger RL. The influence of systemic diseases on oral health care in older adults. J Am Dent Assoc. 2007;138(Suppl 1):7S–14S. [P] Migliorati CA, Madrid C. The interface between oral and systemic health: the need for more collaboration. Clin Microbiol Infect. 2007;13(Suppl 4):11–6.

(continued)

Summary of areas of cross-domain (medical/dental) communication	Dental specialties	Medical subspecialties	References (adding references in progress)
9. Chronic kidney disease (CKD); end state renal disease (ESRD) – periodontal diseases; oral manifestations of renal disease, hemodialysis (HD) and peritoneal dialysis (PD)	General dentist, periodontist	Primary care, nephrologist	Akar H, Akar GC, Carrero JJ, Stenvinkel P, Lindholm B. Systemic consequences of poor oral health in chronic kidney disease patients. Clin J Am Soc Nephrol. 2011;6(1):218–26. Craig RG. Interactions between chronic renal disease and periodontal disease. Oral Dis. 2008;14:1–7. Fisher MA, Taylor GW, Est BT, McCarthy ET. Bidirectional relationship between chronic kidney and periodontal disease: a study using structural equation modeling. Kidney Int. 2011;79:347–55. Fisher MA, Taylor GW, Shelton BJ, Jamerson KA, Rahman M, Ojo AO, Sehgal AR. Periodontal disease and other nontradititional risk factors for CKD. Am J Kidney Dis. 2008;51(1):45–52. Gavaldá C, Bagán JV, Scully J, Silvestre FJ, Milián MA, Jiménez J. Renal hemodialysis patients: oral, salivary, dental and periodontal findings in 105 adult cases. Oral Dis. 1999;5(4):299–302. doi: 10.1111/j.1601-0825.1999.tb00093.x. Grubbs V, Plantinga LC, Crews DC, Bibbins-Domingo K, Saran R, Heung M, Patel PR, Burrows NR, Ernst KL, Powe NR. Centers for disease control and prevention CKD Surveillance Team. Clin J Am Soc Nephrol. 2011;6:711–7. Kshirsagar AV, Craig RG, Moss KL, et al. Periodontal disease adversely affects the survival of patients with end-stage renal disease. Kidney Int. 2009;75:746–51. Nunn JH, Sharp J, Lambert HJ, Plant ND, Coulthard MG. Oral health in children with renal disease. Pediatr Nephrol. 2000;14(10–11):997–1001. doi: 1007/s004670050061. Shultis WA, Weil EJ, Looker HC, Custis JM, Shlossman M, Genco RJ, Knowler WC, Nelson RG. Effect of periodontitis on overt nephropathy and end-stage renal disease in type 2 diabetes. Diabetes Care. 2007;30(2):306–11.

10. Organ failure patients and transplant candidates – oral health care	All specialties Transplant surgeon, corresponding organ specialist	Guggenheimer J, Eghtesad B, Stock DJ. Dental management of the (solid) organ transplant patient. Oral Surg Oral Med Oral Pathol Oral Radiol Endod. 2003;95(4):383–9. Guggenheimer J, Eghtesad B, Close JM, Shay C, Fung JJ. Dental health status of liver transplant candidates. Liver Transpl. 2007;13(2):280–6. NICDR. Dental management of the organ transplant patient. 2011. http://www.nidcr.nih.gov/OralHealth/Topics/OrganTransplantationOralHealth/OrganTransplantProf.htm. Accessed 2 May 2011.
11. Oral health – stillbirth, low birth weight (LBW), prenatal care [Dsptd]	General dentist Primary care, obstetrician/gynecologist	Bobetsis YA, Barros SP, Offenbacher S. Exploring the relationship between periodontal disease and pregnancy complications. J Am Dent Assoc. 2006;137:7S–13S Geist R. Oral health management of pregnant dental patients, MedEdPORTAL. 2009. http://services.aamc.org/30/mededportal/servlet/s/segment/mededportal/?subid=4056. Accessed 17 June 2011. Han YW, Redline RW, Li M, Yin L, Hill GB, McCormick TH. *Fusobacterium nucleatum* induces premature and term stillbirths in pregnant mice: implication of oral bacteria in preterm birth. Infect Immun. 2004;72(4):2272–9. Han YW, Fardini Y, Chen C, Iacampo KG, Peraino VA, Shamonki JM, Redline RW. Term stillbirth caused by oral fusobacterium nucleatum. Obstet Gynecol. 2010;115(2):442–5. Kushtagi P, Kaur G, Kukkamalla MA, Thomas B. Periodontal infection in women with low birth weight neonates. Int J Gynecol Obstet. 2008;101:296–8. Polyzos NP, Polyzos IP, Mauri D, Tzioras S. Effect of periodontal disease treatment during pregnancy on preterm birth incidence: a metaanalysis of randomized trials. Am J Obstet Gynecol. 2009;200(3):225–32. Vergnes J-N, Sixou M. Preterm low birth weight and maternal periodontal status: a meta-analysis. Am J Obstet Gynecol. 2007;196:135.e1–j135.e7.

(continued)

Summary of areas of cross-domain (medical/dental) communication	Dental specialties	Medical subspecialties	References (adding references in progress)
12. Mental health – eating disorder screening	General dentist	Primary care, gastroenterologist, psychiatrist, psychologist	Hague AL. Eating disorders: screening in the dental office. JADA. 2010;141(6):675–8. Hazelton LR, Faine MP. Diagnosis and management of eating disorder patients. Int J Prosthodont. 1996;9(1):65–73. Milosevic A, Brodie DA, Slade PD. Dental erosion, oral hygiene, and nutrition in eating disorders. Int J Eat Disord. 1998;21(2):195–9. Morgan JF, Reid F, Lacey JH. The SCOFF questionnaire: assessment of a new screening tool for eating disorders. BMJ. 1999;319:1467. National Eating Disorders Association (NEDA). Dental complications of eating disorders: information for dental practitioners, NEDA. 2002. http://www.nationaleatingdisorders.org/nedaDir/files/documents/handouts/DentCmps.pdf. Accessed 17 June 2011. National Eating Disorders Association (NEDA). Eating concerns and oral health, NEDA. 2005. http://www.nationaleatingdisorders.org/nedaDir/files/documents/handouts/OralHlth.pdf. Accessed 17 June 2011.
13. Oral health and mental health	General dentist	Primary care, psychologist, psychiatrist	Becker DE. Psychotropic drugs: implications for dental practice. Anesth Prog. 2008;55:89–99. Ponizovsky AM, Zusman SP, Grinshpoon A. Oral health and hygiene among persons with severe mental illness: reply (letter). Psychiatr Serv. 2009;60:1402–3. Rai B. Oral health in patients with mental illness. Internet J Dent Sci. 2008;5(1) http://www.ispub.com/ostia/index.php?xmlFilePath=journals/ijds/vol6n1/mental.xml. Ramon T, Grinshpoon A, Zusman SP, Weizman A. Oral health and treatment needs of institutionalized chronic psychiatric patients in Israel. Eur Psychiatry. 2003;18(3):101–5. See Category 13, eating disorder screening

14. Neurologic topics: dementia, Alzheimer disease, Bell Palsy	General dentist, periocontist	Primary care, neurologist, neuropsychiatrist	Fidanoski B. Bell's Palsy (Facial Paralysis): dental hygiene perspective. 2007. http://www.fidanoski.ca/dentalhygiene/2011/bellspalsy.htm. Accessed 5 May 2011. Gatz M, Mortimer JA, Fratiglioni L, Johansson B, Berg S, Reynolds CA, Pederson NL. Potentially modifiable risk factors for dementia in identical twins, Alzheimer's and Dementia. J Alzheimers Assoc. 2006;2(2):110–7. Watts A, Crimmins EM, Gatz M. Inflammation as a potential mediator for the association between periodontal disease and Alzheimer's disease. Neuropsychiatr Dis Treat. 2008;4:865–76; At: http://www.dovepress.com/inflammation-as-a-potential-mediator-for-the-association-between-perio-peer-reviewed-article. Accessed 10 May 2011.
15. HIV/AIDS – dental Screening	General dentist	Primary care, immunologist, infectious disease	Gerbert B, Badner V, Maguire B. AIDS and dental practice. J Public Health Dent. 1988;48(2):68–73. Gennaro S, Naidoo S, Berthold P. Oral health and HIV/AIDS. MCN Am J Mater Child Nurs. 2008;33(1):50–7. HRSA. HAB HIV performance measures: oral health services, HRSA. 2009. http://hab.hrsa.gov/special/pdf/HABPMsOralHealth.pdf. Accessed 15 June 2011. Kahabuka FK, Fabian F, Petersen PE, Nguvumali H. Awareness of HIV/AIDS and its oral manifestations among people living with HIV in Dar es Salaam, Tanzania. Afr J AIDS. 2007;6(1):91–5.
16. Immunology – Sjögren syndrome and xerostomia– dental screening	All specialties	Primary care, immunologist, ophthalmologist, rheumatologist	Fox PC, Bowman SJ, Segal B, Vivino FB, Murukutla N, Choueiri K, Oale S, McLean L. Oral involvement in primary Sjögren syndrome. J Am Dent Assoc. 2008;139(12):1592–601. Iacopino AM. Sjögren syndrome: reduced quality of life as an oral-systemic consequence. J Can Dent Assoc. 2010;76:a98; http://www.jcda.ca/article/a98. Accessed 15 June 2011.

(continued)

Summary of areas of cross-domain (medical/dental) communication	Dental specialties	Medical subspecialties	References (adding references in progress)
17. Rheumatoid arthritis and oral health	General dentist, periodontist	Primary care, immunologist	Leader D. How Rheumatoid arthritis affects oral health, health and wellness 2007; April 23 2007. http://www.associatedcontent.com/article/214081/how_rheumatoid_arthritis_affects_oral.html?cat. Accessed 10 June 2011. Mercade FB, Marshall RI, Klestov AC, Bartold PM. Relationship between rheumatoid arthritis and periodontitis. J Periodontol. 2001;72(6):779–87.
18. Rheumatology – Ankylosing spondylitis and periodontal disease	General dentist, periodontist	Primary care, rheumatologist	Pischon N, Pischon T, Gülmez E, Kröger J, Purucker P, Kleber B-M, Landau H, Jost-Brinkmann P-G, Schlattermann P, Zernicke J, Burmeister G-R, Bernimoulin J-P, Buttgereit F, Detert J. Periodontal disease in patients with ankylosing spondylitis. Ann Rheum Dis. 2010;69:34–8.
19. Tobacco or betel use cessation (risk factor for oral cancer)	General dentist	Primary care, oncologist	Jette AM, Feldman HA, Tennstedt SL. Tobacco use: a modifiable risk factor for dental disease among the elderly. Am J Public Health. 1993;83(9):1271–6. McDaniel AM, Stratton RM, Britain M. Systems approaches to tobacco dependence treatment. Annu Rev Nurs Res. 2009;27:345–63. Zhang X, Reichart PA. A review of betel quid chewing, oral cancer and precancer in mainland China. Oral Oncol. 2007;43(5):424–30.
20. Oncology –[C] Cancer; [O] Oral cancer screening, oral premalignant lesions [H] Head and neck cancer	General dentist, periodontist	Primary care, oncologist	[H] Cloos J, Spitz MR, Schantz SP, Hsu TC, et al. Genetic susceptibility to head and neck squamous cell carcinoma. J Natl Cancer Inst. 1996;88:530–5. [O] Goodman HS, Yellowitz JA, Yellowitz AM. Oral cancer prevention: the role of family practitioners. Arch Fam Med. 1995;4(7):628–36. [O] Mao L, Lee JS, Fan YH, Ro JY, Batsakis JG, Lippman S, Hittelman W, Hong WK. Frequent microsatellite alterations at chromosomes 9p21 and 3p14 in oral premalignant lesions and their value in cancer risk assessment. Nat Med. 1996;2:682–5. doi:10.1038/nm0696-682. [C] Michaud DS, Joshipura K, Giovannucci E, Fuchs CS. A prospective study of periodontal disease and pancreatic cancer in U.S. male health professionals. J Nat Cancer Inst. 2007;99:1–5.

		[H] Parzuchowski JS, Jordon J, Burgess L, Witsell M, Sobol L, Rontal M, Balaraman S, Ignatius R, Venuturumilli P, Krauss D, Chen P, Fontanesi J, Akervall J. Lead-time from diagnosis to start of radiation shortened by 44% for head and neck cancer when patients go through a multidisciplinary clinic. J Clin Oncol. 2011;29(Suppl):abstre16627.
		[C] Söder B, Yakob M, Meurman JH, Anderson LC, Klinge B, Söder P-Ö. Periodontal disease may associate with breast cancer. Breast Cancer Res Treat. 2010;doi 10.1007/s10549-010-1221-4.
		[C] Uemura N, Okamoto S, Yamamoto S, Matsumura N, et al. *Helicobacter pylori* infection and the development of gastric cancer. N Engl J Med. 2001;345:784–9.
		See Category 19, Tobacco or betel use screening and cessation (risk factor for oral cancer)
21. Bisphosphonate osteonecrosis ([B] BON) and osteoradionecrosis ([R] ORN, postradiation osteonecrosis)	General dentist, oral and maxillofacial surgeon, oral radiologist	[B] Marx RE. Pamidronate (Aredia) and zoledronate (Zometa) induced avascular necrosis of the jaws: a growing epidemic. J Oral Maxillofac Surg. 2003;61:1115–7.
	Primary care, radiologist, orthopedist, oncologist	[B] Migliorati CA. Bisphosphonates and oral cavity avascular bone necrosis. J Clin Oncol. 2003;21:4253–4.
		[O] Rayatt SS, Mureau MAM, Hofer SOP. Osteoradionecrosis of the mandible: etiology, prevention, diagnosis and treatment. Indian J Plast Surg. 2007;40 (21):65–71.
		[B] Ruggiero SL, Mehrotra B, Rosenberg TJ, Engroff SL. Osteonecrosis of the jaws associated with the use of bisphosphonates: a review of 63 cases. J Oral Maxillofac Surg. 2004;62:527–34.
22. Blood disorders, iatrogenic or otherwise: von Willebrand disease, neutropenia, polycythemia, aplastic anemia, sickle cell anemia, hemophilia	All specialties Primary care, hematologist	Cahill MR, Colvin BT. Haemophilia. Postgrad Med J. 1997;73(858):201–6.
		Piccin A, Fleming P, Eakins E, McGovern E, Smith OP, McMahon C. Sickle cell disease and dental treatment. J Ir Dent Assoc. 2008;54(2):75–9.
		Wilde JT, Cook RJ. von Willebrand disease and its management in oral and maxillofacial surgery. Br J Oral Maxillofac Surg. 1998;36(2):112–8.

(continued)

Summary of areas of cross-domain (medical/dental) communication	Dental specialties	Medical subspecialties	References (adding references in progress)
23. Bacterial diseases	General dentist, periodontist	Internist, depends on disease	The U.S. Surgeon General's Report on Oral Health in America (2000) lists: 1. Mucous membrane pemphigoid. 2. Erythema multiforme (Stevens-Johnson) syndrome. [Can be fatal]. 3. Pemphigus vulgaris. Lichen planus
24. Archaeal role in disease	General dentist, periodontist	Primary care physician	Lepp PW, Brinig MM, Ouverney CC, Palm K, Armitage GC, Relman DA. Methanogenic Archaea and human periodontal disease. PNAS. 2004;101:6176–81. doi 10.1073_pnas.0308766101.
25. Fungal diseases	General dentist, periodontist	Internist, depends on disease	The U.S. Surgeon General's Report on Oral Health in America (2000) lists: 1. Candidiasis. 2. Histoplasmosis. [Can be fatal].
26. Viral diseases	General dentist	Internist, depends on disease	Navazesh M, Mulligan R, Kono N, Kumar S, Nowicki M, Alves M, Mack WJ. Oral and systemic health correlates of HIV-1 shedding in saliva. J Dent Res. 2010;89:1074–9. doi: 10.1177/0022034510375290. The U.S. Surgeon General's Report on Oral Health in America (2000) lists: 1. Primary acute herpetic gingivostomatitis (herpes simplex type 1, rarely type 2). 2. Recurrent herpes labialis. 3. Recurrent intraoral herpes simplex. 4. Chicken pox (varicella-zoster virus). 5. Herpes zoster (reactivation of varicella-zoster virus).

Appendix C 383

6. Infectious mononucleosis (Epstein-Barr virus).
7. Warts (HPV, papillomavirus).
8. Herpangina (coxsackievirus A; also possibly coxsackievirus B and echovirus).
9. Hand, foot, and mouth disease (type A cocksackieviruses).
10. Primary HIV infection [Can be fatal].

Regarding HIV See category 16, HIV/AIDS – dental screening.

Brewer JD, Ekdawi NS, Torgerson RR, Camilleri MJ, Bruce AJ, Rogers RS 3rd, Maguire LJ. Lichen planus and cicatricial conjunctivitis: disease course and response to therapy of 11 patients. J Eur Acad Dermatol Venereol. 2011;25(1):100–4.

Bruce AJ, Rogers RS 3rd. Oral manifestations of sexually transmitted diseases. Clin Dermatol. 2004;22(6):520–7.

Bruce AJ, Subtil A, Rogers RS 3rd, Castro LA. Monomorphic Epstein-Barr virus (EBV)-associated large B-cell posttransplant lymphoproliferative disorder presenting as a tongue ulcer in a pancreatic transplant patient. Oral Surg Oral Med Oral Pathol Oral Radiol Endod. 2006;102(4):e24–8.

Sánchez AR, Rogers RS 3rd, Sheridan PJ. Oral ulcerations are associated with the loss of response to infliximab in Crohn's disease. J Oral Pathol Med. 2005;34(1):53–5.

Tanaka T, Satoh T, Yokozeki H. Dental infection associated with nummular eczema as an overlooked focal infection. J Dermatol. 2009;36(8):462–5.

See Categories 23, bacterial diseases, and 26, viral diseases

| 27. Dermatological disease including nummular eczema as a dental focal infection | General dentist, periodontist | Dermatologist |

(continued)

Summary of areas of cross-domain (medical/dental) communication (pediatric)	Dental specialties	Medical subspecialties	References (adding references in progress)
28. Special populations, children (pediatric)	General dentist, pediatric dentist, orthodontist	Primary care, pediatrician	Acs G, Shulman R, Ng MW, Chussid S. The effect of dental rehabilitation on the body weight of children with early childhood caries. Pediatr Dent. 1999;21:109–13. American Academy of Pediatrics. An analysis of costs to provide health care coverage to the child and adolescent population age 0–21. Elk Grove Village: American Academy of Pediatrics; 1998. Griffin SO, Gooch BF, Beltran E, Sutherland JN, Barsley R. Dental services, costs, and factors associated with hospitalization for Medicaid-eligible children, Louisiana 1996–7. J Public Health Dent. 2000;60:21–7. Hellsing E, McWilliam J, Reigo T, Spangfort E. The relationship between craniofacial morphology, head posture and spinal curvature in 8, 11 and 15 years old children. Eur J Orthod. 1987;9:254–64. Kritsineli M, Shim YS. Malocclusion, body posture, and temporomandibular disorder in children with primary and mixed dentition. J Clin Pediatr Dent. 1992;16:86–93. Mouradian WE, Berg JH, Somerman MJ. Addressing health disparities through dental-medical collaboration, part I: the role of cultural competency in health disparities: training primary care medical practitioners in children's oral health. J Dent Educ. 2003;67(8):860–8. Sheller B, Williams BJ, Lombardi SM. Diagnosis and treatment of dental caries-related emergences in a children's hospital. Pediatr Dent. 1997;19:470–5. Slade GD, Rozier RG, Zeldin LP, Margolis PA. Training pediatric health care providers in prevention of dental decay: results from a randomized controlled trial. BMC Health Serv Res. 2007;7(176):1–11. doi:10.1186/1472-6963-7-176. The face of a child: the surgeon general's conference on children and oral health (2001). http://www.nidcr.nih.gov/nr/rdonlyres/ed6fb3b5-cef4-4175-938d-5049d8a74f66/0/sgr_conf_proc.pdf. Accessed 17 June 2011.

		Wehr E, Jameson EJ. Beyond health benefits: the importance of a pediatric standard in private insurance contracts to ensuring health care access for children. Future Child. 1994;4:115–33.
		Westmoreland TM. Innovative management of dental decay for young children enrolled in Medicaid/SCHIP. Health Care Financing Administration. (2011). https://www.cms.gov/smdl/downloads/smd050800.pdf. Accessed 15 June 2011.
		Wysen KH, Hennessy PM, Lieberman MI, Garland TE, Johnson SM. Kids get care: integrating preventive dental and medical care using a public health case management model. J Dent Educ. 2004;68(5):522–30.
29. Special populations: geriatric	All specialties except pediatric dentists	Primary care, gerontologist	Yoneyama T, Hashimoto K, Fukuda H, Ishida M, Arai H, Sekizawa K, Yamaya M, Sasaki H. Oral hygiene reduces respiratory infections in elderly bed-bound nursing home patients. Arch Gerontol Geriatr. 1996;22(1):11–9.

See also Category 6, respiratory diseases |
| 30. Special populations: neurodevelopmental disorder and intellectual disability (ND/ID) | General dentist | Primary care | Farman AG, Horseley B, Warr E, Ianke JL, Hood H. Outcomes of digital X-ray mini-panel examinations for patients having mental retardation and developmental disability. Dentomaxillofac Radiol. 2003;32:15–20.

Oral Health Section of: Mental Retardation and Developmental Disabilities. Section on downs syndrome, The New York City Department of Health and Mental Hygiene 2003. http://www.nyc.gov/html/doh/downloads/pdf/chi/chi22-4.pdf. Accessed 15 June 2011.

Thompson TG. Closing the gap: a national blueprint to improve the health of persons with mental retardation: report of the surgeon general's conference on health disparities and mental retardation. Office of the Surgeon General (US); National Institute of Child Health and Human Development (US); Centers for Disease Control and Prevention (US). Washington (DC): US Department of Health and Human Services. 2002. http://www.ncbi.nlm.nih.gov/books/NBK44344/. Accessed 22 June 2011.

Wolff A, Waldman B, Milano M, Perlman S. Dental students' experiences and attitudes towards individuals with mental retardation. J Am Dent Assoc. 2004;135:353–7.

Zelenski S, Hood H, Holder M. Continuum of quality care series, American Academy of Developmental Medicine and Dentistry. 2008. http://aadmd.org/articles/medicine-i-introduction. Accessed 15 May 2011. |

(continued)

Summary of areas of cross-domain (medical/dental) communication	Dental specialties	Medical subspecialties	References (adding references in progress)
31. Congenital conditions: cleft lip/cleft palate (CL/CP), Hutchinson's teeth, macroglossia	Oral and maxillofacial surgeon(s)	Otolaryngologist, reconstructive surgeon	Bernfeld WK. Hutchinson's teeth and early treatment of congenital syphilis. Br J Vener Dis. 1994 orig. 1971. 47:54. doi: 10.1136/bmj.309.6966.1386. Murthy P, Laing MR. Macroglossia: editorial. BMJ. 1994;309:1386. doi: 10.1136/bmj.309.6966.1386. Salyer KE, Xu H, Portnof JE, Yamada A, Chong DK, Genecov ER. Skeletal facial balance and harmony in the cleft patient: principles and techniques in orthognathic surgery. Indian J Plast Surg. 2009;42 Suppl:S149–67. Tyan ML. Differences in the reported frequencies of cleft lip plus cleft lip and palate in Asians Born in Hawaii and the Continental United States. Exp Biol. 1982;171(1):41–5. doi: 10.3181/00379727-171-41474. Wangsrimongkol T, Jansawang W. The assessment of treatment outcome by evaluation of dental arch relationships in cleft lip/palate. J Med Assoc Thai. 2010;93 Suppl 4:S100–6.
32. Ectodermal dysplasia and severe hypodontia	All specialties trained in genomics and proteomics	Genomic and proteomic researcher (personalized medicine)	Hobkirk JA, Nohl F, Bergendahl B, Storhaug K, Richter MK. The management of ectodermal dysplasia and severe hypodontia. International conference statements. J Oral Rehabil. 2006;33(9):634–7.
33. Breath odor: halitosis	General dentist	Primary care	Bollen CM, Rompen EH, Demanez JP. Halitosis: a multidisciplinary problem. Rev Med Liege. 1999;54(1):32–6. Delanghe G, Ghyselen J, Bollen C, van Steenberghe D, Vandekerckhove BN, Feenstra L. An inventory of patients' response to treatment at a multidisciplinary breath odor clinic. Quintessence Int. 1999;30(5):307–10.

34. Cognitive parameters of reducing disparities in healthcare (including oral health care)	All above or below	Sabbah W, Sheiham A. The relationships between cognitive ability and dental status in a national sample of USA adults. Intelligence. 2010;38:605–10. http://dx.doi.org/10.1016/j.intell.2010.08.003. Accessed 5 June 2011. Sabbah W, Watt RG, Sheiham A, Tsakos G. The role of cognitive ability in socio-economic inequalities in oral health. J Dent Res. 2009;88:351–5. http://jdr.sagepub.com/cgi/content/abstract/88/4/351. Accessed 5 June 2011.
35. Periodontal diseases – systemic inflammation [Rsch]	General dentist, periodontist	Wilson AG. Epigenetic regulation of gene expression in the inflammatory response and relevance to common diseases. J Periodontol. 2008;79(8s):1514–9. Inflammation links periodontal and systemic diseases. DrBicuspid 12/17/08. 2008. Available at: http://www.drbicuspid.com/index.aspx?sec=nws&sub=rad&pag=dis&Itemld=301282. Accessed 17 June 2011.
36. Biofilms: cystic fibrosis, endocarditis, cystitis, dental plaque, indwelling devices and implants. [Rsch]	All specialties trained in genomics and proteomics	Asahi Y, Noiri Y, Igarashi J, Asai H, Suga H, Ebisu S. Effects of N-acyl homoserine lactone analogues on Porphyromonas gingivalis biofilm formation. J Periodontal Res. 2010;45(2):255–61. Donlan RM, Costerton JW. Biofilms: survival mechanisms of clinically relevant microorganisms. Clin Microbiol Rev. 2002;15(2):167–93. Li J, Helmerhorst EJ, Leone CW, Troxler RF, Yaskell T, Haffajee AD, Socransky SS, Oppenheim FG. Identification of early microbial colonizers in human dental biofilm. J Appl Microbiol. 2004;97(6):1311–8. Lynch SV, Dixon L, Benoit MR, Brodie EL, Keyhan M, Hu P, Ackerly DF, Anderson GL, Matin A. Role of the rapA gene in controlling antibiotic resistance of escherichia coli biofilms. Antimicrob Agents Chemother. 2007;51(10):3650–8. http://www.stanford.edu/~amatin/MatinLabHomePage/PDF/RapA%20Lynch%20et%20al.pdf. Accessed 15 June 2011, See also Matin Lab on Biofilm Studies, Available at: http://www.stanford.edu/~amatin/MatinLabHomePage/Biofilm.htm. Accessed 16 June 2011.

(continued)

Summary of areas of cross-domain (medical/dental) communication	Dental specialties	Medical subspecialties	References (adding references in progress)
37. Anesthesia, sedation, and pain or odontalgia management	General dentist, endodontist	Anesthesiologist, nurse anesthetist	Aggarwal V, Joughin A, Zakrzewska J, Crawford F, Tickle M. Dentists' and specialists' knowledge of chronic orofacial pain: results from a continuing professional development survey. Prim Dent Care. 2011;18(1):41–4. Chicago dentists settle out of court in sedation death. DrBicuspid 8/14/08. 2008. Available at: http://www.drbicuspid.com/index.aspx?sec=nws&sub=rad&pag=dis&ItemI d=300843. Accessed 3 May 2009. Kanellis MJ, Damiano PC, Momany ET. Medicaid costs associated with the hospitalization of young children for restorative dental treatment under dental anesthesia. J Public Health Dent. 2000;60:28–32. Kim DS, Cheang P, Dover S, Drake-Lee AB. Dental otalgia. J Laryngol Otol. 2007;121(12):1129–34. Ram S, Teruel A, Kumar SK, Clark G. Clinical characteristics and diagnosis of atypical odontalgia: implications for dentists. J Am Dent Assoc. 2009;140(2):223–8. Rodríguez-Lozano FJ, Sanchez-Pérez A, Moya-Villaescusa MJ, Rodríguez-Lozano A, Sáez-Yuguero MR. Neuropathic orofacial pain after dental implant placement: review of the literature and case report. Oral Surg Oral Med Oral Pathol Oral Radiol Endod. 2010;109(4):e8–12. http://www.oooe.net/article/S1079-2104(09)00918-4/abstract. Accessed 10 May 2011. Spencer CJ, Neubert JK, Gremillion H, Zakrzewska JM, Ohrbach R. Toothache or trigeminal neuralgia: treatment dilemmas. J Pain. 2008;9(9):767–70.

These contact points, some based on oral manifestation(s) of systemic disease, inform the need for **inter-domain communication among medical and dental providers** of a patient to assure quality of care and patient safety.

Relevant resources:

- Cappelli DP, Mobley CC. Prevention in clinical oral health care. St. Louis: Elsevier; 2008.
- NIH. Oral health in America: a report of the Surgeon General. Rockville: U.S. Department of Health and Human Services. Bethesda: National Institute of Dental and Craniofacial Research, National Institutes of Health; 2000.
- Little JW, Falace DA, Miller CS, Rhodus NL. Dental management of the medically compromised patient. 6th ed. St. Louis: Mosby; 2002.

Appendix D

Editorial Team (Editing and Authoring)

- Acharya, Amit

    Amit Acharya, B.D.S, M.S., Ph.D. is general dental surgeon and a computer scientist with expertise in the field of biomedical informatics. **Dr. Acharya's** research focus has been on integration of medical and dental data and clinical systems, design and architecture of electronic health records, developing clinical decision supports and expert systems, information modeling and developing ontologies and terminologies, principles of evidence based practices, knowledge development and representation, and investigating the oral-systemic relationship between periodontal disease and other systemic disease such as diabetes and cardiovascular diseases.

    In his current role as a Dental Informatics Scientist at the Marshfield Clinic Research Foundation's Biomedical Informatics Research Center and the Interim Director of the Marshfield Clinic Research Foundation's Biomedical Informatics Core of the UW Institution for Clinical and Translational Research, his main focus is on the development, implementation and evaluation of clinical information systems by leveraging the field of translational biomedical and dental Informatics. Dr. Acharya also serves on the Management Committee of University of Wisconsin, Madison's Computational and Informatics in Biology and Medicine program which is funded by National Library of Medicine.

    Dr. Acharya has published in many national and international peer-reviewed journals. He has also presented in many national and international conferences and panels. Dr. Acharya has mentored several undergraduate and graduate students as part of the Dental Informatics internship program at Marshfield Clinic. He is also a key member of the American Dental Association's Standard Committee on Dental Informatics and is involved in various national standards development activities. Dr. Acharya played a key role in the development and enhancement of an integrated electronic dental record module within the

Marshfield Clinic's medical EHR system. He has also been involved in the development of a standardized information model for the general dental electronic dental records. As a co-investigator, Dr. Acharya represent Marshfield Clinic's involvement in the HMORN consortium of 12 diverse integrated healthcare systems within US and abroad, collaborating to develop a standardized, multi-system diabetes registry covering over 10 million enrollees and 750,000 members with diabetes mellitus.

- Din, Franklin

Franklin M. Din, D.M.D., M.A. is the Solution Architect for Transactions, Code Sets & Informatics, HP Enterprise Services, Global Healthcare, and is responsible for providing Medical Informatics, Terminology, and other healthcare data standards expertise improve healthcare delivery, costs, outcomes, and future trends. Standardization of data is essential to the Informatics goal of turning massive amounts of data into useful and actionable knowledge.

Frank joined HP in February 2009. In July 2009, he led the Medical Informatics Center of Excellence (MICOE) team successfully partnered with a Title XIX account to seamlessly in-source business analytic work that was previously outsourced at a cost of millions of dollars. In March 2010, he led the MICOE team that successfully delivered an HP proprietary, Medicaid-specific predictive model for diabetes. In November of 2010, Frank successfully designed, prototyped, and demonstrated an approach to perform Medical Term Standardization, Natural Language Processing, and Ontology development, all in Mandarin, for a Nationwide Medical Records Project in China.

Before joining HP, Frank was a Senior Informatics Consultant for Apelon, Inc. He was involved with data standardization for two rounds of the National Health Information Network (NHIN); he led the team that produced a strategy to cross-map discrete medication data streams which resulted in simplified analytics for an academic medical center; he devised a plan to bring SNODENT terminology into compliance with SNOMED CT; he worked on the improvement to the National Cancer Institute's NCI Thesaurus that resulted in the new BioMed GT terminology while simultaneously creating the prototype of a collaborative semantic media wiki that permits remote collaboration on BioMed GT. While working for the VHA in the Salt Lake City Office of Information, Frank created a tool to map concepts in VistA with SNOMED CT for the LDSI (Lab Data Sharing Initiative) which links the VHA and the Department of Defense lab systems; he created an MS Excel mapping tool to convert the Kaiser Permanente ICD-9 based problem list into a SNOMED CT based list. This work became the basis of the FDA's SPL problem list.

Prior to his specialization in Biomedical Informatics, Frank was a practicing dentist, Assistant Clinical Professor of Dentistry at NYU Dental School, and Course Director for Forensics Dentistry at Columbia University School of Dental and Oral Surgery. He currently serves as a member of DMORT (Disaster Mortuary Operational Response Team) to perform Forensic Dental Services at mass disaster sites, with previous deployments to the World Trade Center and Hurricane Katrina.

Frank has active memberships in AMIA (American Medical Informatics Association) and HIMSS (Healthcare Information Management Systems Society). He was a member of HITSP and co-chaired the subcommittee on planning and internal communications for HITSP's Education, Communication, and Outreach (ECO) Committee.

Frank received a BS in Biology from Lehigh University, a DMD from Farleigh Dickinson University, and completed an NLM (National Library of Medicine) post-doctoral fellowship in Biomedical Informatics with an MA from Columbia University.

- Powell, Valerie J.H.

Valerie J. Harvey Powell, Ph.D., M.S., R.T.(R), a native of Racine, Wisconsin, USA, first studied humanities, with a focus on languages, philosophy, and linguistics, then computer science and information systems, and finally radiologic technology. Her undergraduate studies in German and philosophy at Wabash College in Indiana included a year of studies of philosophy and linguistics at the Albert-Ludwigs-Universität, Freiburg im Breisgau, Germany. She then earned a masters degree, and a Ph.D. at the University of Texas at Austin. Her post-doctoral Masters Degree in Computer Science was completed at Texas A&M University in Commerce, Texas. She started teaching at The University of Texas at Austin in the fall of 1959 and has been teaching for over 50 years. She spent a sabbatical semester as a Visiting Scientist in Dynamic Systems at the Software Engineering Institute of Carnegie Mellon University, where the focus of her work was formal modeling of resectorization in the FAA Air Traffic Control system. Dr. Powell's studies in philosophy sensitized her to the properties of classification systems. She feels this foundation helped her question the routine sense of medical care that omitted attention to the stomatognathic system in certain critical respects.

When she began to work with and teach MUMPS (Massachusetts General Hospital Utility Multi-Programming System) in computer science in the early 1980s, she was soon invited to work with the U.S. Department of Veterans Affairs (VA). Her first publications in the field of hospital information systems appeared in the mid 1980s. She taught databases, including clinical databases, for a number of decades (both relational SQL technology and the MUMPS-based VA FileMan database technology of the U.S. Department of Veterans Affairs. She was admitted to the Sigma Xi science research honorary for research leading to a paper presented in Nagoya, Japan, in 1988: "Implications of Non-1NF Extensions to the Relational Database Model for the MUMPS Standard and MUMPS Databases." From 1988 through 1996 she served as a Consulting Scholar in medical computing for IBM Corporation. Dr. Powell carried out a number of projects for the VA (and also for the Indian Health Service (HIS)) over the years through 1999. From 1988 through 1992 she worked with Trident Technical College in Charleston, SC, to add an electronic dental record for patients served by their oral health education programs (dental hygiene and dental assisting).

During this period she also served on software standards committees: X3/DBSSG (Database Systems Study Group), X11 (MUMPS Users Group), NCITS/T3 (OSI Telecommunications), and as chair of NCITS/J21 (model-based formal specification systems), a committee with U.S. Technical Advisory Group (TAG) responsibilities for the Z and VDM international standards. Dr. Powell learned health informatics through collaboration with Dr. Charles J. Austin, author of textbooks on hospital information systems, and Dr. med. Wolfgang Giere, Director, Zentrum für medizinische Informatik, Goethe University, Frankfurt am Main, Germany, and through almost 30 years of experience assisting the U.S. Veterans Health Administration and working with its DHCP (later VistA) electronic health record (EHR) technology. In 1999 she gave invited lectures on health informatics and Year 2000 concerns at the Zentrum für Medizinische Informatik, Goethe University, Frankfurt am Main, Germany. She also lectured on Year 2000 issues at the Brandenburg Technische Hochschule in Cottbus. These lectures were sponsored by the U.S. Embassy in Berlin.

In 2000 she felt she needed clinical experience to do the kind of work in health care informatics she wished to do and completed the prerequisites for a degree in Radiologic Technology, and then the degree itself, passing the ARRT registry exam in 2002. She found this clinical experience valuable in her informatics work. She chose imaging as it would (and did) give her contact with many sub-specialties of medical care as well as first-hand experience in the Emergency Department and with a variety of surgical procedures in the operating room environment. It gave her experience with the workflow of the care setting and the necessary sense of delivering care to an individual patient for which one is responsible and not just for patient data. Since 1999 Dr. Powell has worked with WorldVistA, a non-profit organization making open-source VA VistA EHR technology available domestically and internationally. In 2007 she was invited by the Mexican government agency Instituto Mexicano del Seguro Social (IMSS) to provide technical advice on health information technology (HIT) in Mexico City. She taught health care informatics at Robert Morris University.

In 2007, Pennsylvania Gov. Ed Rendell appointed Dr. Powell to the Governor's Commission on Chronic Care Management, Reimbursement, and Cost Reduction, because of her extensive work with health information technology. With this assignment and facing the question as to whether performance measures proposed for the Commission's strategic plan were adequate, she noticed the omission of "dental referral" from the set of diabetes performance measures. She sought advice from the American Academy of Periodontology research staff in Chicago to learn what she needed to know to evaluate diabetes performance measures. She set about bringing her evaluation to the attention of the American Diabetes Association (ADA) and encouraged the ADA to add "dental referral" to its Standards of Care (SoC) for diabetes. This was done in 2007–2008. In 2008 she started giving lectures on and writing on the need to integrate medical and dental care and patient data. She holds an appointment as University Professor, Computer and Information Systems, at Robert Morris University, Moon Township, Pennsylvania, where she has taught for 20 years. Contact information: powell@rmu.edu

- Torres-Urquidy, Miguel Humberto
  Miguel Humberto Torres-Urquidy, D.D.S., M.S., Ph.D. (candidate) is a dentist who graduated from the National Autonomous University of Mexico. He continued his training with a Masters in Biomedical Informatics at the University of Pittsburgh where he is also finishing his PhD. In addition, he works as Informatics Fellow for the Influenza Division at the Centers for Disease Control and Prevention. He is also Chair of the Dental Informatics Working Groups for both the American Medical Informatics Association and the International Medical Informatics Association. He has published and currently serves as reviewer in several major scientific journals and conferences.

List of Contributing Authors

- Araújo, Filipe Miguel
  Filipe Araújo, D.M.D., M.Sc., is a Masters Degree Lecturer in Dental Medicine of the Health Sciences Department of the Portuguese Catholic University. Born in Coimbra, Portugal, Dr. Araújo was part of the second graduation course in Dental Medicine (2007) in the Health Sciences Department of the Portuguese Catholic University, a state-of-the-art modern dental school incorporating dental new technologies, including an all-in-one concept of clinical equipment, coupled with an advanced interactive ICT-based infrastructure.

  Immediately after his graduation he was invited to start teaching Fixed Prosthodontics and Dental Biomaterials as a Lecturer. In 2010, he completed his Masters Degree in Dental Medicine with research in fixed prosthodontics. In 2011 he was invited to teach also in Dental Informatics, under the supervision of Professor André Correia, Head of this Curricular Unit.

  Dr. Araújo is fully committed to electronic oral-health records and practice management systems, since the University Dental Clinic of the Portuguese Catholic University has electronic support provided by Newsoft Dente®, a leading PMS company in Portugal.

  Dr. Araújo also has a private practice in Dentistry with special dedication to Dental Implants, Biomaterials and Prosthodontics. His research interests included Prosthodontics, Biomaterials, Dental Informatics and Dental Education. He is member of the Portuguese Dental Association, and member of the International Team for Implantology (ITI).

  Contact Information: Universidade Católica Portuguesa – Campus de Viseu, Estrada da Circunvalação 3504–505 Viseu; fmiguel.araujo@gmail.com
- Allen, Mureen
  Mureen Allen, M.D., M.S., M.A., FACP has held a number of positions in the health information technology (HIT) industry and has worked on a variety of HIT initiatives, including solutions directed to physicians. Dr. Allen is committed to the development of HIT solutions that improve the delivery of health care. Her interests include clinical decision support, quality measurement, systems interoperability, usability, and the patient-centered medical home.

Dr. Allen was the Senior Associate for Informatics and Practice Improvement at the American College of Physicians (ACP), providing support for HIT public policy initiatives. Dr. Allen served as a co-chair of the Health Information Technology Standards Panel. As a co-chair she was active in identifying the appropriate standards to support consumer empowerment while using a personal health record, and also supported the identification of standards for consumers to express their preferences for sharing data.

Dr. Allen is board-certified in internal medicine. Beyond her recognition as a Fellow of the American College of Physicians, she is a member of the American Medical Association and the American Medical Informatics Association. Dr. Allen holds master's degrees in Biomedical Informatics and in Technology Management.

Contact information: dr.mallen@yahoo.com

- Boggs, Kelly

Kelly A. Boggs, B.S., M.B.A - Ms. Boggs has recently transitioned to healthcare from a decade long career in sales. As an Academic Administrative Fellow in the Division of Education, serving under the Division Administrator since 2010, she is gaining knowledge of the vision and culture at Marshfield Clinic and working on various special projects. Prior to that she served as a healthcare account executive, at Johnson Controls in their building efficiency division. Ms. Boggs received her Master's Degree from the University of Phoenix in healthcare management, and her undergraduate degree in political science and public administration from the University of Wisconsin Stevens Point. Her interest lies in developing and implementing a new model of education that will bring the practice of medicine and dentistry closer, reduce costs and help streamline the process of delivering healthcare. Ms. Boggs' current projects include the creation of several dental programs including a post-baccalaureate program and dental residency program.

- Casamassimo, Paul

Paul Casamassimo, D.D.S., M.S., is Professor and Chair, Division of Pediatric Dentistry, The Ohio State University College of Dentistry, and Chief of Dentistry, Department of Dentistry, Nationwide Children's Hospital, Department of Dentistry, Columbus, Ohio. He is former Editor-in-Chief of the American Academy of Pediatric Dentistry (AAPD) and its journal, *Pediatric Dentistry*, and also a past-president of AAPD. Dr. Casamassimo is past-president of the Academy of Dentistry for the Handicapped and past editor of the *Journal of Dentistry for the Handicapped* and the *Journal of Dentistry for Children*. Dr. Casamassimo has directed studies addressing early childhood caries and its management and represents the AAPD on projects related to infant oral health, maternal oral health, school health, and dental education. He is currently Interim Director of the AAPD Oral Health Policy Research Center.

- Chaudhari, Monica

Monica Chaudhari, M.S., is a statistician providing methodological, analytical and statistical support to Washington Dental Service. She joined WDS in 2006 after attaining a master's degree in biostatistics from the University of Washington. Her functional areas at WDS include facilitation of medical-dental collaborative research, multi-center provider profiling, dental utilization and costs analysis, and dental treatments and outcomes assessment. Her work has focused on statistical methods for skewed and over-dispersed data, missing data, mixed-effect models, longitudinal – survival joint models, propensity scores and estimation of lifetime cost models. She is also interested in applications of statistical decision theory to evaluate benefit plans and treatment pricing strategy for cost effectiveness with subjective assessments of oral health outcomes. One future goal is to develop new longitudinal models to account for temporal patterns in multistate progression of oral diseases when assessing the overall utility of oral health trajectory.

More recently, **Ms. Chaudhari** and Group Health investigators examined association between diabetes mellitus and periodontal disease in health outcomes and medical costs. They also looked at implications of diabetes in use of dental services and costs. **Ms. Chaudhari** serves as a journal referee and belongs to professional organizations including the International Biometric Society and the American Statistical Association (ASA).

- Cheriyan, Biju

   Biju Cheriyan, M.B.B.S., D.L.O. is an otolaryngologist who has worked as a fellow in a large teaching institution as well as a consultant in private practice in Holy Cross Hospital, Kottiyam and Caritas Hospital, Kottayam in Kerala, India. **Dr. Cheriyan** has rich clinical experience in the management of head and neck infections and tumors and chronic oro-facial pain. His special interests are middle ear reconstruction procedures and microsurgical procedures of the larynx.

- Chyou, Po-Huang

   Currently **Dr. Po-Huang Chyou** is the director of the Biostatistics group at the Marshfield Clinic Research Foundation. He has 22 years of biostatistical application experience in cancer, coronary heart disease, and aging studies. This experience includes seven years with the Kuakini Medical Center, Honolulu, Hawaii, and 15 years with the Marshfield Clinic Research Foundation, Marshfield, Wisconsin. In addition, **Dr. Chyou** has a strong interest in conducting epidemiological research and methodological research in the above-mentioned areas. He has authored or co-authored 90 papers in peer-reviewed journals. Regularly, he gives seminars and presentations to clinicians and scientists. Also, **Dr. Chyou** has many years of work experience using SAS and SUDAAN (Survey Data Analysis) statistical software packages and in helping research clinicians and scientists applying for and receiving research grants.

   Contact information: Po-Huang Chyou, Ph.D., Director/Senior Biostatistician, Biomedical Informatics Research Center, Marshfield Clinic Research Foundation, 1000 North Oak Avenue, Marshfield, WI 54449, Work Phone: (715) 389–4776; Work E-mail: chyou.po-huang@mcrf.mfldclin.edu; Work Fax: (715) 221–6402.

- Correia, Andre

   André Correia, D.M.D., Ph.D., is an Invited Assistant Professor in the Faculty of Dental Medicine of the University of Porto (FMDUP) and in the Health Sciences Department of the Portuguese Catholic University (DCS-UCP).

   Born in Porto, Portugal, Prof. Correia graduated in Dental Medicine in 2003 in FMDUP. In 2004 he was invited to become a Lecturer in the Dental Medicine Graduation Course of the DCS-UCP, a state-of-the-art modern dental school. This School pioneered the inclusion of Dental Informatics in its Curriculum, and Prof. Correia assumed the leadership of the area. From 2005 until now he is Head Professor of this discipline. Due to this commitment, Prof. Correia established formal contacts with Professor Titus Schleyer (Director of the Center for

Dental Informatics of the University of Pittsburgh) and in 2007 he completed an internship in this Center under the supervision of Professor Heiko Spallek, participating in a Project intitled "Proposal for an advanced IT / Informatics Course for Senior Pre-Doctoral Students".

In 2006, he was invited to teach as a Lecturer in FMDUP. In 2009, he achieved a PhD Degree in Dental Medicine (Area of Prosthodontics and Occlusion) in FMDUP. In the same year he became an Invited Assistant Professor in FMDUP and in the DCS-UCP, and also a Researcher in the 'Experimental Mechanics and New Materials' Research Unit.

In 2010, FMDUP invited Prof. Correia to integrate a discipline of Informatics and New Technologies in Dentistry into its PhD Degree and also into the discipline of Dental Medicine, at the Masters Degree level of studies.

Besides his academic activity, Prof. Correia also conducts private practice Dentistry in the Dr. Manuel Neves Dental Clinic, Porto, Portugal, with special dedication to Oral Rehabilitation and to New Technologies applied to Dentistry. His research interests include Dental Informatics, Prosthodontics, Implantology, Oral Biomechanics and Dental Education.

Prof. Correia is fully committed to electronic oral-health records (e-OHR) and practice managements systems (PMS), being a full user of these technologies in the University Dental Clinic and in its Private Practice. He is member of the Portuguese Dental Association, the Portuguese Society of Stomatology and Dental Medicine, and Speaker of the International Team for Implantology (ITI).

Contact Information:
1. Faculdade de Medicina Dentária da Universidade do Porto. Rua Dr. Manuel Pereira da Silva, 4200–393, Porto, Portugal. acorreia@fmd.up.pt
2. Universidade Católica Portuguesa – Campus de Viseu, Estrada da Circunvalação 3504–505 Viseu; andrericardocorreia@gmail.com

- Diehl, Mark

Mark Diehl, D.D.S, is the Director of the Health Informatics program at Misericordia University, Dallas, PA, where he has built a comprehensive undergraduate, graduate, and continuing education program. His research interests include data architecture and modeling, information governance, and the human-system interaction.

Dr. Diehl is member of the US Technical Advisory Group of the International Standards Organization Technical Committee 215 on Health Informatics, chair of the American Dental Association Standards Committee on Dental Informatics Subcommittee 11 on Clinical Informatics, and co-chair of the ASTM subcommittee E31.25 on Healthcare Data Management, Security, Confidentiality, and Privacy. He is the principal author of several health informatics standards such as the ANSI/ADA Specifications 1000, 1027, and 1039, and ASTM standards E2145 and E2436. He has also contributed to standards work in Health Level Seven, serving as the HL7 liaison to the American Dental Association, and has worked on standards activities in the ANSI Health Information Technology Standards Panel and the National Council for Prescription Drug Programs.

Among his degrees, Dr. Diehl received a D. D. S. from Temple University, a MA in Computer Data Management and Health Systems Management from

Webster University, and a MPH in Health Services Administration from the Uniformed Services University.

Contact information: 301 Lake St. Dallas, PA 18612; mdiehl@misericordia.edu.

- Farman, Allan

 Allan G. Farman, B.D.S., Ph.D., M.B.A., D.Sc., Diplomate ABOMR, is a dentist with a current specialty license in Oral and Maxillofacial Radiology in the Commonwealth of Kentucky, current specialty listing in Dental and Maxillofacial Radiology from the General Dental Council, United Kingdom, and a current specialty license in Oral and Maxillofacial Pathology in the Republic of South Africa. He holds earned doctorates both in Oral and Maxillofacial Radiology and in Oral and Maxillofacial Pathology. Dr. Farman is current President of the American Academy of Oral and Maxillofacial Radiology (2009–2011), was 11th President of the International Association of DentoMaxilloFacial Radiology (1994–97), and is founder and organizer of the annual International Congress and exposition Computed Maxillofacial Imaging. He has served as a voting representative to the DICOM Standards Committee for more than a decade and is founding Co-Chair of DICOM Working Group 22 (Dentistry). He is Professor of Radiology and Imaging Science, The University of Louisville School of Dentistry, with concurrent appointments in Anatomical Sciences and Neurobiology, and in Diagnostic Radiology at the Medical School of the same institution. He is Honored Guest Professor to Peking University, Beijing, China. He has contributed to more than 400 journal articles and edited or authored more than 20 books and proceedings, in addition to editorships of a number of scientific journals.

- Foreman, Stephen

 Stephen Foreman, J.D., Ph.D., M.P.A., is Associate Professor of Health Economics at Robert Morris University, Pittsburgh, PA, and in 2008–2009 was a Fulbright Scholar at the Crimea State Medical University, Simferopol, Crimea, where he lectured and conducted research in comparative health policy. CMSU made him an honorary professor and a permanent member of the faculty. He has served as Associate Vice President for Academic Affairs for Robert Morris. He has also been Vice President for Research of the Pennsylvania Medical Society.

 Dr. Foreman has authored reports for and has testified on behalf of the American Medical Association, the American College of Obstetrics and Gynecology, a number of state medical societies, the Attorney General of New York and a number of major national law firms dealing with health care reimbursement and the market for health insurance. He served on Governor Edward Rendell's health care reform task force. He was the author of the 2005, 2007 and 2010 State of Medicine reports published by the Pennsylvania Medical Society.

 Dr. Foreman holds a Ph.D. in Health Economics from the University of California, Berkeley, a J.D. from the University of North Carolina and a Master in Public Administration from Harvard's Kennedy School of Government. Dr. Foreman's research includes the economics of aging and health insurance markets.

 Contact information: foreman@rmu.edu

- Geist, Shin-Mey Rose Yin

  Shin-Mey Rose Yin Geist, **D.D.S.**, **M.S.**, is an Associate Professor in the Departments of Biomedical and Diagnostic Sciences and Patient Management at the University of Detroit Mercy School of Dentistry. Born and raised in Taiwan, Republic of China, **Dr. Geist** graduated from Dental School in Taiwan in 1974. She specialized in Oral Surgery and was teaching in the University Hospital when she found her passion for Oral Medicine. She completed her master's degree in Oral Diagnosis/Oral Medicine at the Indiana University School of Dentistry in 1985 and then studied and worked in Molecular Biology and DNA cloning research at the medical schools at Indiana University and Wayne State University. Dr. Geist received her DDS degree in 1990 from University of Detroit and has been teaching oral diagnosis and oral medicine at UDM since that time. She has been course director of the advanced oral medicine course for graduate students in Periodontics and advanced General Dentistry. **Dr. Geist** served as Chair of the Oral Diagnosis and Oral Medicine section of the American Dental Education Association (ADEA) and is presently serving on the editorial review board of the Journal of Dental Education, the official journal of ADEA. She was recently appointed as a member of the content analysis working group of MedEdPORTAL Oral Health in Medicine Model Curriculum. MedEdPORTAL is a peer-reviewed online publication of the Association of American Medical Colleges (AAMC), partnered with ADEA.

  Dr. **Geist** has held a Diplomate of the American Board of Oral Medicine since 1992 and has special interest in medically complex dental patient management. She is committed to improving the interface between medical and oral health care. Her research interests include the efficiency in teaching and service in providing comprehensive coordinated care. Contact information: geistsh@udmercy.edu

- Glaizel, Jeff

  Jeffrey R. Glaizel, **D.D.S.**, developed, designed, implemented and is currently President and CEO of myDDSnetwork.com, a secure web based dental referral and consultation network. The myDDSnetwork platform has been utilized in a project in Ontario to facilitate the secure electronic transfer of patient information from hospitals to medical doctors' offices. Dr. Glaizel has also been contracted to provide consulting services to the health care industry in Ontario. He maintains a private practice dental office in Toronto and is a consultant to the insurance industry with respect to dental claims.

  Dr. Glaizel is a member of the Royal College of Dental Surgeons of Ontario (provincial regulatory body) working group for electronic dental records, a member of the American Medical Informatics Association, American College of Legal Medicine, American Association of Dental Consultants, Ontario Dental Association, Canadian Dental Association, American Dental Association and the Canadian Association for People Centred Health. He lectures and consults groups on electronic record keeping privacy and security, health care workflow and interoperability of health care records. Dr. Glaizel received his Doctorate of Dental Surgery from the University of Toronto in 2001. Contact information: (e) drjeff@myddsnetwork.com ; (w) www.myddsnetwork.com

Appendix D

- Gounot-Bertaud, Valerie
  Valerie Bertaud-Gounot, Ph.D., is Associate Professor at the University Psychiatric Hospital of Rennes in France. She obtained her bachelor's degree in computer engineering and subsequently her dental degree. She later obtained a PhD in Biomedical Informatics followed by a Masters in Statistics. She teaches preventive medicine, biostatistics, evidence-based medicine and dental informatics. In addition, she continues her clinical activities providing care for patients at the Dental Emergencies Facility of the University Hospital and the Dental Office of the Psychiatric Hospital of Rennes.
- Holder, Matt
  Matthew Holder, M.D., M.B.A., is an international leader in the emerging field of Developmental Medicine, Dr. Holder advocates on behalf of people with neurodevelopmental disorders and intellectual disabilities (ND/ID) for better health services. Dr. Holder currently serves as the Global Medical Advisor for Special Olympics International, the Executive Director for the American Academy of Developmental Medicine and Dentistry, and is the Chief Executive Officer of the Underwood and Lee Clinic in Louisville, Kentucky – a clinic whose mission is to serve the medical, dental and behavioral health needs of people with ND/ID. Over the course of his career, Dr. Holder has advocated at local, state, national and internal levels for better healthcare for people with ND/ID. To this end, Dr. Holder has authored numerous policy statements, research papers and educational curricula.
- Hood, Henry
  Henry Hood, D.M.D., is Director of the Underwood and Lee Clinic, and he is also a Clinical Associate Professor in the Department of Orthodontic, Pediatric and Geriatric Dentistry, University of Louisville School of Dentistry, Louisville, Kentucky. Dr. Hood is Co-Founder and Immediate Past President of the American Academy of Developmental Medicine and Dentistry and Chief Clinical Officer for the CHYRON Management Corporation.
- Johnson, Bruce
  Bruce A. Johnston, M.L.S. is an Associate Professor of Learning Resources and Health Sciences Librarian at Robert Morris University, Pittsburgh, PA. In these roles, he is actively involved in the development and provision of library services, information, and instruction to faculty and students in the School of Nursing and Health Sciences. In addition, he serves on several University-wide committees and is co-chairperson of the Robert Morris University Institutional Review Board (IRB). A 1979 graduate of the University of Pittsburgh School of Library and Information Sciences, he has held several positions at the University of Pittsburgh Medical Center (UPMC) including Director, Blair-Lippincott Library/Learning Resource Center at the Eye & Ear Hospital of Pittsburgh (1979–1996). He presently also serves as Administrative Librarian for the Department of Otolaryngology, University of Pittsburgh School of Medicine. He has co-authored several papers in the field of library science, the most recent of which examined publication misrepresentation rates among Otolaryngology resident applicants.

- Kilsdonk, Joseph

  Joseph Kilsdonk, **AuD**, has served as the Administrator for Marshfield Clinic's Education Division since 2004. The Division oversees the largest community health center based training programs in the State of Wisconsin. Prior to that he served as an associate dean overseeing health career's for a public college, served as an executive for a national ancillary health care service corporation, served on the management team of a multi-specialty physician group practice and a community hospital, taught as an assistant professor, and founded and managed hospital and community based outreach practices.

  Dr. Kilsdonk was the lead author on the Clinic's dental education feasibility study leading to its current efforts in dental education resulting in a public – private partnership for rural dental education expansion. He has presented locally, regionally, and nationally on a number of health care and practice management topics. Most recently he has presented to the "National Health Policy Forum on Oral Health; 10 Years after the Surgeon's General Report" in Washington DC. He has served on Wisconsin's Dental Education Feasibility Study Advisory Committee and presently serves on the Advisory Committee for the Wisconsin Academy for Rural Medicine, the Committee for the Wisconsin Rural Physician Residency Assistance Program, and the Chancellor's Advisory Committee for University of Wisconsin at Stevens Point. He has been a manuscript reviewer for the Journal of Dental Education since 2009. **Dr. Kilsdonk** received his doctorate in audiology for the Arizona School of Health Sciences, a Masters Degree from the University of Wisconsin Oshkosh, and his undergraduate degree in communicative disorders from the University of Wisconsin Stevens Point.
- Klein, W Ted

  W. Ted Klein, **M.S.**, Klein Consulting, Inc. Vocabulary Co-chair, HL7 International.

  Contact Information: tk_cmrc@tklein.com
- Kovaric, Jessica

  Jessica Kovarik, **B.A.**, is currently an ophthalmology resident at the University of Pittsburgh School of Medicine. She received her BA in philosophy at Cornell and then pursued her MD at the University Of Miami Miller School Of Medicine. Her current interests include delivery of eye care in underserved populations.
- Leite, Filipa Almeida

  Filipa Almeida Leite, **M.D.**, is a final-year resident in a Pediatric Training Program in S. Teotónio Hospital, in Viseu, Portugal. Born in Santa Maria da Feira, Portugal, Dr. Leite pursued her Medical Degree in the Faculty of Medical Sciences in the New University of Lisbon, the capital of the country, achieving graduation in 2004. From 2005 to 2006 she completed a General Internship in S. Sebastião Hospital in Santa Maria da Feira, and in 2006 she entered a Pediatric Training Program in the S. Teotónio Hospital, in Viseu, which she will finish in June 2011. In this PTP she performed Clinical Attending through different Pediatric Departments during which she developed several publications in the form of papers, abstracts, posters and oral communications, winning a first prize for the Best Oral Presentation in the 58th Congress of the Spanish Society of Pediatrics, in 2009.

Dr. Leite is totally committed to electronic health records, due to her experience in different departments of various hospitals, where she has worked with Alert® (a leading clinical system in Portugal, with contracts in 12 countries), Medtrix EPR, a third prize awarded software by the XI Microsoft Health Users Group developed in S. Sebastião Hospital and SAM (electronic health record of the Portuguese Health System Central Administration).

Following a special interest in Neurology, Dr. Leite completed an observership in the Department of Neurology of the Children's Hospital, Boston, Massachusetts, USA, under the supervision of Prof. David Urion, in 2010. Besides the Clinical Training and a pediatric private practice, Dr. Leite had a Secondary Appointment as a Clinical Instructor of Pediatrics in the Medical Program of the Jean Piaget University of Angola. Dr. Leite is member of the Portuguese Medical Association and the Portuguese Society of Pediatrics. Contact information: filipasoaresleite@gmail.com

- Liceaga, Rodrigo

Rodrigo Licéaga-Reyes, D.D.S., Ph.D., has been working since 2000 at the Juarez Hospital in Mexico City in the Department of Oral and Maxillofacial Surgery and he has been Associate Professor since 2004. His prominent work at Juarez Hospital made him an invited professor in oral and maxillofacial surgery from other programs of trainees in Mexico, Peru and the Dominican Republic.

Dr. Licéaga-Reyes has authored publications in different areas including oral surgery, oral and maxillofacial pathology, orthognathic surgery, maxillofacial trauma, temporomandibular joint dysfunction, reconstructive surgery and dental stem cells. He is member of the Mexican College and Association of Oral and Maxillofacial Surgery, and is certified by the Mexican Board of Oral and Maxillofacial Surgery.

Dr. Licéaga-Reyes holds a Ph.D. in Oral and Maxillofacial Surgery from the Juarez Hospital and the National Autonomous University of Mexico (UNAM); He is currently Associate Professor or Oral Surgery at Technological University of Mexico (UNITEC). He is committed to improving the relationship between oral and medical health care systems as well as the medical and surgical education of the dental students. He also holds a DDS from the National Autonomous University of Mexico.

Dr. Licéaga-Reyes has been a speaker in Mexico, the USA, South America, Central America and the Caribbean. His private practice is established in Mexico City, limited to oral and maxillofacial surgery.

Contact Information: Tlaxcala 177–606, Col. H Condesa, Mexico, DF, Mexico 06170; r_liceaga@hotmail.com

- Mahnke, Andrea

Andrea Mahnke, B.S., is a Usability Analyst for Biomedical Informatics Research Center of the Marshfield Clinic Research Foundation. Andrea's research focus is in health communication and emerging media technologies. Currently she is a usability analyst in the Interactive Clinical Design Institute (ICDI). ICDI features the Interaction Laboratory where she observes, records and analyzes people interacting with health care computer hardware and software interfaces. The understanding gained from these studies guides design of new computer systems that will be faster, easier to use and reduce medical errors. Andrea also mentors summer undergraduate and graduate intern students. She has presented posters at several national conferences. Andrea is currently pursuing her Master of Science degree.

Contact information: Andrea Mahnke, B.S., Usability Analyst, Biomedical Informatics Research Center, Marshfield Clinic Research Foundation, 1000 North Oak Avenue, Marshfield, WI 54449; 715-389-4474; mahnke.andrea@marshfieldclinic.org

- Marques, Tiago Miguel

Tiago Marques, **D.M.D.**, **M. Sc.**, is a Masters Degree Lecturer in Dental Medicine of the Health Sciences Department of the Portuguese Catholic University.

Born in Viseu, Portugal, Dr.Marques was part of the second graduation course in Dental Medicine (2007) in the Health Sciences Department of the Portuguese Catholic University, a state-of-the-art modern dental school incorporating dental new technologies, including an all-in-one concept of clinical equipment, coupled with an advanced interactive ICT-based infrastructure.

Immediately after his graduation, in 2007, he was invited to start teaching Periodontology and Gerodontology in this Department. In 2008, he successfully completed a post-graduation in Oral Surgery at the Universidad La Habana, Cuba. In 2010, he completed his Masters Degree in Dental Medicine in the Health Sciences Department of the Portuguese Catholic University with a research on Periodontology. In 2011 he was invited to teach also in Dental Informatics, under the supervision of Professor André Correia, Head of this Curricular Unit.

Currently, he is the Clinician responsible for private appointments at the Portuguese Catholic University. Dr. Marques is fully committed to electronic oral-health records and practice managements systems, since this University has an electronic support provided by Newsoft Dente®, leading PMS company in Portugal.

Dr. Marques also practices private Dentistry with special dedication to Periodontology, Dental Implants, Prosthodontics. His research interests include Dental Informatics, Periodontology, Biomaterials and Dental Education. He is member of the Portuguese Dental Association of the International Team for Implantology (ITI).

Contact Information: Universidade Católica Portuguesa – Campus de Viseu, Estrada
   da Circunvalação 3504–505 Viseu; tiagomiguelmarques@gmail.com
- Mishra, Sushma

Sushma Mishra, **M.B.A..Ph.D.**, is an assistant professor of computer information systems at Robert Morris University. She has a MBA degree from India and a PhD in information systems from Virginia Commonwealth University. **Dr. Mishra's** research interests include information security, information assurance issues in health care information systems, systems auditing and systems development methodologies. **Dr. Mishra** has been published in several conference proceedings, book chapters and journal articles on these topics. She teaches information security and decision support systems. Contact information: mishra@rmu.edu

- Nash, David A

  David A. Nash, D.M.D., M.S., Ed.D., is the William R. Willard Professor of Dental Education, and professor of pediatric dentistry, at the College of Dentistry of the University of Kentucky. He holds joint appointments as professor of behavioral science in the College of Medicine, and professor of public health ethics in the College of Public Health. From 1987–1997, Nash was dean of the College of Dentistry at Kentucky. Nash's primary contributions to the literature are on the themes of dental education, professional ethics, and the oral health care workforce. He has served as a visiting professor at over one-half of the nation's dental schools in the United States, and at several institutions internationally. He has been a prime advocate of integrating dental education with medical education, and has called for the creation and adoption of an "oral physician" curriculum. He has also been a leader in advocating adding a new member to the dental team, a "pediatric oral health therapist," to help address the problem of access to oral health care for children. Nash has been named by the American Student Dental Association as one of its *"visionaries"* in American dentistry. He has been acknowledged by students with several outstanding teaching awards.

- Nycz, Gregor

  Greg Nycz is Director of Family Health Center of Marshfield, Inc., (FHC) a federally funded community health center. Greg has been involved with the planning and operation of FHC for over 36 years. The Family Health Center of Marshfield, Inc./Marshfield Clinic partnership has been a model of how a health care delivery system can be developed to meet needs of rural, medically underserved populations. It was formally recognized as such by the Clinton Administration in 1999. Greg, who completed a U.S. Public Health Service Primary Care Policy Fellowship in 1997, has been a co investigator and/or project director for numerous research projects related to providing health care services to underserved rural areas and economically disadvantaged individuals and families.

  Nycz also has been invited to attend, participate and make presentations at local, state and national conferences on such issues as the future of family health centers, mental health services in rural populations, Medicare and Medicaid services, health insurance for the uninsured, health care financing, research opportunities in rural settings and public and private efforts to improve public health. Greg has served on numerous state and national advisory groups and committees, including recent appointments to the NIH Director's Council of Public Representatives and the State of Wisconsin's Special Committee on Health Care Access. Greg is a member of the University of Wisconsin, School of Medicine and Public Health's (UWSMPH) Oversight and Advisory Committee and Medical Education and Research Committee. He also serves on the Advisory Board for the University of Wisconsin Population Health Institute.

  Among many recognitions, Greg has been honored with the American Dental Association Access Recognition Award in 1995, the National Association of

Community Health Centers Advocacy Award for outstanding work to advance the legislative agenda of the health center movement in 1996, the Wisconsin Rural Health Association's "2000 Rural Health Achievement Award" for leadership, innovation and service for rural health in Wisconsin, and the National Network for Oral Health Access, Oral Health Champion Award, October 26, 2010.

Contact information: Greg Nycz, Director, Family Health Center of Marshfield, Inc., 1000 North Oak Avenue, Marshfield, WI 54449; 715-387-9137; nycz.greg@marshfieldclinic.org

- Piraino, Beth

Beth Piraino, **M.D.**, received her bachelor's of science from the University of Pittsburgh. She attended medical school at the Medical College of Pennsylvania, and graduated magna cum laude. She did her subsequent training in Internal Medicine and Nephrology at the University of Pittsburgh Health Center, after which she joined the faculty of the University of Pittsburgh School of Medicine, rising through the ranks over the years to her current position as tenured Professor of Medicine and Associate Dean of Admissions and Financial Aid.

Dr. Piraino's major research interest has been to improve outcomes of patients on peritoneal dialysis. She has published widely in the area of peritoneal dialysis, with numerous presentations at national and international meetings. She received the prestigious Life Time Achievement Award at the 24th Annual Dialysis Conference in 2004 for contributions to the care of peritoneal dialysis patients. She has received the Gift of Life Award from the NKF of Western Pennsylvania. She is the President Elect of the National Kidney Foundation. She is yearly listed in 'Best Doctors,' by Pittsburgh magazine. Contact information: 412-383-4899.

- Schleyer, Titus K

Titus Schleyer, **D.M.D.**, **Ph.D.**, is currently Associate Professor and Director of the Center for Dental Informatics (http://di.dental.pitt.edu) at the University of Pittsburgh. He holds DMD degrees from the University of Frankfurt, Germany, and Temple University, Philadelphia, as well as a PhD degree in molecular biology from the University of Frankfurt and an MBA degree in Health Administration from Temple University. Dr. Schleyer has been active in dental informatics research since 1989, conducting seminal research on electronic dental records, and Internet applications, workflow and human-computer interaction in dentistry. Since 1997, Dr. Schleyer has been a recipient of a training grant for dental informatics from the National Institute of Dental and Craniofacial Research. As a co-director of the Biomedical Informatics Training Program of the School of Medicine, he is responsible for the dental informatics concentration, in which he typically mentors several PhD and MS students. Dr. Schleyer also teaches dental informatics in the School of Dental Medicine predoctoral program and is a clinical instructor in general dentistry. Dr. Schleyer's research on dental computer applications is primarily funded by the National Institutes of Health. He publishes regularly on dental informatics topics in major journals, such as the Journal of the American Dental Association and the Journal of the American Medical Informatics Association. Dr. Schleyer is a member of the American Dental Association's Standards Committee for Dental Informatics. In 2009, he was

Appendix D

elected to the American College of Medical Informatics. More information about Dr. Schleyer is available at http://about.me/titusschleyer.
- Schrodi, Stephen J

Steven J. Schrodi, Ph.D., Associate Research Scientist – Genetics, Center for Human Genetics, 1000 North Oak Avenue – MLR, Marshfield, WI 54449.

Dr. Steven J. Schrodi is currently an Associate Research Scientist at the Marshfield Clinic Research Foundation in the Center for Human Genetics. His primary research interests lie in complex disease genetics, genetics theory, applied probabilistic models, and population genetics. He is a principal investigator in the University of Wisconsin Institute for Clinical and Translational Research and a member of the Wisconsin Genomics Initiative. **Dr. Schrodi's** research has led to several patents and 28 publications in leading scientific journals. He holds a doctoral degree from the University of California and has previously conducted research at the Celera Corporation, The Institute for Theoretical Dynamics, and NASA Ames Research Center. **Dr. Schrodi** is a member of the American Society of Human Genetics, the International Society of Bayesian Analysis, and the American Association for the Advancement of Science. He has also served on the Scientific Advisory Board of DNA Sciences. His experimental studies have resulted in novel discoveries of genes involved in susceptibility to rheumatoid arthritis, neurodegeneration, liver fibrosis, and psoriasis, thereby highlighting key biological pathways responsible for these diseases. **Dr. Schrodi** has also developed Bayesian mapping methods, extended linkage disequilibrium theory, robust experimental design methods, and has made advancements in theoretical molecular evolution. His work has been awarded the Applera Demonstrated Noteworthy Achievement Award in 2007 and the Top 10 Arthritis Advancement Award of 2004 from the Arthritis Foundation.

Dr. Schrodi's laboratory currently focuses on finding genetic variants that predispose individuals to chronic, systemic inflammation, infectious diseases, differential response to pharmaceuticals, neurodevelopmental traits, periodontal disease, and metabolic dysfunction. Additional efforts are placed on large-scale computer simulations, statistical genetic methods, and testable theoretical models.

Contact information: 1-715-221-6443; schrodi.steven@mcrf.mfldclin.edu
- Shoemaker, Wells

Wells Shoemaker, M.D., is the medical director of the California Association of Physician Groups (CAPG), representing 150 medical groups which serve approximately 18 million Californians in prepaid, comprehensive care, PPO, and governmentally funded care. His work emphasizes quality improvement on the population level, primary care rejuvenation, health disparities, and employer-group health coordination…all of which figure prominently as success factors for healthcare reform. He oversees CAPG's annual Standards of Excellence Survey, which serves as a substantial blue print for the infrastructure to support a successful ACO.

Dr. Shoemaker also serves as the co-Chair of the California Quality Collaborative, a 10 year old purchaser/payor/provider organization. Previously,

Dr. Shoemaker served as medical director of a Medi-Cal managed care Plan, an IPA, as well as multiple community based initiatives in Santa Cruz County. He was the principal investigator for an AHRQ funded community wide diabetes registry project 2004–2007. Before focusing entirely upon system based care, **Dr. Shoemaker** practiced primary care pediatrics for 25 years, including 7 years teaching in a family practice residency.

Contact information: 915 Wilshire Blvd #1620, Los Angeles, CA 90017; wshoemaker@CAPG.org.

- Thyvalikakath, Thankam

  Thankam Thyvalikakath, B.D.S., M.D.S., M.S., D.M.D., is Assistant Professor at the University of Pittsburgh, School of Dental Medicine. **Dr. Thyvalikakath**, a researcher and a clinician, holds dental degrees from the University of Kerala, India and University of Pittsburgh, Pittsburgh as well as specialty degree in Oral and Maxillofacial Surgery from the University of Calicut, India and an MS degree in Biomedical Informatics from the University of Pittsburgh. She also has a certificate in Clinical Research from the University of Pittsburgh. Her current work is focused on clinical applications of dental practice management systems, especially relating to usability and clinical decision-making. Dr. Thyvalikakath has designed novel interfaces for chairside applications that support clinicians' decision-making and thus improve patient outcomes. Through a K08 grant funded by the NIDCR in 2009, she is implementing and evaluating informatics-based interventions for risk assessment of periodontal disease in general practice. **Dr. Thyvalikakath's** long-term research interests include, visualizing clinical data to support the cognitive needs of clinicians during patient care, developing decision support tools that identify high-risk patients for chronic oral diseases and implementation and evaluation of informatics-based interventions to help clinicians deliver improved patient care efficiently and effectively.

- Walls, AWG

  Angus W.G. Walls, B.D.S., Ph.D., FDSRCS (England and Edinburgh). **Dr. Walls** is currently Professor of Restorative Dentistry and Director of Research, School of Dental Sciences, Newcastle University and Honorary Consultant in Restorative Dentistry to the Newcastle Hospitals NHS Foundation Trust. He is Vice Dean of the Faculty of Dental Surgery, RCS England. His research interests are the oral health needs of the older population, particularly the oral and dental problems of older people with natural teeth. In 2003 **Dr. Walls** received the Distinguished Scientist Award from the International Association for Dental Research (IADR), which observes that **Dr. Walls'** work "has furthered the understanding of oral health care needs of the ageing population and in particular the association between oral health status and nutrition (BDJ, 2003)." He has more than 100 publications to his credit and has presented many of these findings at major conferences worldwide. **Dr. Walls** is the principal contact for the Oral and Dental Research Trust, which makes awards to support investigations of clinical relevance, particularly in the field of preventive care. *British Dental Journal*, doi:10.1038/sj.bdj.4810377

- Walji, Muhammad F

    Muhammad Walji, Ph.D. is an Assistant Professor at the University of Texas Dental Branch at Houston focused on dental informatics research. He received a B.S. in Biology in 2001 from the University of Texas at Dallas, and a M.S and Ph.D. in Health Informatics from University of Texas School of Health Information Sciences in December 2003, and December 2006 respectively. From 2003 to 2006, he was a National Library of Medicine (NLM) funded pre-doctoral fellow. He joined the Department of Diagnostic Sciences at the UT Dental Branch in January 2007. **Dr. Walji** currently serves as Principal Investigator of a NLM funded grant to develop an Inter-university Oral Health Data Repository from EHR data that will allow end users to directly explore and extract information to support their specific research or decision making needs. In addition, he serves as co-investigator on the NICDR funded project seeking to apply a cognitive approach to refine and enhance use of a Dental Diagnostic Terminology and user interface in EHRs. **Dr. Walji** is also a Project Leader for Project 1: Work-Centered Design of Care Process Improvements in HIT, which is part of the National Center for Cognitive Informatics and Decision Making in Healthcare (NCCD). He has also done extensive work in consumer-health informatics where he has presented and published numerous papers on issues relating to E-health. Contact: muhammad.f.walji@uth.tmc.edu

- Waxman, Evan

    Evan (Jake) Waxman, M.D., Ph.D. is currently Assistant Professor and Vice Chair for Education at the University Of Pittsburgh Department Of Ophthalmology. His medical degree is from the Mount Sinai School of Medicine in New York. His PhD in Biomedical Sciences is from the City University of New York. He received his ophthalmology training at the University of California, Davis. **Dr. Waxman** maintains a busy comprehensive ophthalmology practice in Pittsburgh. Since 1999 he has directed ophthalmology medical student education at the University of Pittsburgh. In addition, since 2001 has served as the ophthalmology residency program director. He is the recipient of numerous medical student and resident teaching awards. He is currently Vice President for Information Technologies for the Association of University Professors in Ophthalmology Medical Student Educators Council. His current areas of focus include the use of interactive fiction in the creation of virtual patients for training health care providers and research into delivery of eye care in underserved populations.

- Yoder, Natalie F.

    Natalie F. Yoder, B.S., is a usability analyst at the Biomedical Informatics Research Center of Marshfield Clinic Research Foundation. Ms. Yoder earned a bachelor's degree in Psychology with a Human Services Emphasis from the University of Wisconsin-Stevens Point. In addition to her course work, her undergraduate studies included an internship in clinical psychology and research in applied psychology and co-authoring an article in *Teaching of Psychology*. In the last few years Ms. Yoder has presented research posters at various conferences including the Midwestern Psychological Association and the American

Medical Informatics Association. Her current research focus is in investigating the usability of health information technology to facilitate improvements and innovative approaches in the design of electronic medical and dental records.

Contact information: Natalie Yoder, Biomedical Informatics Research Center, Marshfield Clinic Research Foundation, 1000 North Oak Avenue, Marshfield, WI 54449; (715) 221-6439; yoder.natalie@mcrf.mfldclin.edu

Appendix E – List of Resources with URLs

American Academy for Pediatrics (AAP): http://www.aap.org/ – Oral Health Initiative: http://www.aap.org/oralhealth/
American Academy for Periodontology (AAP): http://www.perio.org/
American Academy of Pediatric Dentistry: http://www.aapd.org/
American Dental Association (ADA): http://www.ada.org/
American Dental Education Association (ADEA): http://www.adea.org/Pages/default.aspx
American Diabetes Association (ADA): http://www.diabetes.org/
American Medical Informatics Association (AMIA): https://www.amia.org/ and Oral Health: http://www.idf.org/diabetes-and-oral-health
BiomedGT Collaborative Ontology Development Wiki: http://biomedgt.nci.nih.gov/wiki/index.php/Main_Page
Bring Research in Diabetes to Global Environments and Systems (BRIDGES): http://www.idf-bridges.org/
Canadian Paediatric Society (CPS): http://www.cps.ca/
Code on Dental Procedures and Nomenclature (CDT): http://www.ada.org/3027.aspx
Dental Informatics Virtual Global Community (DIOC):http://www.dentalinformatics.com/
HHS/HRSA Strategic Plan: http://www.hrsa.gov/about/strategicplan.html
International Classification of Diseases (ICD), International: http://www.who.int/classifications/icd/en/ – USA: http://www.cdc.gov/nchs/icd.htm – UK National Health Service: http://www.connectingforhealth.nhs.uk/systemsandservices/data/clinicalcoding/codingstandards/icd10
International Health Terminology Standards Development Organization (IHTSDO): http://www.ihtsdo.org/
International Medical Informatics Association (IMIA): http://www.imia.org/
Journal of the Canadian Dental Association (JCDA): http://www.jcda.ca/
Logical Observation Identifiers Names and Codes (LOINC®): http://loinc.org/
National Diabetes Education Program (NDEP): http://ndep.nih.gov/ – Working Together to Manage Diabetes: A Guide for Pharmacists, Podiatrists, Optometrists, and Dental Professionals: http://www.ndep.nih.gov/media/PPODprimer_color.pdf
National Diabetes Information Clearinghouse (NDIC): http://diabetes.niddk.nih.gov/dm/pubs/complications_control/
National Institute of Dental and Cranio-Facial Research (NICDR): http://www.nidcr.nih.gov/ – Dental Management of the Organ Transplant Patient http://www.nidcr.nih.gov/OralHealth/Topics/OrganTransplantationOralHealth/OrganTransplantProf.htm – Oral Complications of Cancer Treatment: What the Dental Team Can Do, http://www.nidcr.nih.gov/OralHealth/Topics/CancerTreatment/OralComplicationsCancerOral.htm.
RxNorm of the Unified Medical Language System® (UMLS®): http://www.nlm.nih.gov/research/umls/rxnorm/
Scottsdale Project – The Report of the Independent Panel of Experts of the Scottsdale Project: http://downloads.pennnet.com/pnet/gr/scottsdaleproject.pdf
SNODENT: http://www.ada.org/2060.aspx
World Dental Federation (IDF): http://www.fdiworldental.org/

Index

A
Accountable Care Organization (ACO), 184
Advanced Education General Dentistry
 (AEGD), 278
Advancing Clinico-Genomic Trials (ACGT), 56
Agency for Healthcare Research and Quality
 (AHRQ), 140–141
Aggressive dental treatment plan
 costs of, 177–181
 potential benefits of, 177
American Academy of Pediatricians (AAP), 6
American Association of Critical Care Nurses
 (AACCN), 358
American Association of Medical Colleges
 (AAMC), 10, 11
American Recovery and Reinvestment Act
 (ARRA), 65, 68, 145
American Society for Testing and Materials
 (ASTM), 41
Antibiotic prophylaxis (AP), 89, 90
Arizona School of Dentistry and Oral Health
 (ASDOH), 274
Atherosclerosis Risk in Communities
 (ARIC) study, 206
Australian Council on Healthcare Standards
 (ACHS), 141, 143
Autoimmune diseases (AD), 81

B
Bad breath, 213–214
Basic Formal Ontology (BFO), 59
Betel quid (BQ) chewing, 14
BFO. *See* Basic Formal Ontology (BFO)
Biosurveillance and dentistry
 background, 229
 and bioterrorism, 230–231
 COHR and computer ownership, 231–232
 dental organizations, 238
 detection algorithms and evaluation,
  237–238
 hypothetical case, 233–235
 privacy and confidentiality, 237
 proposed system, 232–233
 public health systems, 229–230
 security and redundancy, 237
 software architecture, 235–236
 source of information against
  bioterrorism, 232
 standards, 236
 system design, 235
 in US, 230
Bioterrorism
 and dentistry, 230–231
 source of information against, 232
Bisphosphonate-associated osteonecrosis
 (BON), 83
Bleeding time (BT), 95
Branch retinal artery occlusion, 209

C
Canada
 barriers for integration, 300
 CIHI and CCIH, 302
 governance model, 300–301
 OHS, 302
 RCDSO, 301
Canadian Council on Integrated Health Care
 (CCIH), 302
Canadian Institute for Health Information
 (CIHI), 302
Candidate gene studies, 263–264
Candidiasis, 78–79

Caries, 256
Cathepsin C, 264
CCHIT. *See* Certification Commission for Health Information Technology (CCHIT)
CDS. *See* Clinical decision support (CDS)
Central retinal vein occlusion, 209
Cerebral palsy, 216, 217
Certification Commission for Health Information Technology (CCHIT), 65, 71
Chronic graft-*versus*-host disease (CGVHD), 83
Chronic kidney disease (CKD), 79, 92–93
Cleft palate/cleft lip, 211
Clinical attachment level (CAL), 144
Clinical Data Interchange Standards Consortium (CDISC), 242
Clinical decision support (CDS)
 clinical drivers, 111–113
 DART, 112
 historical drivers, 111
 PALM version
  AppForge application, 120
  CPU, 120
  display, 119
  hardware considerations, 118, 119
  high risk patient selection, 128
  high risk patient warning, 128
  hyperthyroid warning, 123, 124
  medical history, 121
  memory, 119–120
  prophylactic antibiotic dosing, 126, 127
  prophylactic antibiotic warning, 126
  prosthetic health valve selection, 125
  prosthetic health valve warning, 125
  thyroid problem selection, 122
  thyroid problem sub-type selection, 123
 PC version, 129
Clinical quality measure (CQM)
 asthma, 150
 cancer, 150
 diabetes, 149
 heart disease, 150
COHR. *See* Computer-based oral health record (COHR)
Commercial-off-the-shelf (COTS) products, 30, 38
Community Health Center (CHC), 143
 CHC model, 273–274
 CHC placement, 278
 interrelationship with CHC, 282
Community Periodontal Index of Treatment Needs (CPITN), 144

Comparative effectiveness research (CER), 243
Computer-based oral health record (COHR), 231–232
Computerized Physician Order Entry (CPOE), 148, 153
 medication orders, 148–153
Cost benefit analysis
 aggressive dental treatment plan
  costs of, 177–181
  potential benefits of, 176
 costs *vs.* benefits, 181
 dental insurance and coverage in US, 169–170
 dental problems and chronic illness, 171–172
 expanded dental insurance coverage, 181–182
 implications for health policy, 172–176
CQM. *See* Clinical quality measure (CQM)
C-reactive protein (CRP) concentrations, 171
Current Procedural Terminology (CPT), 20, 21

D

Decayed, missing, and filled surfaces (DMFS), 144
Decayed, missing, and filled teeth (DMFT), 144
De novo mutations, 261–262
Dental education
 concerns, 280–282
 at crossroads, 268–269
 economics, equity, and education converge, 273–275
 FQHC model, 276–277
 future of, 275–276
 IOM recommendations, 269–273
 Surgeon General's Report, 270–271
 training
  Accountable Care Organization, 279–280
  Advanced Education General Dentistry, 278
  RMED program, 277
  WARM program, 277–278
Dental insurance coverage
 aggressive dental treatment plan
  benefits of, 177
  costs of, 177–181
 cost *vs.* benefits, 181
 dental problems and chronic illness, 171–172
 expanded, 181–182

Index 411

implications for health policy, 172–176
in United States, 169–170
Dentists and otolaryngologists
  halitosis (bad breath), 213–214
  headache, 211
  nasal sinuses tumor, 212
  oral cavity ulcers, 212
  refered otalgia (earache), 213
  temporomandibular joint disorders, 212–213
  trigeminal neuralgia, 211–212
Dentogingival epithelial surface area (DGES), 11, 12
Department of Defense (DoD), 16
Department of Health and Human Service (HHS), 7, 71
Description logics (DLs), 55–56
Descriptive Ontology for Linguistics and Cognitive Engineering (DOLCE), 59
DGES. See Dentogingival epithelial surface area (DGES)
Diabetes mellitus (DM), 78
Diagnostic aid resource tool (DART), 112
Digital Imaging and Communications in Medicine (DICOM), 27, 63, 64
Disease gene mapping, 258–261

E
Earache, 213
Early childhood caries (ECC), 197–198, 200
Economics
  of clinical data integration
    economic impact, 189–191
    increased efficiency and patient safety, 188–189
    insurance industry studies, 186–187
    integrated decision making, 183–185
  dental insurance coverage
    aggressive dental treatment plan, benefits of, 177
    aggressive dental treatment plan, costs of, 177–181
    cost vs. benefits, 181
    dental problems and chronic illness, 171–172
    expanded, 181–182
    implications for health policy, 172–176
    in United States, 169–170
  of integrated decision making, 183–185
EDR. See Electronic dental record (EDR)
EHR. See Electronic health record (EHR)
EHT. See Electronic healthcare technologies (EHT)

Electronic data capture, 240–241
Electronic dental record (EDR)
  communication between EMR and, 250–251
  current use of, 247–249
Electronic financial systems, 247–249
Electronic healthcare technologies (EHT)
  context-specific delivery, 105–107
  totality of data, 109–110
  usability, 108–109
Electronic health record (EHR)
  accountability, 71
  audit controls and monitoring, 76
  authorization policies, 75
  authorization techniques, 72–73
  clinical quality measures
    asthma, 150
    cancer, 150
    diabetes, 149
    heart disease, 150
  cohort selection and patient recruitment, 242
  common language for, 241–242
  comparative effectiveness research, 243
  consumers and providers, 75
  data access mechanisms, 72–73
  data storage and handling, 73
  dental records, 76–77
  disaster recovery plan, 76
  disaster recovery preparation, 73–74
  economic benefits of, 188–189
  economic impact relative to, 189–191
  and electronic data capture, 240–241
  health outcomes policy, 145–146
  inter-organizational agreements, 75
  Marshfield Clinic
    community health centers, 336–338
    dentists' dashboard application, 335
    expert panel discussion analysis, 344–350
    Family Health Center of Marshfield, Inc., 338–344
    Marshfield Clinic Health Center Complex, 333
    physicians' dashboard application, 334
  objectives, 146–149
  patient consent, 71–72, 74
  patient information, 72
  patient registries, 244
  physical security, 76
  policies, procedures and controls, 76
  privacy rule
    ARRA, 68
    CCHIT, 68–69
    collection, use and disclosure limitations, 70

Electronic health record (EHR) (cont.)
    correction, 69
    data quality and integrity, 70
    individual access, 69
    individual choice, 70
    openness and transparency, 69
    safeguards principle, 70
    system complexity, 70
  rating and ranking, 358
  secondary use of, 242–243
  security rule, 67–68
  standard access control, 75
  standardization and interoperability, 75
state privacy laws, 74
  United States Dental School adoption survey, 245–246
Electronic medical record (EMR), 250–251
End stage renal disease (ESRD), 15, 16
Epigenetics, 262–263
Evidence-based integrated care plan (EBICP), 187

F
Federally qualified health center (FQHC), 274–277, 279–280
Federally qualified health centers (FQHCs), 274, 276–277, 280
Fragile X syndrome, 222–225

G
Gardner syndrome, 84–85
Gastro esophageal reflux disorder (GERD), 214, 220
General medical practitioners (GMP), 14
Genetics
  de novo mutations, 261–262
  epigenetics, 262–263
  genetic technologies and disease gene mapping, 258–261
  heritability, 257–258
  oral disease
    candidate gene studies, 263–264
    future of, 266–268
    genome-wide association studies, 266
    linkage studies, 264–265
  site frequency spectrum, 261–262
  structural variants, 261–262
Genetic technologies, 258–261
Genome-wide association studies, 266
Genome-wide linkage studies, 264–265
Genomics
  modern genetics
    de novo mutations, 261–262

    epigenetics, 262–263
    genetic technologies and disease gene mapping, 258–261
    heritability, 257–258
    site frequency spectrum, 261–262
    structural variants, 261–262
  oral disease genetics
    candidate gene studies, 263–264
    future of, 266–268
    genome-wide association studies, 266
    linkage studies, 264–265
  oral disease phenotypes
    caries, 256
    chronic inflammation, metabolic dysfunction, and infection, 253–254
    oral cancers, 256–257
    periodontitis, 254–256
  technological progress in, 261
  transformative developments, 252
GERD. *See* Gastro esophageal reflux disorder (GERD)
GLT6D1, 266
Graft-Versus-Host Disease (GVHD), Chronic, 83
Group Health Cooperative (GH), 100–104

H
Halitosis (bad breath), 213–214
Headache, 211
Head and Neck Cancer (HNC), 84
Health Effectiveness Data and Information Set (HEDIS®), 140–143
Health Information Exchange (HIE), 69, 73–75, 77
Health Information Technology for Economic and Clinical Health (HITECH), 66, 145, 245
Health information technology (HIT)
  American National Standards
    ANSI/ADA Specification 1000, 46–48
    ANSI/ADA Specification 1039, 42–46
    clinical investigation design, 51
    codes and nomenclature, 51
    communications, 49
    health care events, 49–50
    health care materiel, 50
    health services objects, 50
    health services provider, 50
    individual characteristics, 49
    living arrangement and physical characteristics, 49

Index

modeling process, 41–42
organizations, 49
patient health condition diagnosis, 51
patient health facts, 50
patient specimen, 50
patient treatment plan, 51
population characteristics, 49
population health condition diagnosis, 51
population health facts, 50
population outcome reference, 51
provider credentials and privileges, 50
autoimmune diseases, 81
bisphosphonate-associated osteonecrosis, 83
cancer, 82–83
candidiasis, 78–79
chronic graft-*versus*-host disease, 83
chronic kidney disease, 79
cooperation and collaboration, 358
data standards and coded terminologies
  benefits, 37
  bleeding control, 36
  brand names, 32
  caries, 35
  CDT and ICD-9, 38
  clinical terminologies, 32–33
  dental examination, 34
  dental information, 38–39
  extensiveness of code, 36
  hypothetical treatment, 30–31
  medical history of liver disease, 34
  MO amalgam, 35
  patient's complaints, 35
  prescription, 36
  prognosis, 36
  purpose, 30
  SNOMED CT and LOINC, 37–38
diabetes mellitus, 78
early CDS application
  background, 116–118
  PALM version, 119–128
  PC version, 129
efficient structured communication
  bisphosphonate therapy, 97
  chemotherapy/radiation therapy, 98
  illegibility, 98
  implementation, 99
  principles of, 96
  time and manpower, 99
  transmission methods, 98
electronic decision support
  application areas, 114
  clinical drivers, 111–113
  diagnosis, 113
  diagnostic information, 115
  education, 115
  health care delivery system, 116
  historical drivers, 111
  inference mechanisms, 114–115
  justification, 115–116
  workflow, 116
electronic healthcare technologies
  context-specific delivery, 105–107
  totality of data, 109–110
  usability, 108–109
electronic health record
  accountability, 71
  audit controls and monitoring, 76
  authorization policies, 75
  authorization techniques, 72–73
  consumers and providers, 75
  data access mechanisms, 72–73
  data storage and handling, 73
  dental records, 76–77
  disaster recovery plan, 76
  disaster recovery preparation, 73–74
  inter-organizational agreements, 75
  patient consent, 71–72, 74
  patient information, 72
  physical security, 76
  policies, procedures and controls, 76
  privacy rule, 68–70
  security rule, 67–68
  standard access control, 75
  state privacy laws, 74
frequent dental infections, 78–79
Gardner syndrome, 84–85
head and neck cancer, 84
hemophilia, 80–81
HIV infection and AIDS, 80
and informatics
  communication between EMR and EDR, 248–251
  dental school and health system relationship, 250
  department/center for, 246–247
  electronic dental records, 247–249
  electronic financial systems, 247–249
  Medicaid meaningful use incentive program, 249
  United States dental school EHR adoption survey, 245–246
Health information technology (HIT)
  knowledge representation and ontologies
    bottom-up approach, 59
    components and structure, 54
    construction process, 60

Health information technology (HIT) (*cont.*)
        content, 61, 62
        definitions, 53–54
        dental emergencies, 60, 61
        dentistry, 57
        description logics, 55–56
        diverse data, 56
        evaluation, 61
        exchanging data, 56
        integrating data, 56
        intelligent system, 58
        medical/dental care, 61
        Ogden-Richardson semiotic triangle, 52–53
        top-down approach, 59
        types of, 54
        web ontology language, 54–55
    oral healthcare providers, 85
    oral health inclusion, 63–64
patient identification, 100–104
    physicians' needs for dental records, 77–78
    role of standards
        content standards, 26, 27
        HL7 Messaging Standard, 27
        interchange standards, 26
        stop sign and road sign, 28–29
    Sjögren syndrome, 81–82
    standardized/structured communication messages
        antiplatelets, 94
        bleeding time and PFA-100, 95
        cancer patient management, 95
        chronic kidney disease, 92–93
        consultation/referral, 86
        coronary artery stent, 91–92
        diabetes, 91
        heart murmurs and antibiotic prophylaxis, 89, 90
        hypertension, 87, 89
        implantable cardioverter-defibrillator, 93–94
        limitations, 96
        oral anticoagulants, 94
        organic heart murmurs, 90–91
        permanent pacemaker, 93–94
        renal dialysis, 93
    systemic lupus erythematous, 82
    xerostomia, 78–79
Health Insurance Portability and Accountability Act (HIPAA), 65, 66
    accountability, 71
    data storage and handling, 73
    patient information, 72
    PHI, 66, 67
    privacy rule, 68–70
    security rule, 67
Health Resources Services Administration (HRSA), 7–8
    strategic plan calls for integration of oral health into primary care, 9–10, 135
    patient-centered medical-dental home (PCM-DH), 8
    diabetes measure, 143
Health Resources and Services Administration (HRSA), 7, 10, 143
Hemodialysis (HD), 16
Hemophilia, 80–81
Hemophilia treatment centers (HTCs), 80
Heritability, 257–258
Highly Active Anti-Retroviral Therapy (HAART), 80
HIT. *See* Health information technology (HIT)
Hutchinson's teeth, 211
Hypertensive optic neuropathy, 210
Hypertensive retinopathy, 208

I

Implantable cardioverter-defibrillator infections, 93–94
Indian Health Service (IHS), 6, 20
Infective Endocarditis (IE), 89, 97
Institute of Medicine (IOM) report, 4, 10
Institute of Security and Social Services for State Workers, 308
International Classification of Diseases (ICD), 27
International perspectives
    Canada
        barriers for integration, 300
        CIHI and CCIH, 302
        governance model, 300–301
        OHS, 302
        RCDSO, 301
    Mexico
        ambulatory treatments, 305
        communication technologies, 310
        electronic health records, 309
        General Health Law, 303
        governmental medical treatment services, 306
        hospital treatments, 305

Institute of Security and Social Services for State Workers, 308
Mexican Health Ministry, 304
Mexican Institute for Social Security, 306–307
National Health Program, 304
private medical and dental care, 308–309
Portugal
dental education and practice, 314–326
medical care to population, 313–314
medical schools, 312
perspectives and comparisons, 310–311
private health insurance, 311–312
regulation of medical practice, 312
United Kingdom, 326–327
Inter-organizational agreements (IOAs), 75

K
Kidney disease, 203–204
Kidney Disease: Improving Global Outcomes (KDIGO), 92, 93
Kidney Disease Outcomes Quality Initiative (KDOQI), 92

L
Leeds abdominal pain system, 111–112
Linkage disequilibrium, 260
Linkage studies, 264–265

M
MacColl Chronic Care Model (MacColl CCM), 4, 5
Macroglossia, 211
Macy study, 271–272
Marshfield Clinic
additional staff, 158–159
CattailsDental, 335
community health centers, 336–338
dentists' dashboard application, 335
electronic medical record, 158
environmental challenges, 156–157
expert panel discussion analysis
blended health care team model, 346–347
clinical decision support, 347
combined electronic medical and dental record, 345
comprehensive patient care, 346
diagnostic codes and standardized terminology, 347–348
health insurance cooperation, 349–350
integrated dental-medical education model, 348–349
patient education and privacy concerns, 349
themes, 345
Family Health Center of Marshfield, Inc.
clinical training space, 341
dental patients, 342
Health Resources and Services Administration, 341
Ladysmith Dental Center, 339, 340, 343
information overload, 158
Marshfield Clinic Health Center Complex, 333
medications requirements, 156
non-representation of dental practice, 159
patient resistance, 157
physicians' dashboard application, 334
role, 158
staff and patients, data availability, 159
time/priorities, 157
Meaningful Use (MU), 145–160
core objectives, 147–148
how does meaningful use requirement affect dentistry, 150–155
menu objectives, 148–149
potential measures, 155
stage 1, 154, 156–159
Medicaid dental coverage, 170
Medical and dental data
AAP, 6
Aetna's Dental/Medical Integration Program, 5
American Diabetes Association, 6
CIGNA's Oral Health Integration Program[SM], 5–6
clinical vs. medical, 356
clinician vs. physician, 356
consistent and ongoing training, 357
data inconsistency, 16–17
data standards, 20–21
data standards development, 355
Medical and dental data
dental and medical students, 359
EDR certification, 354–355

Medical and dental data (cont.)
  fundamental healthcare delivery
      model, 8–9
  healthcare domains, 1–4
  healthcare education and preventive care,
      9–11
  health information technology, 357–358
  Healthy People 2020, 7
  IHS, 6
  implementation experiences, 357
  informatics consultants and vendors, 358
  Institute of Medicine, 4
  insurance claim, 17–18
  MacColl CCM, 4, 5
  oral health dimension
    clinical research design, 359
    quality measures, 358–359
  patient-centered care
    bisphosphonate caused
        osteonecrosis, 13
    cardiovascular disease, 11–12
    diabetes, 11–12
    eating disorders screening, 14
    kidney disease, 15–16
    low birth weight, 12
    oral cancer prevention, 13–14
    oral cancer screening, 13–14
    oral hygiene and respiratory
        infections, 15
    pediatric care, 14
    periodontal disease, 11–12, 15–16
    post radiation osteonecrosis, 13
    prenatal care, 12
    tobacco and betel use screening, 13–14
  patient data, 18–20
  patient experiences, 360–361
  rating and ranking, 358
  recording of dental diagnoses, 356–357
Medical and dental data
  Scottsdale Project, 6
  timeline, 8
  Wisconsin Diabetes Advisory Group, 5
Metrics and measurements
  ACHS, 141, 143
  annual dental visits, 140
  DMFT, 144
  electronic health records
    clinical quality measures, 146, 149–151
    health outcomes policy, 145–146
    objectives, 146–149
  HEDIS®, 140–143
  HRSA, 143
  Marshfield Clinic Dental Centers
    additional staff, 158–159
    electronic medical record, 158
    environmental challenges, 156–157
    information overload, 158
    medications requirements, 156
    non-representation of dental
        practice, 159
    patient resistance, 157
    role, 158
    staff and patients, data availability, 159
    time/priorities, 157
  meaningful use requirement
    certified EHR, 150
    clinical decision support, 151
    EDR compliance, 151–153
    exchange key clinical information, 155
    patient reminders, 154–155
    potential measures, 155
    quality improvement and public
        reporting, 154
    up-to-date problem list, 154
  NCQA, 141–143
  periodontal disease, 160–163
  totality of healthcare, 142
  WCHQ, 142–144
  WDAG, 143
Mexican Institute for Social Security,
    306–307
Mexico
  ambulatory treatments, 305
  communication technologies, 310
  electronic health records, 309
  General Health Law, 303
  governmental medical treatment
      services, 306
  hospital treatments, 305
  Institute of Security and Social Services
      for State Workers, 308
  Mexican Health Ministry, 304
  Mexican Institute for Social Security,
      306–307
  National Health Program, 304
  private medical and dental care, 308–309
Microarray gene expression data (MGED)
    ontology, 56

N
Nasal sinuses tumor, 212
Nasopharyngeal carcinoma (NPC), 84
National Association of Community Health
    Centers, 338
National Call to Action, 337
National Committee on Quality Assurance
    (NCQA), 141–143

National Dental EDI Council (NDEDIC), 76
National Electronic Disease Surveillance
    System (NEDSS), 229–230
National Program for Oral Health Promotion
    (PNPSO), 319
National Quality Measures Clearinghouse
    (NQMC), 139–140
NCQA. *See* National Committee on Quality
    Assurance (NCQA)
NEDSS. *See* National Electronic Disease
    Surveillance System (NEDSS)
Neurodevelopmental disorders and intellectual
    disabilities
  interdisciplinary solutions for
    interdisciplinary problems, 225–228
  and phenytoin-induced gingival
    enlargement, 221–225
  primary complications, 215–219
  surveying the landscape, 214–215
  and undiagnosed GERD, 220
  and undiagnosed syphilis, 219
Newsoft Dente® odontogram, 324
Newsoft Dente® periogram, 325
Novigest® e-agenda, 326
Novigest® odontogram, 325

O

Office of National Coordinator
    (ONC), 65, 69, 145
Ontario Health Study (OHS), 302
Ophthalmic imaging, integrating
  ARIC study, 206
  branch retinal artery occlusion, 209
  central retinal vein occlusion, 209
  EHR, 205
  hypertensive optic neuropathy, 210
  hypertensive retinopathy, 208
  nonproliferative diabetic retinopathy, 208
  retinal imaging, 206
  retinal macroaneurysm, 210
Oral and Systemic Health Research Project
    (OSHRP), 190–191
Oral Cancer Foundation (OCF), 13
Oral cancers, 256–257
Oral cavity ulcers, 212
Oral disease
  genetics
    candidate gene studies, 263–264
    future of, 266–268
    genome-wide association studies, 266
    linkage studies, 264–265
  phenotypes

caries, 256
chronic inflammation, metabolic
    dysfunction, and infection, 253–254
oral cancers, 256–257
periodontitis, 254–256
Oral disease pathogenesis, 267–268
OSHRP. *See* Oral and Systemic Health
    Research Project (OSHRP)
Osteonecrosis of the jaws (ONJ), 13
Osteoradionecrosis (ORN), 13

P

Patient-centered medical home (PCMH), 184
Patient Protection and Affordable Care Act, 338
Patient records and clinical research
  cohort selection and patient
    recruitment, 242
  common language, 241–242
  electronic data capture, 240–241
  electronic health records, 240–241
  patient registries, 244
  practice-based research networks, 243–244
  secondary use of EHR data, 242–243
Patient registries, 244
PCI. *See* Percutaneous coronary intervention
    (PCI)
Pectus excavatum, 223
Pediatric medical and dental care
  childhood caries prevention, 199–200
  children's oral health, 194–195
  intervention model, 196–199
  oral health characteristics, 193–194
  paper *vs.* EHR, 200–203
Percutaneous coronary intervention (PCI), 91
Periodontal disease, 203–204
Periodontitis, 254–256
Permanent pacemaker (PPM), 93–94
Phenomics. *See* Genomics
Phenytoin-induced gingival enlargement,
    221–225
Physician data query (PDQ), 95
Picture Archiving and Communication
    Systems (PACS), 64
Plan-Do-Study-Act (PDSA), 4
Platelet function assay-100 (PFA-100), 95
Portugal
  dental education and practice
    e-health record, 321–323
    e-oral health record, 323–326
    health information network, 322
    health services, 321
    higher education, 314–316

Portugal
    PNPSO, 319
    Portuguese Dental Association, 314–316
    health subsystems, 311, 312
    medical education and practice
        medical care to population, 313–314
        medical schools, 312
        regulation of, 313
    perspectives and comparisons, 310–311
Post radiation osteonecrosis (PRON), 13
Practice-based research networks (PBRN), 243–244
Practice management system (PMS), 323, 324
Previser risk calculator (PRC), 161–163
Primary care physician (PCP), 2, 3
Privacy and Security Framework (PSF), 70
Protected health information (PHI), 66, 67
Proteomics. *See* Genomics
Public health systems, 229–230

R
Registered Dental Hygienist (RDH) xx, 64
Resource description framework (RDF), 55
Retinal macroaneurysm, 210
Risk assessment
    tools for periodontal disease, 160–163
    multi-factorial models, 161
    early childhood caries, 197–198
Role-Based Access Control (RBAC), 64
Royal College of Dental Surgeons of Ontario (RCDSO), 301

S
Significant Caries Index (SiC), 136, 144
Sjögren syndrome (SS), 81–82
Social security number (SSN), 100, 101, 104
Society for Imaging Informatics in Medicine (SIIM), 64
Standards Committee on Dental Informatics (SCDI), 40
Support physician activities (SAM), 321, 322
Swedish Oral Medicine Web (SOMWeb) system, 57

Systematized Nomenclature of Dentistry (SNODENT), 21, 34, 35, 36, 154, 242, 297
Syphilis, 216, 219
Systematized Nomenclature of Medicine (SNOMED), 21
    clinical Terms – CT, 239
Systemic lupus erythematous (SLE), 82

T
Temporomandibular joint disorders, 212–213
Trigeminal neuralgia, 211–212
Trisomy 21, 216, 217

U
Ulcers, oral cavity, 212
United States Dental School EHR adoption survey, 245–246
User interface (UI), 108
US illnesses, chronic, 173

V
Veterans Affairs, Department of (VA; also Veterans Health Administration or VHA), xii, xxix, 18, 75, 188, 358

W
Washington Dental Service (WDS), 100–104
Web ontology language (OWL), 54–55
WHO Global Oral Health Programme, 2
Wisconsin Academy for Rural Medicine (WARM program), 277–278
Wisconsin Collaborative for Health Quality (WCHQ), 142–144
Wisconsin Diabetes Advisory Group (WDAG), 5, 143
World Health Organization (WHO), 2

X
Xerostomia, 78–79

MIX
Papier aus verantwortungsvollen Quellen
Paper from responsible sources
FSC® C105338

If you have any concerns about our products,
you can contact us on
ProductSafety@springernature.com

In case Publisher is established outside the EU,
the EU authorized representative is:
**Springer Nature Customer Service Center GmbH
Europaplatz 3, 69115 Heidelberg, Germany**

Printed by Libri Plureos GmbH
in Hamburg, Germany